Progress in
Cancer Research and Therapy
Volume 23

MATURATION FACTORS AND CANCER

Progress in Cancer Research and Therapy

Progress in
Cancer Research and Therapy
Volume 23

Maturation Factors and Cancer

Editor

Malcolm A. S. Moore, D. Phil.
Memorial Sloan–Kettering Cancer Center
New York, New York

Raven Press ■ New York

Raven Press, 1140 Avenue of the Americas, New York, New York 10036

Made in the United States of America

International Standard Book Number 0–89004–596–8
Library of Congress Catalog Number 80–5836

Preface

This volume represents the proceedings of a workshop on Maturation (Differentiation) Factors in Cancer sponsored by the Biological Response Modifier Program of the Division of Cancer Treatment, National Cancer Institute, U.S.A. Its purpose was to review the role of regulatory factors influencing the proliferation and differentiation of neoplastic cell populations.

Biological response modifiers refer to the agents or approaches which will modify the relationship between tumor and host by modifying a host's biological response to tumor cells with resultant therapeutic benefit. The subjects and speakers reflected the current state of interest and activity in this area. Special emphasis is placed on the observation that the apparent maturation block associated with neoplastic transformation in various cell systems can be a reversible phenomenon. Terminal differentiation can be induced by a variety of factors, both physiological and pharmacological and attention is being paid to translating *in vitro* studies to *in vivo* experimental and clinical trials. Where investigated in depth, the proliferation and/ or differentiation of renewing cell populations has been shown to be controlled by specific growth regulatory factors, generally of a glycoprotein or polypeptide nature. Contrary to earlier beliefs, most transformed cells retain some dependence upon growth regulatory factors of exogenous or endogenous origin, and thus manipulation of production or action of growth and maturation factors has a role to play in cancer therapy.

In some cell systems, growth factors induce proliferation of target cells without inducing further differentiation. Inappropriate production of such mitogenic factors by neoplastic cells or the production of functionally similar molecules following viral transformation confers a proliferative advantage upon the transformed cell. A number of therapeutic strategies are discussed in this volume, some based on blocking the synthesis and/or release of the growth factor upon which tumor proliferation depends, others based upon modulation or blocking receptors for growth factors using synthetic peptide antagonists or monoclonal antibodies.

Recognition and appreciation of the clinical potential of biological response modification has occurred slowly but it is to be hoped that the rapid advances in our understanding of cellular control mechanisms will provide a solid scientific basis for evolving rational therapy for cancer. This book will be of interest to all researchers in oncology and cell biology as well as those involved in cancer therapy.

Malcolm A. S. Moore

Contents

Contributors

D. Aden
The Wistar Institute
Philadelphia, PA 19104

Miloslav Beran
Department of Developmental
Therapeutics
The University of Texas System Cancer
Center
M. D. Anderson Hospital and Tumor
Institute
Houston, TX 77030

Leslie Brandeis
Department of Pathology
New York University Medical School
New York, NY 10016

Theodore R. Breitman
Laboratory of Tumor Cell Biology
Department of Health and Human
Services
National Cancer Institute
National Institutes of Health
Bethesda, MD 20205

Ronald N. Buick
Ontario Cancer Institute
Toronto, Ontario M4X 1K9, Canada

Edith R. Butler-Gralla
Molecular Biology Institute and
Laboratory of Nuclear Medicine and
Radiation Biology
UCLA Center for the Health Sciences
Los Angeles, CA 90024

Paul Calabresi
Department of Medicine
Roger Williams General Hospital
Rhode Island Hospital and
Section of Medicine
Division of Biology and Medicine
Brown University
Providence, RI 02912

Cecilia Caramatti
Department of Medicine
Montefiore Hospital
University of Pittsburgh School of
Medicine
Pittsburgh, PA 15213

Daniel B. Cawley
Department of Biological Chemistry and
Laboratory of Nuclear Medicine and
Radiation Biology
UCLA Center for the Health Sciences
Los Angeles, CA 90024

Richard K. Cheney
Immunobiology Laboratories
Departments of Pathology and Medicine
University of New Mexico School of
Medicine
Albuquerque, NM 87131

Gerald W. Crabtree
Section of Biochemical Pharmacology
Division of Biology and Medicine
Brown University
Providence, RI 02912

Michael Daley
Immunobiology Laboratories
Departments of Pathology and Medicine
University of New Mexico School of
Medicine
Albuquerque, NM 87131

C. Damsky
The Wistar Institute
Philadelphia, PA 19104

Daniel L. Dexter
Department of Medicine
Roger Williams General Hospital and
Section of Medicine
Division of Biology and Medicine
Brown University
Providence, RI 02912

David End
Section on Intermediary Metabolism
Laboratory of Developmental
  Neurobiology
National Institute of Child Health and
  Human Development
National Institutes of Health
Bethesda, MD 20205

Robert C. Gallo
Laboratory of Tumor Cell Biology
Department of Health and Human
  Services
National Cancer Institute
National Institutes of Health
Bethesda, MD 20205

Kathleen M. Gilbert
Memorial Sloan-Kettering Cancer Center
New York, NY 10021

Steven Gillis
Basic Immunology Program
Fred Hutchinson Cancer Research Center
Seattle, WA 98104

Arvin S. Glicksman
Department of Radiation Oncology
Rhode Island Hospital and
Section of Radiation Medicine
Division of Biology and Medicine
Brown University
Providence, RI 02912

Allan L. Goldstein
Department of Biochemistry
The George Washington University
School of Medicine and Health Sciences
Washington, DC 20037

Rosanne Goodman
Department of Pediatrics
University of Pennsylvania
Joseph Stokes, Jr. Research Institute
The Children's Hospital of Philadelphia
Philadelphia, PA 19104

R. M. Gorczynski
Ontario Cancer Institute
Toronto, Ontario M4X 1K9, Canada and
Department of Medicine
Sunnybrook Medical Centre
University of Toronto
Toronto, Ontario, Canada

Pamela Gorin
Department of Neurobiology
Stanford University School of Medicine
Stanford, CA 94305

Denis Gospodarowicz
Cancer Research Institute and
The Department of Medicine M 1282
University of California Medical Center
San Francisco, CA 94143

Gordon Guroff
Section on Intermediary Metabolism
Laboratory of Developmental
  Neurobiology
National Institute of Child Health and
  Human Development
National Institutes of Health
Bethesda, MD 20205

Harvey R. Herschman
Department of Biological Chemistry
Molecular Biology Institute and
Laboratory of Nuclear Medicine and
  Radiation Biology
University of California Los Angeles
  Center for the Health Sciences
Los Angeles, CA 90024

Michael K. Hoffmann
Memorial Sloan-Kettering Cancer Center
New York, NY 10021

C. A. Izaguirre
Ontario Cancer Institute
Toronto, Ontario M4X 1K9, Canada

Eugene Johnson
Department of Pharmacology
Washington University Medical School
St. Louis, MO 63110

Benjamin Koziner
Memorial Sloan-Kettering Cancer Center
New York, NY 10021

B. Lange
Children's Hospital
Division of Oncology-Hematology
Philadelphia, PA 19104

Lewis L. Lanier
Immunobiology Laboratories
Departments of Pathology and Medicine
University of New Mexico School of
*   Medicine*
Albuquerque, NM 87131

D. Lebman
The Wistar Institute
Philadelphia, PA 19104

John T. Leith
Department of Radiation Oncology
Rhode Island Hospital and
Section of Radiation Medicine
Division of Biology and Medicine
Brown University
Providence, RI 02912

Jay Lilliquist
Laboratory of Tumor Biology
Sidney Farber Cancer Institute and
Laboratory of Microbiology and
*   Molecular Genetics*
Harvard Medical School
Boston, MA 02115

Kathryn L. Locatell
Department of Pediatric Hematology-
*   Oncology*
Sidney Farber Cancer Institute and
Children's Hospital Medical Center
Harvard Medical School
Boston, MA 02115

Brian I. Lord
Paterson Laboratories
Christie Hospital and Holt Radium
*   Institute*
Manchester M20 9BX, England

Teresa L. K. Low
Department of Biochemistry
The George Washington University
School of Medicine and Health Sciences
Washington, DC 20037

E. A. McCulloch
Ontario Cancer Institute
Toronto, Ontario M4X 1K9, Canada

Roland Mertelsmann
Memorial Sloan-Kettering Cancer Center
New York, NY 10021

Steven B. Mizel
Department of Microbiology, Cell
*   Biology,*
Biochemistry and Biophysics
The Pennsylvania State University
University Park, PA 16802

Malcolm A. S. Moore
Sloan-Kettering Institute for Cancer
*   Research*
Walker Laboratory
Rye, NY 10580

Ilona Nakoinz
Sloan-Kettering Institute for Cancer
*   Research*
Walker Laboratory
Rye, NY 10580

Herbert F. Oettgen
Memorial Sloan-Kettering Cancer Center
New York, NY 10021

Patricia Osborne
Department of Pharmacology
Washington University Medical School
St. Louis, MO 63110

Robert E. Parks, Jr.
Section of Biochemical Pharmacology
Division of Biology and Medicine
Brown University
Providence, RI 02912

John Pearson
Department of Pathology
New York University Medical School
New York, NY 10016

G. Pegoraro
Istituto di Medicina Interna
University of Torino
Cso Polonia 14
Torino, Italy

B. Perussia
The Wistar Institute
Philadelphia, PA 19104

Giuseppe Pigoli
Department of Medicine
Montefiore Hospital
University of Pittsburgh School of
* Medicine*
Pittsburgh, PA 15213

Bernard J. Poiesz
Laboratory of Tumor Cell Biology
National Cancer Institute
National Institutes of Health
Bethesda, MD 20205

Gerald B. Price
Ontario Cancer Institute
Toronto, Ontario M4X 1K9, Canada and
Department of Medicine
Sunnybrook Medical Centre
University of Toronto
Toronto, Ontario, Canada

Peter Ralph
Sloan-Kettering Institute for Cancer
* Research*
Walker Laboraty
Rye, NY 10580

William C. Raschke
The Salk Institute for Biological Studies
La Jolla, CA 92037

Giovanni Rovera
The Wistar Institute
Philadelphia, PA 19104

Francis W. Ruscetti
Laboratory of Tumor Cell Biology
National Cancer Institute
National Institutes of Health
Bethesda, MD 20205

Charles D. Scher
Department of Pediatric Hematology-
* Oncology*
Sidney Farber Cancer Institute and
* Children's Hospital Medical Center*
Harvard Medical School
Boston, MA 02115

J. S. Senn
Ontario Cancer Institute
Toronto, Ontario M4X 1K9, Canada and
Department of Medicine
Sunnybrook Medical Centre
University of Toronto
Toronto, Ontario, Canada

Richard K. Shadduck
Department of Medicine
Montefiore Hospital
University of Pittsburgh School of
* Medicine*
Pittsburgh, PA 15213

Alice Patricia Sheridan
Sloan-Kettering Institute for Cancer
* Research*
Walker Laboratory
Rye, NY 10580

Joseph M. Sorrentino
*Department of Biological Chemistry and
Laboratory of Nuclear Medicine and
    Radiation Biology
UCLA Center for the Health Sciences
Los Angeles, CA 90024*

Gary Spitzer
*Department of Developmental
    Therapeutics
The University of Texas System Cancer
    Center
M. D. Anderson Hospital and Tumor
    Institute
Houston, TX 77030*

Charles D. Stiles
*Laboratory of Tumor Biology
Sidney Farber Cancer Institute and
Laboratory of Microbiology and
    Molecular Genetics
Harvard Medical School
Boston, MA 02115*

Corrado Tarella
*Litton Bionetics
Kensington, MD 20795*

George J. Todaro
*Department of Health and Human
    Services
Laboratory of Viral Carcinogenesis
Division of Cancer Cause and Prevention
National Cancer Institute
National Institutes of Health
Bethesda, MD 20205*

G. Trinchieri
*The Wistar Institute
Philadelphia, PA 19104*

J. Vartikar
*The Wistar Institute
Phildelphia, PA 19104*

Dharmvir S. Verma
*Department of Developmental
    Therapeutics
The University of Texas System Cancer
    Center
M. D. Anderson Hospital and Tumor
    Institute
Houston, TX 77030*

I. Vlodavsky
*Cancer Research Institute and the
    Department of Medicine
University of California, Medical Center
San Francisco, CA 94143*

Abdul Waheed
*Department of Medicine
Montefiore Hospital
University of Pittsburgh School of
    Medicine
Pittsburgh, PA 15213*

Edwin Walker
*Immunobiology Laboratories
Departments of Pathology and Medicine
University of New Mexico School of
    Medicine
Albuquerque, NM 87131*

Noel L. Warner
*Immunobiology Laboratories
Departments of Pathology and Medicine
University of New Mexico School of
    Medicine
Albuquerque, NM 87131*

James Watson
*Department of Medical Microbiology
California College of Medicine
University of California at Irvine
Irvine, CA 92717*

Eric G. Wright
*University of St. Andrews
Fife KY16 9TS
Scotland, U. K.*

Maturation Factors and Cancer,
edited by Malcolm A. S. Moore.
Raven Press, © New York 1982.

Use of an Autoimmune Approach to Study the Biological Role of Nerve Growth Factor

*Eugene Johnson, **Pamela Gorin, *Patricia Osborne,
†Leslie Brandeis, and †John Pearson

*Department of Pharmacology, Washington University Medical School,
St. Louis, Missouri 63110; **Department of Neurobiology, Stanford University
School of Medicine, Stanford, California 94305; †Department of Pathology,
New York University Medical School, New York, New York 10016*

Nerve growth factor (NGF) is perhaps the best characterized of all of the "growth factors." However, despite years of intensive study since the original description of Levi-Montalcini and coworkers (for a recent review, see ref. 10), the precise biological role(s) of NGF are far from completely understood. The two primary approaches that have been used to address the question of the biological role of NGF have been (a) to assess the effect of NGF *in vitro* on either explants, dissociated cells, or cell lines; and (b) to deprive an experimental animal of NGF *in vivo* by administration of antibodies prepared against mouse NGF (anti-NGF). Studies using anti-NGF have demonstrated that mammalian sympathetic neurons of the para- and prevertebral ganglia die (immunosympathectomy) if deprived of NGF during the neonatal period (13). Death of other cell types has not been seen.

The usefulness of heterologous antiserum-induced NGF deprivation is limited by problems associated with its repeated administration (e.g., serum sickness) and by difficulties in administering it to prenatal animals. In an effort to overcome the inherent limitations in the administration of heterologous anti-NGF, we explored an alternative "autoimmune" approach by determining whether an animal immunized with 2.5 S mouse NGF (2) makes antibody with some degree of cross-reactivity with its own NGF. This is indeed the case, as shown by the ability of antisera raised in rats against mouse NGF to produce immunosympathectomy in newborn *rats*. Our results therefore repeat the same experiment carried out in rabbits reported by Levi-Montalcini and Booker (13) in the original paper describing immunosympathectomy. More recently, with the availability of guinea pig NGF (9), we have shown that antibodies raised in the guinea pig against mouse NGF will neutralize the effects of guinea pig NGF in the classical dorsal root ganglion bioassay system (5,12). We have proceeded to ask two general questions: (a) What happens to the adult animal (particularly with respect to the sympathetic nervous system) chronically producing antibodies against its own NGF? (b) What happens to the offspring that are exposed to maternal anti-NGF prenatally *in utero* and postnatally in milk? The result of much of this work is reported in a recent series of papers

1

(6–8,11), and what follows is a description of some of the major points made in those papers.

EFFECTS IN ADULT ANIMALS IMMUNIZED AGAINST MOUSE NGF

Adult rats were immunized by the administration 100 μg of 2.5 S NGF (2) in complete Freund's adjuvant (CFA) and boosted at 4- to 6-week intervals with 10 μg of NGF in CFA. Control animals were immunized with horse heart cytochrome C in CFA. Animals immunized with cytochrome C or a variety of other proteins never demonstrated an adverse effect on sympathetic neurons.

It had been shown previously that administration of heterologous anti-NGF to mature animals for 5 days produced atrophy, but not cell death, of sympathetic neurons (1). The major question that we wished to address was whether the much longer exposure to anti-NGF made possible by the autoimmune approach would produce cell death as well as atrophy. Such a result would imply that the mature sympathetic neuron requires NGF, not only for normal function, but for survival. When a large group of adult rats were immunized, animals with varying titers (assessed in the bioassay) were produced. Five months after initial immunization, animals were killed and the superior cervical sympathetic ganglion (SCG; a para-vertebral ganglion) was assayed biochemically for evidence of atrophy. The data in Fig. 1 show that the enzymes involved in norepinephrine synthesis, tyrosine hydroxylase (TOH), and dopamine-β-hydroxylase (DBH) were reduced 60 to 80%. The protein content was also reduced about 30%. Choline acetyltransferase, the enzyme which synthesizes acetylcholine and which is localized in the preganglionic

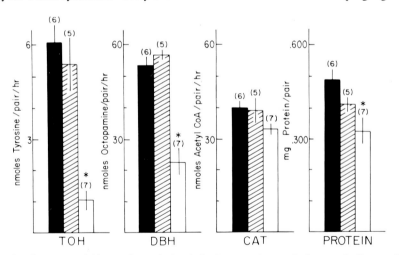

FIG. 1. Enzyme activities and protein levels in the superior cervical sympathetic ganglia of adult rats. Bars represent means ± SEM for unimmunized age-matched controls (solid bars), cytochrome c immunized controls (hatched bars), and NGF-immunized rats (open bars). Immunizations were for a 5-month duration. Number of animals in a group is given in parentheses. $*$, $p < 0.05$. Data taken from ref. (8).

nerve terminals, rather than in sympathetic neurons, was not significantly reduced. No differences were found between unimmunized controls and cytochrome C immunized controls with respect to any parameter. Similar results were seen in the celiac ganglion (a prevertebral ganglion). Subsequent experiments demonstrated that the degree of enzyme decrease correlated well with the serum titers of anti-NGF in an individual animal.

These biochemical results were consistent with the light microscopic appearance of the ganglia, in which marked neuronal atrophy was observed. The critical question as to neuronal death was addressed by carrying out cell counts of SCGs of animals showing the highest serum titers and the greatest degree of biochemical atrophy. In these animals, neuronal numbers were reduced 34% (control 28,180 ± 277, $n = 4$; experimental 18,598 ± 922, $n = 4$ $p < 0.001$). In more recent experiments in rabbits producing anti-NGF for 10 months, decreases in neuronal numbers of up to 85% have been observed (unpublished data). Thus these data strongly suggest that NGF deprivation, although not producing the rapid death seen in the immature neuron, ultimately produces the death of mature sympathetic neurons.

EFFECTS OF EXPOSURE TO MATERNAL ANTI-NGF ON THE NERVOUS SYSTEM OF OFFSPRING

The effects of maternal anti-NGF on developing offspring are determined to a large extent by the properties of passive transfer of antibody from mother to offspring. These vary considerably from species to species (3). Most of our experiments have been carried out in the rat, a species that receives a modest amount of maternal antibody prenatally and considerably more postnatally via the milk. In a series of experiments involving cross-fostered offspring (i.e., newborns switched at birth from an anti-NGF-producing female to a normal female, and vice versa), it was shown that exposure to maternal anti-NGF either prenatally or postnatally destroyed sympathetic neurons, as shown by marked decreases in the size (protein content) and tyrosine hydroxylase activity (Table 1) in the SCG of 2-week-old animals. As expected, 2-week-old animals nursing from an anti-NGF-producing mother had higher titers than the offspring of the female had at birth. Exposure to anti-NGF

TABLE 1. *Effects of prenatal and/or postnatal exposure to maternal anti-NGF on the superior cervical ganglia of 2-week old rats[a]*

Exposure to anti-NGF			Protein	Tyrosine hydrolase
In utero	Milk	*n*	(mg/pair SCG)	activity[b]
−	−	8	0.20 ± 0.01	4.91 ± 0.030
+	−	6	0.08 ± 0.01	1.81 ± 0.37
−	+	8	0.06 ± 0.01	0.22 ± 0.03
+	+	5	0.04 ± 0.01	0.02 ± 0.02

[a]Data taken from ref. (6).
[b]Nmoles tyrosine oxidized/pair SCG/hr ± SEM.

both prenatally and postnatally (i.e., offspring born to and nursed by the NGF-immunized rat) produced more profound effects than those produced by exposure during only one of these time intervals. No decreases in norepinephrine levels were found in brain dissected into major regions or in the vas deferens. Likewise, no morphological or biochemical alterations were seen in the adrenal medulla. Therefore, the only component of the sympathoadrenal nervous system observed to be adversely affected by exposure to maternal anti-NGF were sympathetic neurons.

Despite the dramatic effects of exposure to maternal anti-NGF which were demonstrated above, it was found that there was a great deal of variability among litters, even though the mothers had comparable titers of antibody against mouse NGF. In our experience, only 20 to 30% of immunized female rats produce litters severely affected (as in Table 1) at birth. A likely explanation is that despite comparable antibody titers against *mouse NGF*, there is considerable variability in the cross-reactivity of these antibodies against *rat NGF* (which is not available for direct testing). Consistent with this suggestion is the observation that although there was considerable variability in the effects on offspring in litters from different rats, successive litters from the same female showed a consistent degree of effects. Likewise, there was little variability among rats from the same litter.

In addition to effects on sympathetic neurons, data indicating an effect on dorsal root ganglion (DRG) sensory neurons were obtained. It was found that the protein content of cervical DRGs was permanently reduced by 25 to 40% in rats exposed to maternal anti-NGF prenatally *(in utero)* but, in contrast to sympathetic ganglia, protein content was unaffected by postnatal exposure to maternal anti-NGF (in milk). Likewise, the ability to retrogradely transport ^{125}I-NGF from the periphery to the cell bodies in the DRG was reduced about 70% in animals exposed to maternal anti-NGF prenatally, but not postnatally. These data suggested that a large percentage of sensory neurons in the DRG are sensitive to anti-NGF during prenatal development, but the sensitivity to the antibody is lost by birth. This tentative conclusion was confirmed by carrying out cell counts in the SCG and DRG of adult rats cross-fostered at birth (Table 2). The data show that exposure to maternal anti-NGF either prenatally or postnatally resulted in the death of over 90% of sympathetic neurons in the SCG. In contrast, the number of neurons in the 8th cervical DRG was reduced 70% by *in utero* exposure to antibody but unaltered by postnatal

TABLE 2. *Number of neurons in ganglia of adult rats exposed to maternal anti-NGF prenatally or postnatally[a]*

Exposure to maternal anti-NGF	Neurons/ganglion	
	Superior cervical	8th cervical DRG
None (control)	25,400 ± 1,940 (*n* = 3)	5,650 ± 220 (*n* = 3)
In utero only	1,690 ± 40 (*n* = 3)	1,750 ± 110 (*n* = 3)
In milk only	2,300 ± 270 (*n* = 3)	5,870 ± 220 (*n* = 3)

[a]Data taken from ref. (11).

exposure. The latter result is quantitatively consistent with the decrease in ability of DRG neurons to retrogradely transport NGF.

More profound effects of prenatal exposure to anti-NGF would be expected in a species that receives most of its passive immunity prenatally. This is confirmed by our observations in guinea pigs. Female guinea pigs produced higher titers of antibody against mouse NGF (titers often $> 4,000$) than did female rats (titers usually > 500 but $< 1,000$). Newborn guinea pigs had titers at birth comparable to maternal titers ($> 1,000$), whereas newborn rats had titers of > 10 but < 25 at birth. Consistent with the higher titers observed in the newborn guinea pigs, a greater destruction of sympathetic and DRG neurons was observed (Table 3). The numbers of neurons in the nodose ganglia (10th cranial nerve), which are derived during embryogenesis from placodal rather than neural crest tissue origin, were unaffected. Also, in contrast to the rats, guinea pigs born to NGF-immunized mothers had marked sensory deficits, in that they did not respond to painful mechanical, thermal, and chemical stimuli. All of the newborn guinea pigs born to date (4 litters from 2 animals) have failed to gain weight and have died before 2 weeks of age. The exact reason(s) for their deaths has not been determined as yet.

These data provide the first *in vivo* evidence that sensory neurons of neural crest origin go through a phase of NGF dependence. Therefore, these data provide the *in vivo* correlate for the observed NGF dependence *in vitro* of embryonic dorsal root ganglia (4,14,15) neurons for survival in culture and indicate that most, if not all, DRG neurons go through a phase of dependence on NGF.

POTENTIAL OF THE EXPERIMENTAL APPROACH

The autoimmune approach has thus provided important information regarding the role of NGF in the life cycle of the sympathetic and sensory neuron. In the future, it offers the potential for examining the role of NGF in various cell types *in utero*, for determining the time of NGF dependence, for determining the embryonic origin (neural crest vs placodal) of neurons in cranial ganglia, and for

TABLE 3. *Number of neurons in ganglia of newborn guinea pigs exposed to maternal anti-NGF[a]*

| | Neurons/ganglion | | |
Group	Superior cervical	8th cervical DRG	Nodose
Control	57,600 ± 5,080 (n = 3)	15,500 ± 96 (n = 3)	15,900 ± 980 (n = 3)
Anti-NGF exposure			
Litter 1	280 ± 130 (n = 5)	3,120 ± 96 (n = 3)	15,500 ± 1,530 (n = 3)
Litter 2		2,280 ± 156 (n = 3)	

[a]Data taken from ref. (11).

determining the secondary effects of destruction of most of the peripheral sensory nervous system.

The general "autoimmune" approach may be applied to other proteins, many of which have been classified as "growth factors" largely on the basis of their ability to affect cell growth or multiplication *in vitro*. The autoimmune approach offers a possible method to deprive a developing organism *in vivo* of a putative growth factor. The applicability of the approach to other polypeptide factors depends on the antigenicity of the peptide, the accessibility of the antibody to its synthetic sources and storage sites prior to and during the developmental event of interest, and the cross-reactivity of the antibody for the polypeptide in the particular species under study.

ACKNOWLEDGMENTS

The authors would like to thank Dr. Ralph Bradshaw for his help during the course of this work, and Drs. John Russell and Arthur Loewy for their many helpful discussions. This work was supported by the March of Dimes Birth Defects Foundation, the Familial Dysautonomia Foundation, NIH grants HL-20604 and HD-12260, and NIH training grant 5T32 HL-07275. E. Johnson is an Established Investigator of the American Heart Association.

REFERENCES

1. Bjerre, B., Wiklund, L. and Edwards, D. C. (1975): A study of the de- and regenerative changes in the sympathetic nervous system of the adult mouse after treatment with the antiserum to nerve growth factor. *Brain Res.*, 92:257–278.
2. Bocchini, V., and Angeletti, P. U. (1969): The nerve growth factor: purification as a 30,000 molecular weight protein. *Proc. Natl. Acad. Sci. U.S.A.*, 64:787–794.
3. Bramwell, F. W. R. (1970): The transmission of passive immunity from mother to young. In: *Frontiers of Biology*, Vol. 18, American Elsevier, New York.
4. Crain, S. M., and Peterson, E. R. (1974): Enhanced afferent synaptic functions in fetal mouse spinal cord-sensory ganglion explants following NGF-induced ganglion hypertrophy. *Brain Res.*, 79:145–152.
5. Fenton, E. L. (1970): Tissue culture assay of nerve growth factor and of the specific antiserum. *Exp. Cell Res.*, 59:383–392.
6. Gorin, P. D., and Johnson, E. M. (1979): Experimental autoimmune model of nerve growth factor deprivation: effects on developing peripheral sympathetic and sensory neurons. *Proc. Natl. Acad. Sci. U.S.A.*, 76:5382–5386.
7. Gorin, P. D., and Johnson, E. M. (1980): Effects of exposure to nerve growth factor antibodies on the developing nervous system of the rat: an experimental autoimmune approach. *Dev. Biol.*, 80:313:323.
8. Gorin, P. D., and Johnson, E. M. (1980): Effects of long-term nerve growth factor deprivation on the nervous system of the adult rat: an experimental autoimmune approach. *Brain Res.*, 198:27–42.
9. Harper, G. P., Barde, Y. A., Burnstock, G., Carstairs, J. R., Dennison, M. E., Suda, K., and Vernon, C. A. (1979): Guinea pig prostate is a rich source of nerve growth factor. *Nature*, 279:160–162.
10. Harper, G. P., and Thoenen, H. (1980): Nerve growth factor: biological significance, measurement and distribution. *J. Neurochem.*, 34:5–16.
11. Johnson, E. M., Gorin, P. D., Brandeis, L. O., and Pearson, J. (1980): Dorsal root ganglion neurons are destroyed by *in utero* exposure to maternal antibody to nerve growth factor. *Science*, 210:916–918.

12. Levi-Montalcini, R., Meyer, H., and Hamburger, V. (1954): *In vitro* experiments on the effects of mouse sarcomas 180 and 37 on the spinal and sympathetic ganglia of the chick embryo. *Cancer Res.*, 14:49–57.
13. Levi-Montalcini, R., and Booker, B. (1960): Destruction of the sympathetic ganglia in mammals by an antiserum to a nerve growth protein. *Proc. Natl. Acad. Sci. U.S.A.*, 46:384–391.
14. Levi-Montalcini, R., and Angeletti, P. U. (1963): Essential role of the nerve growth factor in the survival and maintenance of dissociated sensory and sympathetic embryonic nerve cells *in vitro*. *Dev. Biol.*, 7:653–659.
15. Varon, S., Raiborn, C., and Tyszka, E. (1973): *In vitro* studies of dissociated cells from newborn mouse dorsal root ganglia. *Brain Res.*, 54:51–63.

Maturation Factors and Cancer, edited by
Malcolm A. S. Moore.
Raven Press, © New York 1982.

Nerve Growth Factor and Epidermal Growth Factor Responsiveness of Pheochromocytoma Cells

*David End and *Gordon Guroff

*Section on Intermediary Metabolism, Laboratory of Developmental Neurobiology,
National Institute of Child Health and Human Development, National Institutes of Health,
Bethesda, Maryland 20205*

There are now 20 or 30 "factors" reported in the literature. Of these, nerve growth factor is probably the most fully characterized, and a reasonable amount of information is also available about epidermal growth factor. But about fibroblast growth factor, mesenchymal growth factor, glial factor, glial maturation factor, sarcoma growth factor, and all the rest, information is quite incomplete. The chemistry of most of these others is unknown. The overall actions are also unknown. The methodology for the study of most of these is tedious and cumbersome, at least in biochemical terms. Even the fundamental biological significance of most of the factors is not firmly established.

Since information about nerve growth factor is fairly extensive, it may be useful to discuss it as a prototype of the growth and maturation factors. Nerve growth factor was discovered in the late 1940s by Bueker (13,14). His experiments involved the implantation of small fragments of certain tumors, among them the Sarcoma 180, into chick embryos. The perhaps unexpected result of these manipulations was the enlargement of portions of the peripheral nervous system. When Levi-Montalcini and Hamburger repeated these experiments, but placed the tumor fragments on the chorioallantoic membrane so that they were physically separated from the embryo (41,42), the results were essentially the same. The interpretation of these latter studies was that the effect of the tumor on the peripheral nervous system was due to something diffusing from the tumor across the membrane. Cohen tried to purify this diffusable factor from the tumor (17,18) using, in the process, snake venom as a lytic agent. He found that the venom contained more of this factor than the tumor itself. His survey of tissues comparable in function to the venom-producing gland in the snake led to the observation that the richest source of the factor was the submaxillary gland of the mature male mouse. The biological significance of the high concentration of factor in this source is not known, but the gland remains a most useful biological laboratory reagent. Levi-Montalcini and Booker (39) provided a most persuasive argument for the biological significance of the factor by preparing an antibody against it and showing that this antibody, when injected into

9

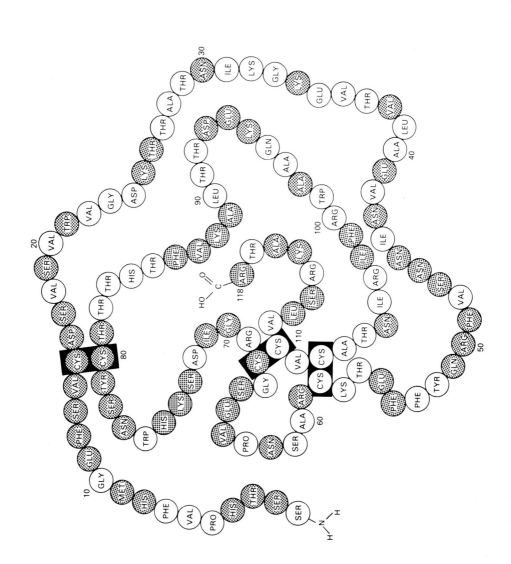

young animals, deprived them of their sympathetic nervous system, a procedure now known as "immunosympathectomy." The biological relevance of the factor for the development of the sensory nervous system has recently been strongly confirmed through the work of Johnson and his colleagues (38) on the autoimmune model.

A great deal of information about nerve growth factor is now available (11,29,66). Thus after some 30 years of work in many laboratories, it is known that nerve growth factor is a small, basic protein with a molecular weight of 13,500 and that it exists as a noncovalently linked dimer of molecular weight about 27,000. This dimer can be isolated as such from the salivary gland in a form known as the 2.5S (10). The dimer can also be isolated as part of a larger molecule called the 7S (63). In this case, the noncovalently linked dimer is called the β subunit and is accompanied by two other kinds of subunits, the α subunits, the functions of which are unknown, and the γ subunits, which have proteolytic action and seem to be involved in the processing of nerve growth factor from some larger precursor. The 2.5S and the β subunit are identical except for some minor proteolytic degradation, which appears to take place during the isolation of the 2.5S. The larger 7S molecule contains Zn^{2+}, and it falls apart when the Zn^{2+} is removed. The biological significance of the 7S is not firmly established, but there are suggestions that it serves to store and protect the active β subunit. Only the β subunit is active, and the activity of the 7S is, on a molar basis, identical with that of the 2.5S. The linear sequence of the β subunit has been worked out by Bradshaw and his colleagues (5) (Fig. 1), and they have observed that it bears a resemblance to the linear sequence of proinsulin (23). Whether the correlation found in the linear sequences will, indeed, also be found in the secondary and tertiary structures is still not clear. It is clear, however, that this line of research has given new direction to the studies of these proteins.

The methodology for the quantitation of nerve growth factor leaves much to be desired. The original assay developed by Levi-Montalcini and her coworkers (40) involves the explanting of dorsal root ganglia from chick embryos into a semisolid medium. The presence of increasing amounts of nerve growth factor (Fig. 2) leads to a so-called "halo" response, which can be scored semiquantitatively to give an estimate in the nanogram range. The apparent inhibition seen at higher levels of nerve growth factor is now known to be simply a reorientation of the fibers and not a lessening of the overall outgrowth. The assay is sensitive and specific and is used in most laboratories engaged in the study of the factor. But it remains semiquantitative, slow, and tricky. Modifications of the "halo" assay using single neurons or PC12 cells are available. There are radioimmunoassays based on one-site or

---

FIG. 1.   The linear sequence of mouse nerve growth factor and its homology with proinsulin. The darkened residues are those which are either the same as corresponding residues in human proinsulin or are considered to be favored amino acid substitutions. (Adapted from the work of Frazier et al., ref. 23.)

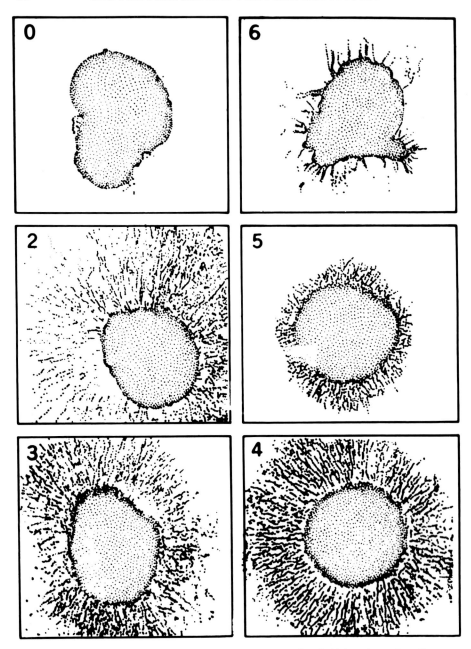

FIG. 2. Fiber outgrowth from explanted dorsal root ganglia of chick embryo. Ganglia were cultured for 20 hr in the presence of no (0) nerve growth factor or increasing amounts (2 to 6) of nerve growth factor. Phase contrast magnification ×100. (Adapted from Varon, ref. 61a.)

on two-site principles, and a complement fixation assay has been published. There is a receptor assay, a rocket immunoelectrophoresis assay, and an assay based on the recombination of the various subunits of the 7S. None of these methods has been widely enough accepted, nor is free enough of problems, to have become the method of choice. The most promising of the new methods is the radioimmunoassay developed by Thoenen and his colleagues (59). This method, which makes use of highly purified nerve growth factor antibody (56,61), appears to avoid some of the criticisms leveled at earlier radioimmunoassays and may provide a valuable addition to the nerve growth factor methodology.

Nerve growth factor is made by any number of cells in culture (12). So many cell types have been shown to produce the factor that the general feeling is that all cells in the body produce nerve growth factor in small amounts. The details of this biosynthesis have been studied most extensively by Shooter and his colleagues using explants of mouse saliva gland (8,9). These explants will make nerve growth factor, and it can be shown that the biosynthesis occurs by the proteolytic processing of larger peptides to the final nerve growth factor monomer. These studies have also produced evidence that this processing can be carried out by the proteolytic activity of the γ subunit of the 7S nerve growth factor. The manner in which nerve growth factor biosynthesis is regulated is unknown, but there is evidence that the amounts of nerve growth factor produced by various cells can be increased by certain steroid hormones (50) and by β-adrenergic agonists (53).

There are receptors for nerve growth factor on the plasma membranes of its target cells (7,24,35). These receptors are specific for nerve growth factor and have been solubilized from the membrane (6). They have high affinity for nerve growth factor and appear in no way different than the receptors for other peptide hormones. There is evidence that the receptors for nerve growth factor on PC12 cells can be internalized (69). There are also receptors on the nuclei of various target cells (1,69), although there is some disagreement as to the exact subnuclear localization of these receptors. Finally, there is evidence that there are receptors at the synaptic ending of the various neurons sensitive to nerve growth factor. This evidence comes from the retrograde transport experiments of Hendry, Thoenen, and their colleagues (34,49,57,58). The data involved show that nerve growth factor, administered to the organs innervated by nerve growth factor-sensitive neurons, will enter those neurons at the synaptic ending and progress in a retrograde fashion up the axon to the cell body. The data indicate that the process is specific, and that the specificity resides in receptors for nerve growth factor at the synaptic ending. There is no information as yet as to which of these receptors, membrane, nuclear, or synaptic, is involved in initiating the action(s) of nerve growth factor on its target cells.

The classical target cells for nerve growth factor are certain of the sympathetic and sensory neurons. Currently it is thought that the sympathetic neurons require nerve growth factor throughout their lifetime; the responsive sensory neurons appear to require nerve growth factor only during a specific, early developmental period. There is some evidence, although not entirely persuasive, that adrenal medullary

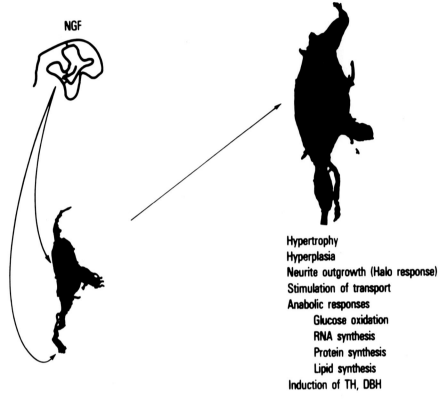

NGF

Hypertrophy
Hyperplasia
Neurite outgrowth (Halo response)
Stimulation of transport
Anabolic responses
    Glucose oxidation
    RNA synthesis
    Protein synthesis
    Lipid synthesis
Induction of TH, DBH

FIG. 3. The actions of nerve growth factor on sympathetic ganglia.

cells respond to nerve growth factor, and there is some, albeit even less convincing, evidence that the central nervous system contains nerve growth factor-responsive cells. But basically, among the normal cells, the nerve growth factor-responsive neurons are in the sympathetic and the sensory nervous systems. There are, however, a number of tumors which respond in various ways. A number of human melanomas have large numbers of nerve growth factor receptors (22) but exhibit no change in growth rate or alteration in morphology. A few of the neuroblastomas show changes in morphology when in the presence of nerve growth factor (51,68). The F98 glioma shows changes in growth rate and alterations in morphology when given nerve growth factor (67). Finally, the various clones of rat pheochromocytoma respond in different ways. The PC-G2 shows induction of tyrosine hydroxylase (25), and the PC12 exhibits remarkable alterations in many of its properties, changes that will be discussed in detail below.

The actions of nerve growth factor on its target cells (Fig. 3) include increases in the uptake of metabolites (46,62) and the extrusion of Na^+ (55), alterations in the conformation of the membrane (19), and alterations in the adhesiveness of cells (52,64,65). Hypertrophy has been seen in many nerve growth factor-responsive

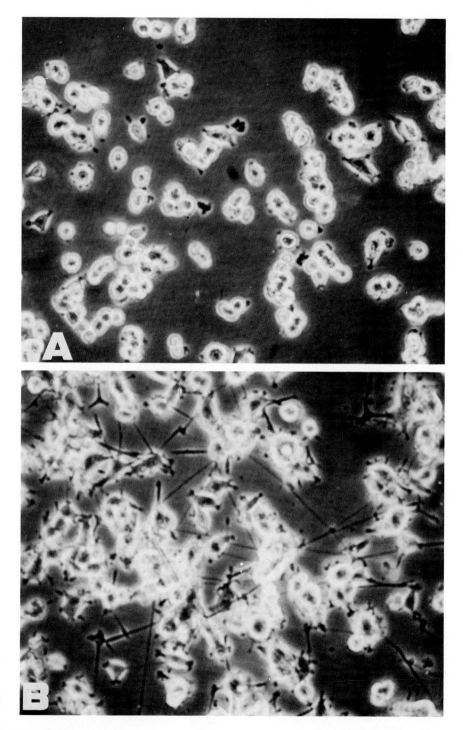

FIG. 4. PC12 cells **(A)** minus nerve growth factor and **(B)** plus 50 ng/ml 2.5S nerve growth factor for 7 days.

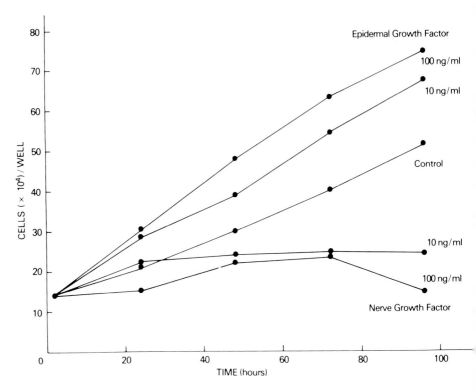

FIG. 5.   Proliferation of PC12 cells treated with nerve growth factor or epidermal growth factor.

cells (20,31,41), but hyperplasia, originally thought to be a consequence of nerve growth factor treatment (33,41), is now thought to be unlikely (32). Neurite outgrowth, of course, is the most recognized consequence. Frequently, there are increases in a number of anabolic processes (2–4,43,44), and an induction of certain enzymes, notably those involved in the synthesis of transmitter (21,25,60). In culture, nerve growth factor is frankly required for the survival of its target neurons. Indeed, the multitude of effects caused by nerve growth factor has complicated studies on its mechanism of action and led to the feeling that there is more than one site of action within the cell.

Although the exact mechanism of action of nerve growth factor is still not known, there is good evidence that the factor initiates two classes of events within the cell. The membrane effects are rapid and include changes in morphology of the membrane, increases in metabolite and ion transport, and increased cellular adhesiveness. Another class of events depends upon transcriptional actions in the cells and includes the induction of transmitter-synthesizing enzymes (45), process formation in unprimed cells (15), and perhaps the anabolic increases and the hypertrophy. It has been suggested by Bradshaw (11) and by others that the combination of nerve growth factor with its receptor initiates the rapid membrane effects seen in target

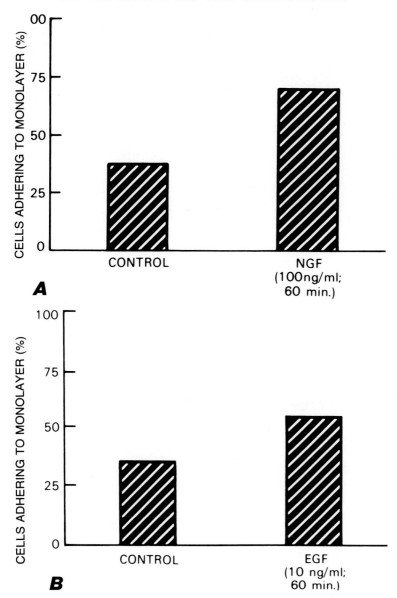

FIG. 6. Adhesion of labeled PC12 cells to a monolayer of unlabeled PC12 cells in the presence of **(A)** nerve growth factor (100 ng/ml) or **(B)** epidermal growth factor (150 ng/ml).

cells. An internalization of the nerve growth factor followed by its combination with the nuclear receptor could serve to trigger the transcriptionally mediated actions. Alternatively, the generation of a second messenger, such as cAMP, for which there is some evidence (47,48,52,54), could serve as the intracellular signal. In either case, nuclear events, such as the increased phosphorylation of nuclear

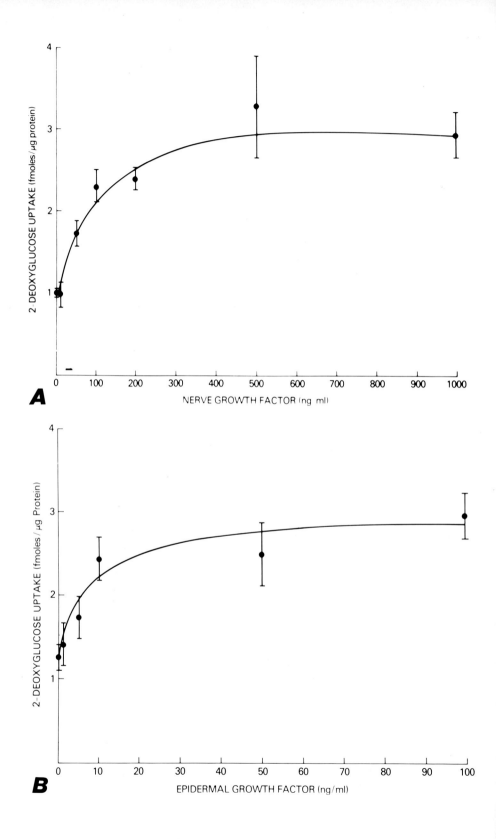

proteins (70,71), could initiate the transcriptional events. Definitive evidence upon which to decide the correct pathway is still lacking, but it is clear that both membrane and nuclear events are required to explain all the actions of nerve growth factor on its target cells.

Since nerve growth factor is required for the survival of sympathetic and sensory neurons in culture, *in vitro* studies on the mechanism of nerve growth factor actions have been complicated. Obviously, any effects observed due to the addition of nerve growth factor could be simply due to the fact that the controls were dying. Thus it has been very difficult to devise experiments in which the discrete effects of nerve growth factor on biochemical processes could be separated from its effects on survival. The development of several nerve growth factor-responsive tumor lines has provided a new avenue for such studies. As mentioned earlier, there are several tumor lines which respond in various ways to the addition of nerve growth factor. The most useful and the most used of these has been the PC12 clone.

The PC12 clone, derived from a tumor of the rat adrenal medulla, has been developed largely by Greene and his colleagues (20,27,28,30). When placed in culture, it grows as a rounded, unremarkable cell (Fig. 4A). Upon the addition of nanogram amounts of nerve growth factor, it exhibits a rapid and profuse outgrowth of neurites (Fig. 4B). Along with this profound morphological alteration, the cells develop excitable membranes, and will form synapses with appropriate cells in culture. They stop dividing and, overall, differentiate, albeit reversibly, into a sympathetic neuron. They exhibit massive membrane changes (19), increases in metabolite transport (46), hypertrophy (20), and a number of the other effects seen when nerve growth factor impinges on its normal target cells. Indeed, the PC12 has been used extensively as a model for the action of nerve growth factor, and even more, as a tool by which to dissect the various different actions of nerve growth factor, since there are some nerve growth factor-induced changes in sympathetic neurons, e.g., the induction of tyrosine hydroxylase, which are not seen in PC12.

From a different vantage point, these cells can be viewed as a model of neuronal differentiation. Using nerve growth factor, then, one can perhaps observe changes in the cells at some early point in the decision to become neurons. In this regard, we were surprised to find, in collaboration with Drs. Rosanne Goodman and Harvey Herschman, that the PC12 cells also respond to epidermal growth factor. Epidermal growth factor, although usually isolated from the same source as nerve growth factor, the submaxillary gland of the mature male mouse, is completely different in size and sequence. Our interest in this observation stems from the fact that nerve growth factor is a terminal differentiator in this system, while epidermal growth factor, in most of its responsive cells, is a potent mitogen (16,26). We have,

FIG. 7. Stimulation of [³H]2-deoxy-D-glucose uptake into PC12 cells by **(A)** nerve growth factor or **(B)** epidermal growth factor.

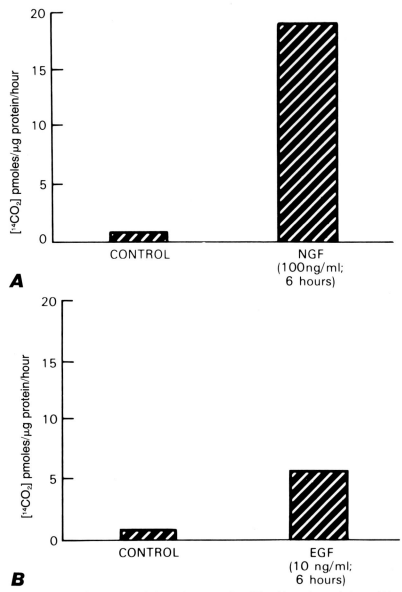

FIG. 8. Effect of **(A)** nerve growth factor (100 ng/ml) or **(B)** epidermal growth factor (10 ng/ml) on ornithine decarboxylase activity in PC12 cells.

therefore, explored the relationship between these two seemingly antagonistic peptides (36,37).

The overall effects of these two growth-regulating peptides on the cells are quite different. Nerve growth factor stimulates neurite outgrowth, induces hypertrophy, and inhibits cell proliferation. Epidermal growth factor causes little outgrowth, no

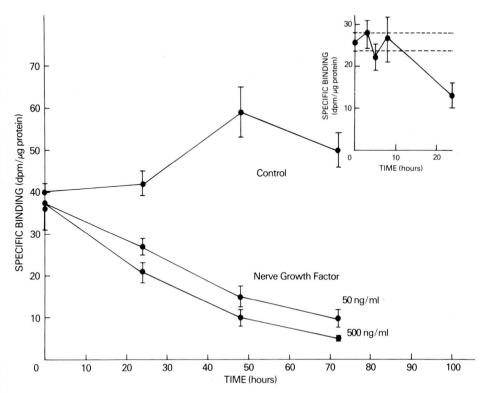

FIG. 9. Time course of nerve growth factor-induced loss of epidermal growth factor binding to PC12 cells.

TABLE 1. *The effect of epidermal growth factor on ornithine decarboxylase levels in nerve growth factor-treated and control PC12 cells*

Cells	Treatment	Ornithine decarboxylase activity (nmoles $^{14}CO_2$ released/mg protein per hr)
Control	None	1.22
	EGF	7.56
NGF-treated	None	1.01
	EGF	2.31

hypertrophy, and produces a modest increase in cell proliferation (Fig. 5). Although the increase in cell numbers caused by epidermal growth factor is not a convincing demonstration of mitogenicity, it is clear that the effect is different than that of nerve growth factor. The small effect on cell numbers may be due to the richness of the medium in which the cells are grown.

Surprisingly, although the two peptides are different in their ultimate effect on the cells, they promote some of the same intracellular responses. For example, both

TABLE 2. *The binding of ^{125}I-epidermal growth factor to nerve growth factor-treated and control PC12 cells*

Cells	Specific binding of epidermal growth factor (cpm/μg protein)	
	Experiment 1	Experiment 2
Control	762	416
NGF-treated	131	81

peptides increase the adhesiveness of the cells (Fig. 6). Both increase the uptake of the model sugar, 2-deoxyglucose (Fig. 7). Both produce an induction of the enzyme ornithine decarboxylase (Fig. 8). Whether these peptides alter these parameters by the same mechanism is not known. However, preliminary evidence suggests that both cell adhesiveness and ornithine decarboxylase induction are greater in the presence of maximal amounts of the two peptides together than of either alone, indicating that in these two cases, at least, the changes may be brought about by different mechanisms.

It was of interest to know what happens if the two factors are added to the cells at the same time. The answer is that the cells respond to nerve growth factor as if the epidermal growth factor were not present. That is, the cells form neurites, stop dividing, and look, outwardly, the same as cells treated with nerve growth factor alone. In other words, the action of nerve growth factor appears to predominate and overrides the modest effects of epidermal growth factor on cell proliferation.

In order to find out if this morphological predominance was reflected in biochemical events in the cells, we used ornithine decarboxylase as a probe. The experiments involved treating the cells with nerve growth factor until they were well differentiated and then inspecting their response to epidermal growth factor. In such an experiment, it was observed that the normal induction of ornithine decarboxylase caused by epidermal growth factor in untreated cells was much attenuated in cells previously treated with nerve growth factor (Table 1). That the cells were not simply refractory for ornithine decarboxylase induction was shown by the fact that the induction produced by treatment with dBcAMP was the same in nerve growth factor-treated cells as it was in controls. Consistent with the morphological predominance of nerve growth factor, the induction of ornithine decarboxylase by nerve growth factor was the same whether the cells had been treated with epidermal growth factor or not. Thus cells differentiated with nerve growth factor respond to dBcAMP, but not to epidermal growth factor, but cells treated with epidermal growth factor respond normally to nerve growth factor.

Inquiring into the molecular mechanism of the nerve growth factor-induced attenuation of the ornithine decarboxylase response led us to inspect the epidermal growth factor receptors on the cells. These receptors are easy to measure and have straightforward properties. They are saturable with a K_d of approximately 10^{-9}M. They are specific for epidermal growth factor; nerve growth factor does not compete for binding. The amount of binding does not change with the density of the culture.

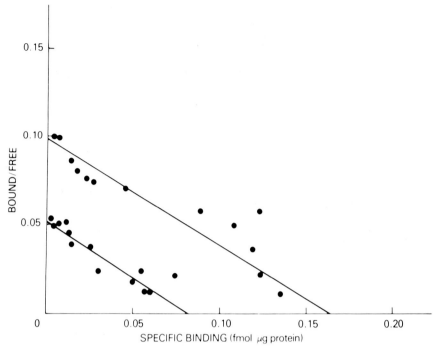

FIG. 10. Scatchard analysis of the nerve growth factor-induced decrease in epidermal growth factor binding.

The binding of epidermal growth factor to nerve growth factor-treated cells is much lower than the binding to untreated cells (Table 2). About 80% of the binding is lost within 72 hr of the addition of nerve growth factor. Even recalculating on the basis of cell number to take into account the hypertrophy of the cells under the influence of nerve growth factor shows at least 60% loss of binding per cell. The time course of the loss of binding (Fig. 9) shows that the response is fairly slow, paralleling roughly the morphological alterations. This would suggest that the change in binding is not due to rapid alterations in the membrane, which are seen within seconds, but rather to long-term, perhaps transcriptional, alterations within the cells. Finally, Scatchard analysis, done after 24 hr of treatment, since the loss of binding after 72 hr is so profound as to be difficult to analyze in this fashion, reveals that the number of receptors on the cells decreases from about 80,000 to about 40,000 per cell, but that the affinity of these receptors for epidermal growth factor remains about the same (Fig. 10).

The results lend themselves to interpretation at several different levels. Very simply, the results suggest that nerve growth factor limits the response of PC12 cells to epidermal growth factor by limiting their synthesis of the epidermal growth factor receptor. A mild extrapolation of this suggestion would be that this diminution of receptors is part of the mechanism by which nerve growth factor causes the PC12 cells to differentiate, i.e., by preventing their response to this and perhaps to other mitogens. A bolder interpretation is that this is part of the way in which neurons in general differentiate, by a reduced response to mitogens, and that this action of nerve growth factor is a fundamental route by which maturation factors act. Experiments by which to test this hypothesis in normal cells are in progress.

ACKNOWLEDGMENT

David End was the recipient of a National Research Service Award (1-F32-HD05905-01).

REFERENCES

1. Andres, R. Y., Jeng, I., and Bradshaw, R. A. (1977): Nerve growth factor receptors: identification of distinct classes in plasma membranes and nuclei of embryonic dorsal root neurons. *Proc. Natl. Acad. Sci. U.S.A.*, 74:2785–2789.
2. Angeletti, P. U., Gandini-Attardi, D., Toschi, G., Salvi, M. L., and Levi-Montalcini, R. (1965): Metabolic aspects of the effect of nerve growth factor on sympathetic and sensory ganglia: protein and ribonucleic acid synthesis. *Biochim. Biophys. Acta*, 95:111–118.
3. Angeletti, P. U., Luizzi, A., and Levi-Montalcini, R. (1964): Stimulation of lipid biosynthesis in sympathetic and sensory ganglia by a specific nerve growth factor. *Biochim. Biophys. Acta*, 84:778–781.
4. Angeletti, P. U., Luizzi, A., Levi-Montalcini, R., and Gandini-Attardi, D. (1964): Effect of a nerve growth factor on glucose metabolism by sympathetic and sensory nerve cells. *Biochim. Biophys. Acta*, 90:445–450.
5. Angeletti, R. H., and Bradshaw, R. A. (1971): Nerve growth factor from mouse submaxillary gland: amino acid sequence. *Proc. Natl. Acad. Sci. U.S.A.*, 68:2417–2420.
6. Banerjee, S. P., Cuatrecasas, P., and Snyder, S. H. (1976): Solubilization of nerve growth factor receptor of rabbit superior cervical ganglia. *J. Biol. Chem.*, 251:5680–5685.
7. Banerjee, S. P., Snyder, S. H., Cuatrecasas, P., and Greene, L. A. (1973): Binding of nerve growth factor in sympathetic ganglia. *Proc. Natl. Acad. Sci. U.S.A.*, 70:2519–2523.
8. Berger, E. A., and Shooter, E. M. (1977): The biosynthesis and processing of pro β-NGF, a biosynthetic precursor to β-nerve growth factor. *Proc. Natl. Acad. Sci. U.S.A.*, 74:3647–3651.
9. Berger, E. A., and Shooter, E. M. (1978): The biosynthesis of β-nerve growth factor in mouse submaxillary gland. *J. Biol. Chem.*, 243:804–810.
10. Bocchini, V., and Angeletti, P. U. (1969): The nerve growth factor: purification as a 30,000-molecular-weight protein. *Proc. Natl. Acad. Sci. U.S.A.*, 64:787–794.
11. Bradshaw, R. A. (1978): Nerve growth factor. *Ann. Rev. Biochem.*, 47:191–216.
12. Bradshaw, R. A., and Young, M. (1976): Nerve growth factor—recent developments and perspectives. *Biochem. Pharmacol.*, 25:1445–1449.
13. Bueker, E. D. (1948): Implantation of tumors in the hind limb field of the embryonic chick and the developmental response of the lumbosacral nervous system. *Anat. Record*, 102:369–390.
14. Bueker, E. D. (1952): Hypertrophy and hyperplasia of sympathetic and spinal ganglia in the chick embryo induced by sarcoma 180. *Anat. Record*, 102:317.
15. Burstein, D. E., and Greene, L. A. (1978): Evidence for both RNA-synthesis dependent and independent pathways of stimulation of neurite outgrowth by nerve growth factor. *Proc. Natl. Acad. Sci. U.S.A.*, 75:6059–6063.
16. Carpenter, G. (1978): The regulation of cell proliferation: advances in the biology and mechanism of action of epidermal growth factor. *J. Invest. Dermatol.*, 71:283–287.
17. Cohen, S. (1959): Purification and metabolic effects of a nerve growth-promoting protein from snake venom. *J. Biol. Chem.*, 234:1129–1137.
18. Cohen, S. (1960): Purification of a nerve growth promoting protein from the mouse salivary gland and its neurocytotoxic antiserum. *Proc. Natl. Acad. Sci. U.S.A.*, 46:302–311.
19. Connolly, J. L., Greene, L. A., Viscarello, R., and Riley, W. D. (1979): Rapid sequential changes in surface morphology of PC12 pheochromocytoma cells in response to nerve growth factor. *J. Cell Biol.*, 82:820–827.

20. Dichter, M. A., Tischler, A. S., and Greene, L. A. (1977): Nerve growth factor-induced increase in electrical excitability and acetylcholine sensitivity of a rat pheochromocytoma cell line. *Nature*, 268:501–504.

21. Edgar, D. H., and Thoenen, H. (1978): Selective enzyme induction in a nerve growth factor-responsive pheochromocytoma cell line (PC12). *Brain Res.*, 154:186–190.

22. Fabricant, R. N., DeLarco, J. E., and Todaro, G. J. (1977): Nerve growth factor receptors on human melanoma cells in culture. *Proc. Natl. Acad. Sci. U.S.A.*, 74:565–569.

23. Frazier, W. A., Angeletti, R. H., and Bradshaw, R. A. (1972): Nerve growth factor and insulin. *Science*, 176:482–488.

24. Frazier, W. A., Boyd, L. F., and Bradshaw, R. A. (1974): Properties of the specific binding of ^{125}I nerve growth factor to responsive peripheral neurons. *J. Biol. Chem.*, 249:5513–5519.

25. Goodman, R., and Herschman, H. R. (1978): Nerve growth factor-mediated induction of tyrosine hydroxylase in a clonal pheochromocytoma cell line. *Proc. Natl. Acad. Sci. U.S.A.*, 75:4587–4590.

26. Gospodarowicz, D., and Moran, J. S. (1976): Growth factors in mammalian cell culture. *Ann. Rev. Biochem.*, 45:531–558.

27. Greene, L. A., and Rein, G. (1977): Synthesis, storage, and release of acetylcholine by a noradrenergic pheochromocytoma cell line. *Nature*, 268:349–351.

28. Greene, L. A., and Rein, G. (1977): Release, storage, and uptake of catecholamines by a clonal cell line of nerve growth factor (NGF) responsive pheochromocytoma cells. *Brain Res.*, 129:247–263.

29. Greene, L. A., and Shooter, E. M. (1980): The nerve growth factor: biochemistry, synthesis, and mechanism of action. *Ann. Rev. Neurosci.*, 3:353–402.

30. Greene, L. A., and Tischler, A. S. (1976): Establishment of a noradrenergic clonal line of rat adrenal pheochromocytoma cells which respond to nerve growth factor. *Proc. Natl. Acad. Sci. U.S.A.*, 73:2424–2428.

31. Hendry, I. A. (1976): A method to correct adequately for the change in neuronal size when estimating neuronal numbers after nerve growth factor treatment. *J. Neurocytol.*, 5:337–349.

32. Hendry, I. A. (1977): Cell division in the developing sympathetic nervous system. *J. Neurocytol.*, 6:299–309.

33. Hendry, I. A., and Campbell, J. (1976): Morphometric analysis of rat superior cervical ganglion after axotomy and nerve growth factor treatment. *J. Neurocytol.*, 5:351–360.

34. Hendry, I. A., Stoeckel, K., Thoenen, H., and Iversen, L. L. (1974): The retrograde axonal transport of nerve growth factor. *Brain Res.*, 68:103–121.

35. Herrup, K., and Shooter, E. M. (1973): Properties of the NGF receptor of avian dorsal root ganglia. *Proc. Natl. Acad. Sci. U.S.A.*, 70:3884–3888.

36. Huff, K. R., End, D., and Guroff, G. (1981): Nerve growth factor-induced alteration in the response of PC12 pheochromocytoma cells to epidermal growth factor. *J. Cell Biol.*, 88:189–198.

37. Huff, K. R., and Guroff, G. (1979): Nerve growth factor-induced reduction in epidermal growth factor responsiveness and epidermal growth factor receptors in PC12 cells: an aspect of cell differentiation. *Biochem. Biophys. Res. Commun.*, 89:175–180.

38. Johnson, E. M., Jr., Gorin, P. D., Brandeis, L. D., and Pearson, J. (1980): Dorsal root ganglion neurons are destroyed by in utero exposure to maternal antibody to nerve growth factor. *Science*, 210:916–918.

39. Levi-Montalcini, R., and Booker, B. (1960): Destruction of the sympathetic ganglia in mammals by an antiserum to the nerve growth protein. *Proc. Natl. Acad. Sci. U.S.A.*, 46:384–391.

40. Levi-Montalcini, R., Mayer, H., and Hamburger, V. (1954): In vitro experiments on the effects of mouse sarcoma 180 and 37 on the spinal and sympathetic ganglia of the chick embryo. *Cancer Res.*, 14:49–57.

41. Levi-Montalcini, R., and Hamburger, V. (1951): Selective growth-stimulating effects of mouse sarcoma on the sensory and sympathetic nervous system of the chick embryo. *J. Exp. Zool.*, 116:321–362.

42. Levi-Montalcini, R., and Hamburger, V. (1953): A diffusable agent of mouse sarcoma producing hyperplasia of sympathetic ganglia and hyperneurotization of viscera in the chick embryo. *J. Exp. Zool.*, 123:233–288.

43. Luizzi, A., Angeletti, P. U., and Levi-Montalcini, R. (1965): Metabolic effects of a specific nerve growth factor (NGF) on sensory and sympathetic ganglia: enhancement of lipid biosynthesis. *J. Neurochem.*, 12:705–708.

44. Luizzi, A., Pocchiari, F., and Angeletti, P. U. (1968): Glucose metabolism in embryonic ganglia: effect of nerve growth factor (NGF) and insulin. *Brain Res.*, 7:452–458.
45. MacDonnell, P., Tolson, N., and Guroff, G. (1977): Selective de novo synthesis of tyrosine hydroxylase in organ cultures of rat superior cervical ganglia after in vivo administration of nerve growth factor. *J. Biol. Chem.*, 252:5859–5863.
46. McGuire, J. C., and Greene, L. A. (1979): Rapid stimulation by nerve growth factor of amino acid uptake by clonal PC12 pheochromocytoma cells. *J. Biol. Chem.*, 254:3362–3367.
47. Narumi, S., and Fujita, T. (1978): Stimulatory effects of substance P and nerve growth factor (NGF) on neurite outgrowth in embryonic chick dorsal root ganglia. *Neuropharmacology*, 17:73–76.
48. Nikodijevic, B., Nikodijevic, D., Yu, M. W., Pollard, H., and Guroff, G. (1975): The effect of nerve growth factor on cyclic AMP levels in superior cervical ganglia of the rat. *Proc. Natl. Acad. Sci. U.S.A.*, 72:4679–4771.
49. Paravicini, U., Stoeckel, K., and Thoenen, H. (1975): Biological importance of retrograde axonal transport of nerve growth factor in adrenergic neurons. *Brain Res.*, 84:279–291.
50. Perez-Polo, J. R., Hall, K., Livingston, K., and Westlund, K. (1977): Steroid induction of nerve growth factor synthesis in cell culture. *Life Sci.*, 21:1535–1544.
51. Reynolds, C. P., and Perez-Polo, J. R. (1975): Human neuroblastoma: glial induced morphological differentiation. *Neurosci. Lett.*, 1:91–97.
52. Schubert, D., and Whitlock, C. (1977): Alteration of cellular adhesion by nerve growth factor. *Proc. Natl. Acad. Sci. U.S.A.*, 74:4055–4058.
53. Schwartz, J. P., Chuang, D. M., and Costa, E. (1977): Increases in nerve growth factor content of C_6 glioma cells by the activation of a β-adrenergic receptor. *Brain Res.*, 137:369–375.
54. Skaper, S. D., Bottenstein, J. E., and Varon, S. (1979): Effects of nerve growth factor on cyclic AMP levels in embryonic chick dorsal root ganglia following factor deprivation. *J. Neurochem.*, 32:1845–1851.
55. Skaper, S. D., and Varon, S. (1979): Sodium dependence of nerve growth factor-regulated hexose transport in chick embryo sensory neurons. *Biochem. Biophys. Res. Commun.*, 88:563–568.
56. Stoeckel, K., Gagnon, C., Guroff, G., and Thoenen, H. (1976): Purification of nerve growth factor (NGF) antibodies by affinity chromatography. *J. Neurochem.*, 26:1207–1211.
57. Stoeckel, K., Guroff, G., Schwab, M., and Thoenen, H. (1976): The significance of retrograde axonal transport for the accumulation of systemically administered nerve growth factor (NGF) in the rat superior cervical ganglion. *Brain Res.*, 109:271–284.
58. Stoeckel, K., Paravicini, U., and Thoenen, H. (1974): Specificity of the retrograde axonal transport of nerve growth factor. *Brain Res.*, 76:413–421.
59. Suda, K., Barde, Y. A., and Thoenen, H. (1978): Nerve growth factor in mouse and rat serum: correlation between bioassay and radioimmunoassay determinations. *Proc. Natl. Acad. Sci. U.S.A.*, 75:4042–4046.
60. Thoenen, H., Angeletti, P. U., Levi-Montalcini, R., and Kettler, R. (1971): Selective induction by nerve growth factor of tyrosine hydroxylase and dopamine-β-hydroxylase in rat superior cervical ganglia. *Proc. Natl. Acad. Sci. U.S.A.*, 68:1598–1602.
61. Tomita, J. T., and Varon, S. (1971): Preparation of antibodies to the three subunits of mouse 7S nerve growth factor. *Neurobiology*, 1:176–190.
61a. Varon, S. (1972): In: *Methods of Neurochemistry*, Vol. 3, edited by R. Fried. Marcel Dekker, New York.
62. Varon, S., and Horii, Z. (1977): Nerve growth factor action on membrane permeation to exogenous substrates in dorsal root ganglionic dissociates from the chick embryo. *Brain Res.*, 124:121–135.
63. Varon, S., Nomura, J., and Shooter, E. M. (1967): The isolation of the mouse nerve growth factor protein in a high molecular weight form. *Biochemistry*, 6:2202–2209.
64. Varon, S., Raiborn, C., and Burnham, P. A. (1974): Selective potency of homologous ganglionic non-neuronal cells for the support of dissociated ganglionic neurons in culture. *Neurobiology*, 4:231–252.
65. Varon, S., Raiborn, C., and Burnham, P. A. (1974): Comparative effects of nerve growth factor and ganglionic non-neuronal cells on purified mouse ganglionic neurons in culture. *J. Neurobiol.*, 5:355–391.
66. Vinores, S., and Guroff, G. (1980): Nerve growth factor: mechanism of action. *Ann. Rev. Biophys. Bioeng.*, 9:223–257.
67. Vinores, S. A., and Koestner, A.: The effect of nerve growth factor on undifferentiated glioma cells. *Cancer Lett. (in press).*

68. Waris, T., Rechardt, L., and Waris, P. (1973): Differentiation of neuroblastoma cells induced by nerve growth factor in vitro. *Experientia*, 29:1128–1129.
69. Yankner, B. A., and Shooter, E. M. (1979): Nerve growth factor in the nucleus: interaction with receptors on the nuclear membrane. *Proc. Natl. Acad. Sci. U.S.A.*, 76:1269–1273.
70. Yu, M. W., Hori, S., Tolson, N., Huff, K., and Guroff, G. (1978): Increased phosphorylation of a specific nuclear protein in rat superior cervical ganglia in response to nerve growth factor. *Biochem. Biophys. Res. Commun.*, 81:941–945.
71. Yu, M. W., Tolson, N., and Guroff, G. (1980): Increased phosphorylation of specific nuclear proteins in superior cervical ganglia and PC12 cells in response to nerve growth factor. *J. Biol. Chem.*, 255:10481–10492.

Maturation Factors and Cancer,
edited by Malcolm A. S. Moore.
Raven Press, © New York 1982.

Pheochromocytoma Cells as Neuronal Models: Effects of EGF and NGF

*R. Goodman and **H. R. Herschman

*Department of Pediatrics, University of Pennsylvania, and Joseph Stokes, Jr., Research Institute, The Children's Hospital of Philadelphia, Philadelphia, Pennsylvania 19104; **Department of Biological Chemistry and Laboratory of Nuclear Medicine and Radiation Biology, University of California, Los Angeles, School of Medicine, Los Angeles, California 90024*

TUMORS OF THE NERVOUS SYSTEM

Tumors of the nervous system, while representing only a small proportion of all cancers, are of interest because some of these tumors retain a high degree of differentiated function. Among the neuronal tumors derived from neuroectoderm which exhibit differentiated function are the neuroblastomas, retinoblastomas, medulloblastomas, and pheochromocytomas. Little is known about the etiology of these neuronal tumors, but there is increasing evidence that some of them may be genetically related. Familial histories indicate that families or patients exhibiting one of these tumors will show a predilection to develop certain other tumors (30). The occurrence of neuroblastoma cells in the adrenals of young infants autopsied after death from causes unrelated to cancer is 40 times higher than the clinical frequency of neuroblastoma (3). Many of these tumor cells must, therefore, either regress spontaneously or differentiate into mature cells later than the rest of the adrenal medullary cells. One might speculate that the growth and regression or control of these tumor cells is regulated by hormones and/or growth factors.

Since neuronal tumors apparently lose the controlled growth exhibited by normal cells, but often retain much of their differentiated functions, these cells may serve as useful model systems for the study both of the regulation of neuronal functions as well as the relationships between differentiation and growth control. A number of laboratories have utilized a highly differentiated rat pheochromocytoma, a tumor of adrenal medullary origin, to study both regulation of neuronal functions and growth control by several growth factors and hormones. In this review, we summarize the findings of various laboratories concerning regulation of cell division and neuronal differentiation by growth factors in cell lines derived from this transplantable rat pheochromocytoma tumor (53). Both morphological and biochemical

29

aspects of neuronal differentiation have been studied, with the hope of shedding some light upon the mechanism of development and regulation of differentiated functions in the normal and neoplastic neuron.

THE SYMPATHETIC NERVOUS SYSTEM

The peripheral sympathetic nervous system synthesizes the catecholamine neurotransmitters epinephrine and norepinephrine. These neurotransmitters are produced by the cells of the adrenal medulla and by sympathetic ganglion cells. The rate limiting enzyme in catecholamine biosynthesis is the adrenergic enzyme tyrosine hydroxylase (TH) [tyrosine 3-monooxygenase; L-tyrosine, tetrahydropteridine: oxygen oxidoreductase (3-hydroxylating), EC 1.14.16.2]. Any event that affects the levels of TH will ultimately also affect the levels of catecholamines produced. Of course, any manipulations that affect the development of normal functioning of the adrenergic nervous system will also produce changes in the levels of the catecholamines. Sympathetic ganglion cells, represented by the superior cervical ganglion cells, have been shown to exhibit several responses to specific protein and hormonal factors. The best characterized specific responses are to a protein growth factor, nerve growth factor (NGF), which affects the sympathetic nervous system in several ways.

NERVE GROWTH FACTOR

The enhancement of neurite outgrowth in response to nerve growth factor was initially reported by Bueker, who noted that implantation of Sarcoma 180 into chick embryos caused hypertrophy of the sympathetic nervous system (7). Levi-Montalcini and Hamburger subsequently showed that a diffusable factor from the murine tumor caused the sympathetic enlargement (36). Cohen, while purifying this factor from the sarcoma preparation, discovered similar activity in snake venom (10). Led by this finding to study analogous organs in other species, Cohen found that the male mouse salivary gland contained relatively high concentrations of nerve growth factor (11). While most of the laboratory investigations over the past 20 years have been carried out with NGF isolated from mouse salivary glands, recent studies have indicated that NGF can be isolated from several other sources such as human placental tissue (18), human tumors (14,51), and guinea pig prostate gland (27); smaller amounts have been reported in several cell culture lines (28,39,42,43,54). The biologically active subunit of mouse NGF is a basic (IP = 9.1) molecule with a sedimentation of 2.5 S. The amino acid sequence of this molecule has been determined by Angelletti and Bradshaw (2).

There is an absolute requirement for NGF both for the development and maintenance of the sympathetic nervous system *in vivo* as well as *in vitro*. If the active beta subunit of NGF is injected into newborn mice or rats, extensive hypertrophy of the sympathetic ganglia results; the superior cervical ganglia of NGF-treated rodents may have over fivefold the protein content of control animals. Injection of antisera to NGF into neonatal rodents completely supresses the development of the sympathetic nervous system; 92 to 95% of the nerve cell population of the paravertebral and prevertebral ganglia are destroyed. This finding emphasizes the necessity of NGF for development and maintenance of a functional sympathetic nervous system (for reviews, see refs. 32 and 35). Similarly, isolated sympathetic neurons are not viable in dissociated cell culture without NGF (40). However, concentrations of NGF as low as 5 ng/ml (2×10^{-10}M) provide for survival and morphological differentiation of neonatal sympathetic neurons in culture (21,22). This morphological differentiation, characterized by the extension of long neuritic processes, is the basis for most assays of the biological activity of NGF (16,21,23,37). (For a more detailed discussion of NGF assays, see D. End and G. Guroff, *this volume*.) Withdrawal of the NGF leads to degeneration of the cell processes, cell bodies, and ultimately to cell death (34,35,40). Thus NGF is required for the viability and morphological differentiation of the sympathetic nervous system, both *in vivo* and in culture.

NGF INDUCTION OF TH

In addition to its effects on viability and morphology, NGF also elicits a selective induction of the adrenergic enzymes tyrosine hydroxylase (TH) and dopamine β-hydroxylase in the sympathetic ganglia. This NGF-mediated induction of TH has been demonstrated in sympathetic ganglia *in vivo* (33), in organ cultures of sympathetic ganglia (13,44,55), and in a clonal cell line PC-G2 (19), derived from a rat pheochromocytoma tumor. Figure 1 shows the dose-response curve generated by incubating PC-G2 cells with various concentrations of β-NGF. At concentrations of NGF above 0.5 μg/ml, there is a significant increase in the specific activity of TH. The maximal induction is four- to fivefold over the control values at concentrations of NGF above 1 μg per ml. The concentration of NGF necessary to effect the induction of tyrosine hydroxylase in the PC-G2 cells is similar to that necessary to cause induction of TH in cultured sympathetic ganglia, which is also in the μg/ml range ($\sim 10^{-8}$M) (44). In PC-12, another clonal cell line derived from this tumor by Greene and Tischler (26), NGF does not affect the level of the adrenergic enzyme tyrosine hydroxylase, but it does induce a morphological differentiation similar to that seen in cultures of sympathetic neurons of young rodents (40). In contrast, the PC-G2 cell line does not exhibit this morphological response to NGF.

While both of these clonal pheochromocytoma cell lines PC-12 and PC-G2 respond to the same protein, nerve growth factor, and each line exhibits a response characteristic of the sympathetic ganglion cells, each line exhibits a different response. One of the great advantages of utilizing these clonal lines is that the responses have been separated into two different cell lines, so that the mechanism by which NGF elicits one response can be studied in a system that exhibits only that response. Thus the mechanism by which NGF elicits process formation can be studied in the PC-12 cells and separated from the mechanisms by which NGF elicits TH induction. Similarly, in the PC-G2 cells, events involved in the NGF-mediated induction of TH can be examined in the absence of process formation. In this way,

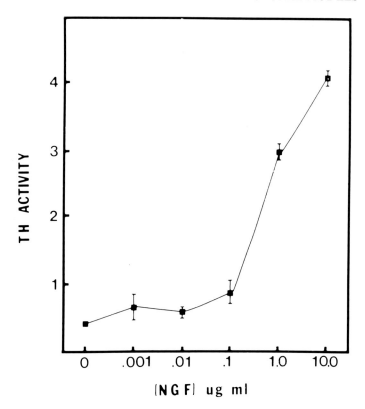

FIG. 1. Induction of tyrosine hydroxylase in PC-G2 cells by NGF. PC-G2 cells were plated at 5 × 10⁵ cells/100 mm dish. NGF was added to the dishes 24 hr later. After 4 days of exposure, the cells were scraped from the dish and assayed for tyrosine hydroxylase activity according to previously published methods (19). Values are means ± SE of triplicate plates. Enzyme activity in control cultures was 0.42 ± 0.03 nmoles DOPA/hr/mg protein. (Reprinted, with permission, from Goodman and Herschman, ref. 19).

the molecular mechanisms for each process can be studied and common or divergent pathways elucidated. Since primary sympathetic neurons are dependent upon NGF for survival in culture and since they have had previous exposure to this protein (as well as other unknown factors) *in vivo*, it has not been possible to study the earliest stages of NGF exposure and of neuritic extension. On the other hand, since the PC-12 cell, in contrast to the sympathetic neuron, does not require the continued presence of NGF for survival in cell culture when there is serum present in the medium, the early events following NGF exposure can be examined. Burnstein and Greene have shown that the stimulation of neuritic extension in PC-12 cells by NGF requires an RNA-synthesis-dependent step, followed by an RNA-synthesis-independent step (8). This first RNA-synthesis-dependent event has not been reported in sympathetic ganglion cells. The differences between the two findings can probably be related to the unavoidable exposure of the ganglion cells to NGF *in vivo*.

SERUM-FREE MEDIA AND THE ROLE OF GROWTH FACTORS IN PHEOCHROMOCYTOMA SURVIVAL

Although the problems of controlling environmental influences are minimized by performing experiments in cell culture rather than *in vivo*, the need for serum in the culture medium still introduces a lack of total environmental control. Since the composition of serum is not defined, the cells are exposed to a multitude of unknown factors whose levels may vary depending on the history of the animal from which the serum is obtained. Several laboratories have attempted to circumvent this problem by utilizing a chemically defined medium. Greene has reported that in a very minimal medium (RPM1 1640), which contains vitamins and amino acids in a balanced salt solution, PC-12 cells do not survive in the absence of either serum or NGF (24). However, the N2 medium devised by Bottenstein and Sato (5), which contains only five other components (selenium, transferrin, progesterone, insulin, and putrescine), in addition to the vitamins and amino acids, will support the growth of PC-12 cells (6). A second chemically defined medium devised by Ambesi-Impiobato et al. (1), which contains an amino acid and vitamin base supplemented with hydrocortisone, somatostatin, insulin, thyrotropin, and glycyl-histidyl-lysine, will also support growth of PC-12 cells. Neither of these media contain either NGF or epidermal growth factor (EGF).

In contrast to the ability of PC-12 cells to grow in these chemically defined media, the PC-G2 cells are unable to survive in the N2 medium unless it is supplemented with EGF (Fig. 2). There is a bell-shaped concentration range of EGF, over which the growth stimulatory effects on PC-G2 cells are observed. Preliminary experiments indicate that NGF will also support the survival of PC-G2 cells in chemically defined medium (data not shown; R. Goodman et al., *manuscript in preparation*). (We are presently exploring this phenomenon further.) Preliminary data suggest that the PC-G2 cells also exhibit the same requirement for either NGF or EGF in order to survive in the chemically defined medium devised by Ambesi-Impiobato et al (1). Thus the pheochromocytoma cell lines cultured in appropriate media should be useful model systems for studying the growth factor dependence exhibited by sympathetic neurons both *in vivo* and in culture.

INDUCTION OF TH BY EGF IN PC-G2 CELLS

The PC-G2 cells depend on either NGF or EGF for their survival in serum-free medium. In addition to the ability of EGF to support the survival of the PC-G2 cells in serum-free medium, EGF also mimics NGF in the ability to induce TH in the PC-G2 cells (Fig. 3). The optimal dose for the EGF-mediated TH induction in PC-G2 cells is in the ng/ml range ($\sim 10^{-10}$M) (far lower than the amount of NGF required to cause the same induction, μg/ml).

While both of these proteins are isolated from the submaxillary glands of male mice, they bear no structural or serological similarity. The amino acid sequences of both proteins have been determined (2,48). NGF is a basic protein (IP = 9.1) and EGF is acidic (IP = 4.5). While EGF has been studied primarily as a mitogen

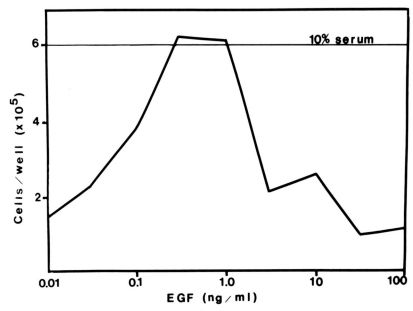

FIG. 2. Growth of PC-G2 cells in defined-free medium. PC-G2 cells were plated at 5×10^4 cells per 16 mm well in N2 medium supplemented with varying concentrations of EGF or with 10% fetal calf serum. Cultures were incubated at 37°C in a humidified atmosphere of 95% air-5% CO_2. The medium was renewed at 3-day intervals. On day 12, the cells were counted. Each data point represents the mean of three replicate cultures.

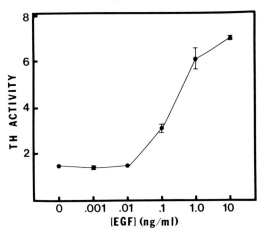

FIG. 3. Concentration dependence of EGF-mediated TH induction in PC-G2 cells. PC-G2 cells were exposed to varying concentrations of EGF for 4 days. Culture conditions are as described in Fig. 1. The cells were then harvested and assayed for TH activity. The TH activity is expressed as nanomoles dopa formed per hr per mg protein. The TH activity of the control cultures was 1.44 ± 0.02 nmoles DOPA/hr per mg protein. Values are means $\pm$ SEM of 3 cultures. (Reprinted, with permission, from Goodman et al., ref. 20).

for fibroblast cells, it has also been shown to affect a variety of differentiated functions, including synthesis of hyaluronic acid in fibroblasts (31), ornithine de-carboxylase synthesis in chick epidermis (52) and PC-12 cells (29), prostaglandin synthesis in canine kidney cells (38), fibronectin expression in fibroblasts (9), secretion of human chorionic gonadotrophin (4), survival of epidermal keratinocytes (47), and prolactin and growth hormone synthesis in cultured rat pituitary cells (49).

The maximal effective dose for EGF-mediated induction of TH in PC-G2 cells is in the ng/ml range, or 500-to-1,000-fold lower than that required for NGF induction of TH. Since both NGF and EGF are isolated from the same source—murine salivary glands—it became important to show that the NGF preparations were not contaminated by EGF. While both NGF and EGF have only one methionine residue, the location of the methionine residue of EGF at position 21 makes the EGF molecule sensitive to cleavage by cyanogen bromide. The biological activity of EGF is destroyed following CNBr cleavage (12), whereas this chemical modi-fication has no effect on the biological activity of NGF (20). CNBr treatment of NGF and EGF resulted in the loss of the TH inductive property of the EGF prep-aration but had no effect on the activity of the NGF preparation (Fig. 4), thus indicating that the TH induction effected by the NGF preparation was not due to low level EGF contaminations.

Our observation that EGF could induce TH in the PC-G2 cells led us to inquire whether or not EGF as well as NGF can induce TH in sympathetic ganglia. We have studied the induction of TH by EGF in organ cultures of superior cervical ganglia. Although the induction of TH by EGF is not as great as that caused by NGF, there is a significant induction of this enzyme over control values in the cultured ganglia in response to EGF (Fig. 5).

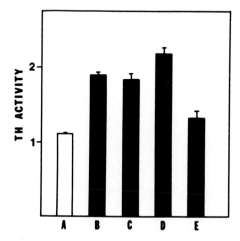

FIG. 4. CNBr sensitivity of NGF and EGF mediated TH induction in PC-G2 cells. PC-G2 cells were exposed to con-trol medium (A), 5 μg/ml of NGF (B), 5 μg ml of CNBr-treated NGF (C), 10 ng/ml of EGF (D), or 10 ng/ml of CNBr-treated EGF (E) for 3 days. The cultures were then harvested and assayed for TH as described in Fig. 1. Data are expressed as in Fig. 1. The TH activity in control cultures was 1.10 ± 0.01 nmoles DOPA/hr per mg protein. Values given represent the means ± SEM of 3 cul-tures. (Reprinted, with permission, from Goodman et al, ref. 20).

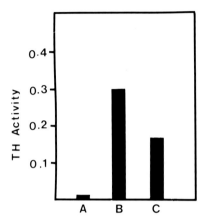

FIG. 5. Induction of TH in organ cultures of superior cervical ganglia by NGF and EGF. Superior cervical ganglia were asceptically removed from 5–8-day-old rats and placed on stainless steel grids in organ culture dishes. The ganglia were incubated in BGJ_b medium (Fitton-Jackson modification) supplemented with 10% fetal calf serum (A), 5 µg/ml NGF (B), or 0.5 ng/ml EGF (C). Cultures were incubated at 37°C in a humidified atmosphere of 5% CO_2-95% air for 48 hr, and then 5 ganglia were pooled and homogenized and assayed for TH as in Fig. 1.

NEUROTRANSMITTER SYNTHESIS IN PHEOCHROMOCYTOMA CELLS

During the past few years, several laboratories have suggested that the cells of the sympathetic nervous system exhibit a plasticity in their commitment to synthesize specific neurotransmitters (17,45,46). Previously, it was accepted that a neuronal cell was "programmed" to synthesize a specific neurotransmitter. Once this "programming" step had occurred, the cell was presumably fixed in the mode to synthesize only this one neurotransmitter. However, it has recently been reported that under various conditions, sympathetic ganglion cells which are normally adrenergic can become cholinergic and switch to the synthesis of acetylcholine, or can even synthesize both adrenergic and cholinergic neurotransmitters simultaneously. Patterson and Chun (45,46) have shown that dissociated sympathetic ganglion cells remain adrenergic when cultured in the absence of nonneuronal cells, but they will exhibit both adrenergic and cholinergic properties if cultured in the presence of nonneuronal cells or in conditioned medium. McLennan et al. have recently demonstrated that the presence of glucocorticoids in the medium prevents the development of cholinergic properties in cultured sympathetic ganglia (41). The same duality of neurotransmitters has been demonstrated in PC-12 cells by several laboratories. The effects of high cell density, conditioned medium, cyclic AMP, NGF, and glucocorticoids on the induction of choline acetyl transferase and the synthesis of acetylcholine in PC-12 cells have been reported by several laboratories (15,25,50). Thus the PC-12 cells mimic the duality of neurotransmitter synthesis shown by the normal sympathetic ganglion cells both *in vivo* and *in vitro*. The pheochromocytoma cell lines should play an important role in the further elucidation of the mechanisms by which these hormonal and growth controlling factors influence the neurotransmitter choice. They may also be of great value in describing other factors that influence the expression of differentiated functions of the normal neurons.

In summary, during the last few years, the use of these clonal pheochromocytoma cell lines has yielded much valuable information regarding neuronal regulation and differentiation. They have also helped to describe new functions for some of the growth factors and hormones that have as their targets neuronal cells.

ACKNOWLEDGMENTS

This work was supported by Department of Energy contract DEAM03 76 SF000 12, National Institutes of Health grant GM 24797, and National Science Foundation grant BNS 791 3827. Rosanne Goodman was the recipient of a National Research Service Award (NINCDS - 5F32 N0558602).

REFERENCES

1. Ambesi-Impiobato, F. S., Parks, L. A. M., and Coon, H. G. (1980): Culture of hormone dependent functional epithelial cells from rat thyroids. *Proc. Natl. Acad. Sci. U.S.A.*, 77:3455–3459.
2. Angeletti, R. H., and Bradshaw, R. A. (1971): Nerve growth factor from mouse submaxillary gland: amino acid sequence. *Proc. Natl. Acad. Sci. U.S.A.*, 68:2417–2420.
3. Beckwith, J. B., and Perrin, E. V. D. (1963): In situ neuroblastomas: a contribution to the natural history of neural crest tumors. *Am. J. Pathol.*, 43:1089–1104.
4. Benveniste, R., Speeg, K. V., Jr., Carpenter, G., Cohen, S., Lindner, J., and Rabinowitz, D. (1978): Epidermal growth factor stimulates secretion of human chorionic gonadotropin by cultured human choriocarcinoma cells. *J. Clin. Endocrinol. Metab.*, 46:169–172.
5. Bottenstein, J. E., and Sato, G. H. (1979): Growth of a rat neuroblastoma cell line in serum-free supplemented medium. *Proc. Natl. Acad. Sci. U.S.A.*, 76:514–517.
6. Bottenstein, J. E., Sato, G. H., and Mather, J. P. (1979): Growth of neuroepithelial-derived cell lines in serum-free hormone-supplemented media. In: *Hormones In Cell Culture*, edited by G. H. Sato and R. Ross, Vol. 6, pp. 531–544. Cold Spring Harbor Conference on Cell Proliferation, Cold Spring Harbor Laboratory, Cold Spring Harbor.
7. Bueker, E. D. (1948): Implantation of tumors in the hind limb field of the embryonic chick and the developmental response of the lumbosacral nervous system. *Anat. Rec.*, 102:369–390.
8. Burstein, D. E., and Greene, L. A. (1978): Evidence for RNA synthesis—dependent and independent pathways in stimulation of neurite outgrowth by nerve growth factor. *Proc. Natl. Acad. Sci. U.S.A.*, 75:6059–6063.
9. Chen, L. B., Gudor, R. C., Sun, T-T., Chen, A. B., and Mosesson, M. W. (1977): Control of a cell surface major glycoprotein by epidermal growth factor. *Science*, 197:776–778.
10. Cohen, S. (1959): Purification and metabolic effects of a nerve growth-promoting protein from snake venom. *J. Biol. Chem.*, 234:1129–1137.
11. Cohen, S. (1960): Purification of a nerve growth-promoting protein from the mouse salivary gland and its neurocytotoxic antiserum. *Proc. Natl. Acad. Sci. U.S.A.*, 46:302–311.
12. Cohen, S., and Savage, C. R., Jr. (1974): II. Recent studies on the chemistry and biology of epidermal growth factor. *Recent Prog. Horm. Res..*, 30:551–574.
13. Coughlin, M. D., Boyer, D. M., and Black, I. B. (1977): Embryologic development of a mouse sympathetic ganglion *in vivo* and *in vitro*. *Proc. Natl. Acad. Sci. U.S.A.*, 74:3438–3442.
14. Cramer, S. F., Bradshaw, R. A., Baglan, N. C., and Meyers, J. A. (1979): Nerve growth factor in medullary carcinoma of the thyroid. *Hum. Pathol.*, 10:731–736.
15. Edgar, D. H., and Thoenen, H. (1978): Selective enzyme induction in a nerve growth factor-responsive pheochromocytoma cell line (PC-12). *Brain Res.*, 154:186–190.
16. Fenton, E. L. (1970): Tissue culture assay of nerve growth factor and of the specific antiserum. *Exp. Cell. Res.*, 59:383–392.
17. Furshpan, E. J., MacLeish, P. R., O'Lague, P. H., and Potter, D. D. (1976): Chemical transmission between rat sympathetic neurons and cardiac myocytes developing in microcultures: evidence for cholinergic, adrenergic, and dual-function neurons. *Proc. Natl. Acad. Sci. U.S.A.*, 73:4225–4229.
18. Goldstein, L. D., Reynolds, C. P., and Perez-Polo, J. R. (1978): Isolation of human nerve growth factor from placental tissue. *Neurochem. Res.*, 3:175–183.

19. Goodman, R., and Herschman, H. R. (1978): Nerve growth factor—mediated induction of tyrosine hydroxylase in a clonal pheochromocytoma cell line. *Proc. Natl. Acad. Sci. U.S.A.*, 75:4587–4590.
20. Goodman, R., Slater, E., and Herschman, H. R. (1980): Epidermal growth factor induces tyrosine hydroxylase in a clonal pheochromocytoma cell line, PC-G2. *J. Cell Biol.*, 84:495–500.
21. Greene, L. A. (1974): A dissociated cell culture bioassay for nerve growth factor. *Neurobiology*, 4:286–292.
22. Greene, L. A. (1977): Quantitative *in vitro* studies on the nerve growth factor requirement of neurons. I. Sympathetic neurons. *Dev. Biol.*, 58:96–105.
23. Greene, L. A. (1977): A quantitative bioassay for nerve growth factor (NGF) activity employing a clonal pheochromocytoma cell line. *Brain Res.*, 133:350–353.
24. Greene, L. A. (1978): Nerve growth factor prevents the death and stimulates the neuronal differentiation of clonal PC-12 pheochromocytoma cells in serum-free medium. *J. Cell Biol.*, 78:747–755.
25. Greene, L. A., and Rein, G. (1977): Synthesis, storage and release of acetylcholine by a noradrenergic pheochromocytoma cell line. *Nature*, 268:349–351.
26. Greene, L. A., and Tischler, A. S. (1976): Establishment of a noradrenergic clonal line of rat adrenal pheochromocytoma cells which respond to nerve growth factor. *Proc. Natl. Acad. Sci. U.S.A.*, 73:2424–2428.
27. Harper, G. P., Barde, Y. A., Burnstock, G., Carstairs, J. R., Dennison, M. E., Suda, K., and Vernon, C. A. (1979): Guinea pig prostate is a rich source of nerve growth factor. *Nature*, 279:160–162.
28. Harper, G. P., Pearce, F. L., and Vernon, C. A. (1976): Production of nerve growth factor by the mouse adrenal medulla. *Nature*, 261:251–253.
29. Huff, K. R., and Guroff, G. (1979): Nerve growth factor-induced reduction in epidermal growth factor responsiveness and epidermal growth factor receptors in PC-12 cells: an aspect of cell differentiation. *Biochem. Biophys. Res. Commun.*, 89:175–180.
30. Knudson, A. G., Jr. (1977): Genetics and etiology of human cancer. In: *Advances in Human Genetics*, Vol. 8, edited by H. Harris and K. Hirshhorn, pp. 1–66. Plenum Press, New York.
31. Lembach, K. J. (1976): Enhanced synthesis and extracellular accumulation of hyaluronic acid during stimulation of quiescent human fibroblasts by mouse epidermal growth factor. *J. Cell Physiol.*, 89:277–288.
32. Levi-Montalcini, R. (1976): The nerve growth factor: its role in growth, differentiation and function of the sympathetic adrenergic neuron. In: *Progress in Brain Research*, Vol. 45, edited by M. A. Corner and D. F. Swabb, pp. 235–256. Elsevier, New York.
33. Levi-Montalcini, R., Aloe, L., Mugnaini, E., Oesch, F., and Thoenen, H. (1975): Nerve growth factor induces volume increase and enhances tyrosine hydroxylase synthesis in chemically axotomized sympathetic ganglia of newborn rats. *Proc. Natl. Acad. Sci. U.S.A.*, 72:595–599.
34. Levi-Montalcini, R., and Angeletti, P. U. (1966): Immunosympathectomy. *Pharmacol. Rev.*, 18:619–628.
35. Levi-Montalcini, R., and Angeletti, P. U. (1968): Nerve growth factor. *Physiol. Rev.*, 48:534–569.
36. Levi-Montalcini, R., and Hamburger, V. (1953): A diffusible agent of mouse sarcoma producing hyperplasia of sympathetic ganglia and hyperneurotization of viscera in the chick embryo. *J. Exp. Zool.*, 123:233–288.
37. Levi-Montalcini, R., Meyer, H., and Hamburger, V. (1954): *In vitro* experiments on the effects of mouse sarcomas 180 and 37 on the spinal and sympathetic ganglia of the chick embryo. *Cancer Res.*, 14:49–57.
38. Levine, L., and Hassid, A. (1977): Epidermal growth factor stimulates prostaglandin biosynthesis by canine kidney (MDCK) cells. *Biochem. Biophys. Res. Commun.*, 76:1181–1187.
39. Longo, A. M., and Penhoet, E. E. (1974): Nerve growth factor in rat glioma cells. *Proc. Natl. Acad. Sci. U.S.A.*, 71:2347–2349.
40. Mains, R. E., and Patterson, P. H. (1973): Primary cultures of dissociated sympathetic neurons I. Establishment of long-term growth in culture and studies of differentiated properties. *J. Cell Biol.*, 59:329–345.
41. McLennan, I. S., Hill, C. E., and Hendry, I. A. (1980): Glucocorticoids modulate transmitter choice in developing superior cervical ganglion. *Nature*, 283:206–207.
42. Murphy, R., Pantazis, M., Arnason, B., and Young, M. (1975): Secretion of a nerve growth factor by mouse neuroblastoma cells in culture. *Proc. Natl. Acad. Sci. U.S.A.*, 72:1895–1898.

43. Oger, J., Arnason, B. G. W., Pantazis, N., Lehrich, J., and Young, M. (1974): Synthesis of nerve growth factor by L and 3T3 cells in culture. *Proc. Natl. Acad. Sci. U.S.A.*, 71:1554–1558.
44. Otten, U., and Thoenen, H. (1977): Effect of glucocorticoids on nerve growth factor-mediated enzyme induction in organ cultures of rat sympathetic ganglia: enhanced response and reduced time requirement to initiate enzyme induction. *J. Neurochem.*, 29:69–75.
45. Patterson, P. H., and Chun, L. L. Y. (1974): The influence of non-neuronal cells on catecholamine and acetylcholine synthesis and accumulation in cultures of dissociated sympathetic neurons. *Proc. Natl. Acad. Sci. U.S.A.*, 71:3607–3610.
46. Patterson, P. H., and Chun, L. L. Y. (1977): The induction of acetylcholine synthesis in primary cultures of dissociated rat sympathetic neurons I. Effects of conditioned medium. *Dev. Biol.*, 56:263–280.
47. Rheinwald, J. G., and Green, H. (1977): Epidermal growth factor and the multiplication of cultured human epidermal keratinocytes. *Nature*, 265:421–424.
48. Savage, C. R., Jr., Inagami, T., and Cohen, S. (1972): The primary structure of epidermal growth factor. *J. Biol. Chem.*, 247:7612–7621.
49. Schonbrunn, A., Krasnoff, M., Westerdorf, J. M., and Tashjian, A. H., Jr. (1980): Epidermal growth factor and thyrotropin-releasing hormone act similarly on a clonal pituitary cell strain. *J. Cell Biol.*, 85:786–797.
50. Schubert, D., Heinemann, S., and Kidokoro, Y. (1977): Cholinergic metabolism and synapse formation by a rat nerve cell line. *Proc. Natl. Acad. Sci. U.S.A.*, 74:2579–2583.
51. Sherwin, S. A., Sliski, A. H., and Todaro, G. J. (1979): Human melanoma cells have both nerve growth factor and nerve growth factor-specific receptors on their cell surfaces. *Proc. Natl. Acad. Sci. U.S.A.*, 76:1288–1292.
52. Stastny, M., and Cohen, S. (1970): Epidermal growth factor. IV. The induction of ornithine decarboxylase. *Biochim. Biophys. Acta*, 204:578–589.
53. Warren, S., and Chute, R. N. (1972): Pheochromocytoma. *Cancer*, 29:327–331.
54. Young, M., Oger, J., Blanchard, M. H., Asdourian, H., Amos, H., and Arnason, B. (1975): Secretion of a nerve growth factor by primary chick fibroblast cultures. *Science*, 187:361–362.
55. Yu, M. W., Nikodijevic, B., Lakshmanan, J., Rowe, V., MacDonnell, P., and Guroff, G. (1977): Nerve growth factor and the activity of tyrosine hydroxylase in organ cultures of rat superior cervical ganglia. *J. Neurochem.*, 28:835–849.

Maturation Factors and Cancer,
edited by Malcolm A. S. Moore.
Raven Press, © New York 1982.

Isolation and Characterization of Variants of 3T3 Cells Deficient in a Proliferative Response to Specific Mitogens

*Harvey R. Herschman, **Joseph M. Sorrentino,
†Edith R. Butler-Gralla, and **Daniel B. Cawley

*Department of Biological Chemistry, Molecular Biology Institute, and Laboratory of
Nuclear Medicine and Radiation Biology; **Department of Biological Chemistry and
Laboratory of Nuclear Medicine and Radiation Biology; †Molecular Biology Institute
and Laboratory of Nuclear Medicine and Radiation Biology, UCLA Center for the Health
Sciences, Los Angeles, California 90024

In a multicellular organism, the individual cells exist in three states with respect to proliferation. Cells such as red blood cells, fused muscle cells, and the bulk of central nervous system neurons are terminally differentiated and are incapable of cell division. They are *postmitotic*. Other cells, such as those of the intestinal crypt villi, are actively dividing. The final class is made up of quiescent, nonproliferating cells with the potential to reenter the cell cycle and divide in response to an appropriate mitogenic signal. The stimulus for recruitment of this latter class of cells to division is dependent on cell type; hepatocytes respond to surgical resection, antibody producing cells to foreign antigen, mammary cells to elevated circulating levels of insulin and prolactin, fibroblasts to wounding, etc. Appropriate initiators, whether exogenous molecules, endogenous hormones and growth factors, or physical injury, evoke cell-type specific stimulation of nonproliferating cells into the division cycle. The regulation of growth control, i.e., the decision to enter or exit the cycle in response to environmental cues, is an intricate and complex phenomenon for which much of the molecular basis is currently unknown.

Our interest lies in the elucidation of the biochemical and physiological events requisite for the transition from the resting to the proliferative state. An extensive literature on the cell cycle (for reviews, see refs. 24,37,56) has suggested the existence of a determinative "Go" resting state (24) or, alternatively, a probabilistic "A" state (56) for the resting cell. Whichever of these models of the nonproliferating state is ultimately correct, our basic interest lies in the elucidation of the necessary biochemical steps for the Go to Gl transition in the deterministic model and/or those molecular events required for the alteration in transition probability from the A to the B state in the stochastic formulation.

THE MODEL SYSTEM

The murine embryo Swiss 3T3 cell line established by Todaro and Green (61) demonstrates growth control in culture. The cells are clonal and have an apparently infinite life span. The saturation density to which Swiss 3T3 cells grow is proportional to the serum concentration in the medium (25). The cells withdraw from the division cycle at a density dependent on serum concentration, but remain in a viable, resting state. If additional serum is added to the culture medium the cells respond, after 8 to 12 hr, by proceeding through a round of DNA synthesis and subsequent cell division. The 3T3 cells thus exhibit growth control, withdrawing from and reentering the division cycle in response to environmental cues. In addition to serum, noncycling 3T3 cells can respond to a wide variety of chemical mitogenic signals (Table 1), including (but not limited to) polypeptide mitogens such as fibroblast growth factor, epidermal growth factor, platelet-derived growth factor and vasopressin, fatty acid derivatives such as prostaglandin F2α, the polycyclic plant derivative 12-0-tetradecanoyl-phorbol-13-acetate (TPA), and the bacterial toxin cholera toxin.

When resting 3T3 cells are exposed to a mitogen, a large number of events, collectively termed the "pleiotypic response" (23), occur during the transition to the proliferating state (Table 2). These include (a) increases in the rates of transport of ions and small molecules, (b) alterations in the rate-limiting steps of several metabolic pathways such as polyamine synthesis and glycolysis, (c) posttranslational modifications of cellular substrates, e.g., phosphorylation reactions, (d) alterations such as down-regulation and internalization of specific receptors, and (e) induction of other enzymes such as plasminogen activator and phospholipase. This list of associated alterations in the mitogenic pleiotypic response grows with each issue of the cell biology and biochemistry journals.

THE MAJOR QUESTIONS TO BE ADDRESSED IN GROWTH CONTROL

Swiss 3T3 cells respond to an embarrassment of riches in the number and diversity of molecules which can stimulate quiescent cells to enter the proliferating pool.

TABLE 1. *Mitogens for 3T3 cells*

Mitogen	Reference
Serum	(24,25)
Platelet derived growth factor (PDGF)	(2,13,38)
Fibroblast growth factor (FGF)	(19)
Epidermal growth factor (EGF)	(43)
Multiplication stimulating activity (MSA)	(32)
Vasopressin (VP)	(47)
Cholera toxin (CT)	(40)
Prostaglandin F2α (PGF2α)	(28)
12-0-Tetradecanoyl-phorbol-13-acetate	(22,55)

TABLE 2. *Components of the pleiotypic response stimulated by mitogens*

Elevated phosphate transport	(20)
Elevated sodium transport	(57)
Elevated potassium transport	(46)
Elevated glucose transport	(3)
Elevated uridine transport	(48)
Altered cyclic nucleotide levels	(52)
Elevated ornithine decarboxylase levels	(32,33)
Elevated phosphofructokinase levels	(51)
Elevated phospholipase levels	(53)
Stimulation of plasminogen activator secretion	(63)
Polysome mobilization	(23)
Receptor internalization (EGF)	(7)
Receptor phosphorylation (EGF)	(9,10)

Structures as distinct as EGF, a 53 amino acid polypeptide obtained from murine salivary glands (49,60), and TPA, a diester of the diterpine alcohol phorbol isolated from the croton plant, are both extremely potent mitogens for Swiss 3T3 cells (22,43,55). Mitogens of such diverse structure might initiate cell division by means of a common pathway. After different mitogens bind to specific receptors, the next step distal to receptor occupancy in the proliferation pathway may be a reaction common to all mitogens (step C in Fig. 1), i.e., a *ubiquitous pathway*. Alternatively, the sequence of events following receptor binding may be *different* and *unique* for various mitogens or mitogen subclasses; i.e., various mitogens may follow *unique pathways*. The latter model predicts that there will be distinct, unique biochemical events in the initial portion of each mitogenic pathway, triggered by individual mitogens after they bind to specific receptors (e.g., steps 1a, 1b, 1c of Fig. 1).

Question 1

Do mitogens of diverse structure stimulate the same set or different sets of causal events distal to receptor occupancy; i.e., are there common or distinct pathways to proliferation for different mitogens?

Studies from our laboratory and others now favor the "unique pathway" model. For example, EGF must be present continuously both to commit resting 3T3 cells to enter S phase and to cause subsequent DNA synthesis and cell division (1). In contrast, platelet-derived growth factor (PDGF) can establish "competence," i.e., cause a commitment of cells to subsequent entry into S phase, in only 2 hr; subsequent DNA synthesis and cell division of PDGF primed cells can occur in the absence of PDGF, as long as appropriate "progression factors" for DNA synthesis and cell division are present (38). EGF cannot substitute for PDGF as a competence factor; nor can it serve as a progression factor (58). Although it is possible to still squeeze these phenomena into a common model, it is easier to think of these two

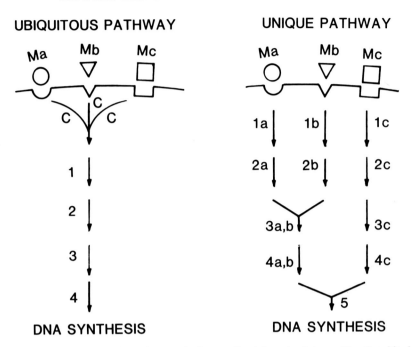

FIG. 1. Alternate models for pathways of mitogen stimulation of cellular proliferation. Ma, Mb, and Mc are chemically distinct mitogens.

mitogens as operating via different pathways. (A moment's reflection on the animal physiology is instructive. EGF is present constantly as a circulating hormone; it is not surprising that it needs to be present continuously in mitogenesis. PDGF is released locally by platelets in response to wounding, then washed away by circulating plasma. One would predict a trigger mechanism for this agent.)

The wide range of transport alterations, metabolic responses, enzyme activations, and additional components of the pleiotypic response (Table 2) provide a plethora of cellular events occurring in response to mitogen stimulation. Although these events are initiated by the mitogenic signal, we do not at present know which mitogen-induced alterations in cellular physiology, biochemistry, and metabolism are essential for the initiation of DNA synthesis.

Question 2

What are the *causal*—as opposed to the *correlative*—events which occur in the transition from a noncycling to a cycling cell in response to mitogens?

It is difficult to distinguish events which merely *accompany* the mitogenic response from changes *requisite* for the response. Increased transport of phosphate was demonstrated to occur in response to several mitogenic stimuli. However, Cunningham and his colleagues (20) have shown that elevated phosphate uptake is not necessary for cells to mount a mitogenic response; i.e., this event is a *correl-*

ative, but not a *causal*, occurrence after exposure to a mitogen. If individual mitogens (or groups of mitogens) have unique pathways (Fig. 1), then the causal versus correlative events must be elucidated on a mitogen-by-mitogen basis. Causal event 1a, occurring in response to mitogen Ma, would be a biochemically distinct event from 1b, occurring in response to mitogen Mb.

SELECTION OF MITOGEN-SPECIFIC NONPROLIFERATIVE VARIANTS OF 3T3 CELLS

In order to approach the questions posed above, we have isolated variants of 3T3 cells which are unable to mount a mitogenic response to specific mitogens. Our selection procedure is a modification of the procedure Vogel et al. (62) used to isolate "flat" variants of transformed 3T3 cells. The selection of mitogen-specific nonproliferative variants is carried out as illustrated in Fig. 2. Cells are grown to their saturation density in medium containing 5% fetal calf serum. The 3T3 cells exit the proliferative phase and enter into a resting, noncycling state. The mitogen for which variants are to be selected is added to the quiescent population, along with sufficient colchicine to arrest mitotic cells. Cells stimulated by the mitogen proceed through the cell cycle and enter mitosis, where they are trapped by the colchicine. Three or four days after the addition of mitogen and colchicine the cells arrested in mitosis, and thus only loosely attached to the plate, are washed from the plate with a stream of medium. The interphase cells, which are tightly attached to the plate, are not washed from the dish by this procedure. After the wash, the cells remaining on the plate are dislodged by trypsin treatment and replated. The cells are once again grown to the point at which they become quiescent, then subjected to another round of selection. The procedure is continued until the population response is reduced to 50% of the parental response. Individual clones are then isolated and tested for their mitogenic phenotype.

EGF NONPROLIFERATIVE 3T3 VARIANTS

The first mitogen we used in this selection procedure was EGF. The protein is easily purified (49), extremely stable, and well characterized chemically (60). Carpenter and Cohen (8) have recently reviewed the EGF literature. A distinct receptor exists for EGF on 3T3 cells and has been identified not only by binding criteria (1) but in biochemical terms (14). Currently, our knowledge of both the interaction of EGF with target cell receptors and the alterations in cells in response to EGF is greater than for any other mitogen active on 3T3 cells.

The first variant isolated by the mitogen-colchicine procedure, using EGF as the selective mitogen, was named 3T3-NR6 (39). (In fact, several other clones were also isolated, but NR6 was selected as representative of these isolates, since the selection procedure did not guarantee isolation of clones arising from independent events.) The 3T3-NR6 cell line is unable to respond to EGF, but does divide in response to TPA, PGF2α, serum (39), and FGF (41). It is thus a mitogen-specific nonproliferative variant.

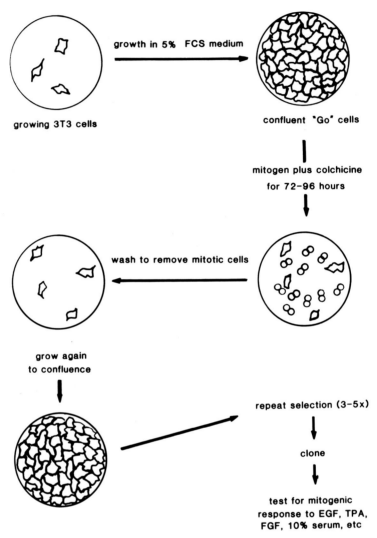

FIG. 2.   Selection protocol for isolation of mitogen-specific nonproliferative 3T3 variants.

The basis for the lack of a proliferative response to EGF in the 3T3-NR6 variant was easily established. This variant is unable to bind ^{125}I-EGF (39); it is missing functional EGF receptors. Although the 3T3-NR6 variant has been useful in several studies concerned with EGF receptor biology (15,42), its utility is limited in answering the two major questions we pose. While this variant does formally demonstrate that the binding of EGF to a cell surface receptor is necessary to initiate the mitogenic response, it does not help to distinguish between the alternative pathways present in Fig. 1, nor does it help to define the causal steps distal to receptor occupancy in EGF stimulation of proliferation. A "receptorless" variant for a specific mitogen is consistent with either the *unique* or *ubiquitous* models of Fig. 1.

TPA NONPROLIFERATIVE 3T3 VARIANTS

Interest in TPA first developed because of its promoting activity in two stage carcinogenesis of mouse skin (4). TPA, derived from the croton plant, is the most active promoter known (21). It is also a powerful mitogen (16,22,55). In addition to its activities as a promoter and as a mitogen, TPA has profound effects on the expression of differentiated functions of cultured cells, inhibiting expression of cell-type specific properties in some cases (13,17,31,44), while inducing expression of differentiated function in other cases (26,27,45,59). More recently, an interesting interaction between EGF and TPA has been reported. Lee and Weinstein (29) described an inhibitory effect of TPA on binding of ^{125}I-EGF to HeLa cells. Later studies showed that, on rodent cells, TPA reduces the affinity of the EGF receptor (i.e., shifts the binding curve to the right) without altering the number of EGF receptors or the binding of other hormones or growth factors (5,12,54).

We chose TPA as our second mitogen for variant selection because of (a) its interesting activity as a promoter, (b) its mitogenic potency on 3T3 cells, (c) its effects on expression of differentiation, (d) its interaction with EGF, and (e) its commercial availability. After we initiated our selections with TPA, Dreidger and Blumberg (18) described specific, high affinity receptors for phorbol esters. Using the same selection procedure described previously (Fig. 1), we have isolated two independent TPA nonproliferative variants from 3T3 cells (6).

Both TPA variants respond to 10% serum (Fig. 3) and, in a separate experiment, to FGF. Neither variant responds to TPA. One of the variants, 3T3-TNR-9, responds to EGF. In contrast, the second variant, 3T3-TNR-2, does not respond to EGF. These data were confirmed by tests employing autoradiographic analyses of [125]-iododeoxyuridine incorporation into DNA, autoradiographic determination of incorporation of ^{3}H-thymidine into nuclei, and time course analysis for stimulation of ^{3}H-thymidine incorporation into DNA. In all cases, wild-type 3T3 cells responded to 10% serum, to EGF, and to TPA. The 3T3-TNR-9 variant retained response to serum and EGF, while the 3T3-TNR-2 cells were no longer responsive to either EGF or TPA (6). The inability of the two variants to respond to TPA is not a quantitative shift; neither variant responds across a range of TPA concentrations (6).

We were surprised to observe the loss of response to EGF in the 3T3-TNR-2 variant, since this cell line was selected for inability to respond to TPA. We could not detect any binding of ^{125}I-EGF to the 3T3-TNR-2 variant (Fig. 4). The 3T3-TNR-9 variant had a reduced number of receptors for EGF when compared to the parental cell, although the apparent affinity of the receptor is the same (Fig. 4, inset). Despite a reduced number of EGF receptors, the 3T3-TNR-9 cell is able to mount a mitogenic response equivalent to wild-type 3T3 cells, by all the assays utilized, in response to 10 ng/ml of EGF (6).

The modulation of EGF binding by TPA (5,12,54) presents a method for examining the interaction of TPA with cells that retain EGF receptors. TPA is able

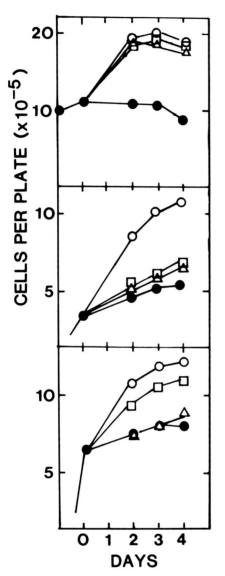

FIG. 3. Mitogenic response of Swiss 3T3 cells (top panel) and the TPA nonresponsive variants 3T3-TNR2 (middle panel) and 3T3-TNR9 (lower panel). Cells were grown in 35 mm dishes. Mitogens were added after cells had ceased division (day 0 of the figure). No addition, ●; EGF (10 ng/ml), □; TPA (100 ng/ml), Δ; 10% serum, ○. Data are from Butler-Gralla and Herschman (6).

to reduce the binding of ^{125}I-EGF not only to 3T3 cells, but also to the TPA nonresponsive 3T3-TNR-9 variant (6). These data suggest (a) that the 3T3-TNR-9 variant, although it no longer has a mitogenic response to TPA, possesses receptors for TPA, and (b) the TPA-receptor complex is able to perform some TPA-induced biological responses in the nonproliferative variant. Recent collaborative ^{3}H-phorbol ester binding experiments with Peter Blumberg at Harvard have demonstrated the presence of TPA receptors on the TPA nonresponsive 3T3-TNR-2 and 3T3-TNR-9 variants.

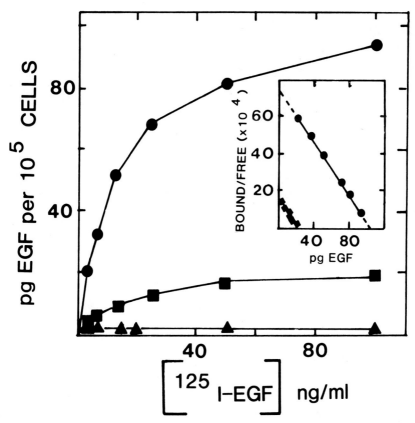

FIG. 4. Binding of EGF to 3T3, 3T3-TNR-2, and 3T3-TNR-9 cells. Binding was performed at 4°C for 90 min. The inset shows the data for 3T3 and 3T3-TNR-9 replotted according to Scatchard (50). 3T3, ●;3T3-TNR-2, ▲; 3T3-TNR-9, ■. Data are from Butler-Gralla and Herschman (6).

TABLE 3. *Properties of mitogen-specific nonproliferative variants*

	Response to serum	Response to FGF	Response to EGF	Response to TPA	Presence of EGF receptors	TPA modulation of EGF binding
3T3	+	+	+	+	+	+
3T3-NR6	+	+	−	+	−	N.A.[a]
3T3-TNR-2	+	+	−	−	−	N.A.
3T3-TNR-9	+	+	+	−	+	+

[a]N.A., not applicable.

SUMMARY OF EXISTING VARIANTS

We have now characterized one EGF variant and two independently isolated TPA variants. The data are summarized in Table 3. There are some interesting—and perhaps surprising—overlaps in the two classes. Thus the EGF-selected variant

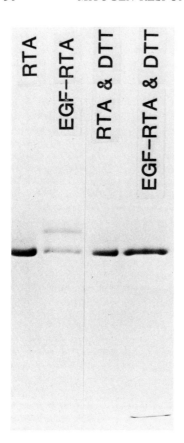

FIG. 5. SDS gel electrophoresis of EGF-ricin A chain conjugate and ricin A chain: cleavage of the conjugate by dithiothreitol. Proteins were incubated for 15 min at 37°C in sample buffer. Reduced samples contained 50 mm dithiothreitol. Electrophoresis was on 15% gels. Protein samples were 8.5 μg of ricin A chain and 22 μg of EGF-ricin A conjugate. The EGF-ricin A samples shown here are from the reaction mixture prior to chromatography to remove unreacted ricin A chain. Data are from Cawley et al. (11).

3T3-NR6 and the TPA-selected variant 3T3-TNR-2 both lack the ability to bind EGF. The relationship between EGF and TPA is complex and currently unresolved. The ability of 3T3-NR6 cells, which lack an EGF binding site, to respond to TPA suggests that these two mitogens bind to distinct physical sites. This conclusion is supported by data describing the effect of TPA on ^{125}I-EGF binding (5,12,54). However, the isolation of a variant (3T3-NR2) in which both TPA and EGF responsiveness have been concomitantly effected suggests that these two elements, the EGF and the TPA recognition sites, may coexist on a common molecular structure, or at least interact in some fashion. In contrast to the complex interrelationships of EGF and TPA in our variants, all respond to fibroblast growth factor.

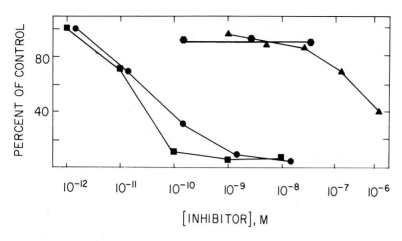

FIG. 6. Inhibition of protein synthesis in 3T3 cells by EGF-ricin A, ricin, and ricin A chain. Cells (8 × 10⁴) were plated in scintillation vials. After 24 hr, the medium was removed and fresh medium containing the toxin was added. After an additional 24 hr, the medium was removed, and the cells were incubated with fresh medium containing 1 μCi of ³H-leucine. Samples were processed for determination of incorporation of radioactivity (30). Ricin, ■; EGF-ricin A chain (purified by gel-filtration chromatography), ●; ricin A chain, ▲; equimolar mixtures of unconjugated EGF and ricin A chain, ● . Data are from Cawley et al. (11).

We now have, in our collection of variants, two independent isolates (3T3-TNR-2 and 3T3-NR6) which are unable to bind EGF. If we can establish a somatic cell genetic analysis of these mutants and others with this phenotype we should, in principle, be able to determine the number of steps required for the synthesis of the EGF receptor. We have two variants which retain TPA receptors but are unable to mount a mitogenic response to TPA. In these variants, a causal step apparently distal to mitogen binding is impaired in the proliferative response. Somatic cell genetic analysis of a collection of such variants should, in principle, allow us to define the minimal number of causal steps in a proliferative pathway.

Analysis of the component parts of the pleiotypic response (Table 2) in our variants should determine those components insufficient for a complete mitogenic response and suggest candidates for causal roles from these many phenomena. We are currently attempting to isolate temperature sensitive mitogen-specific nonproliferating variants to expand this approach to the study of the mechanism of initiation of cellular proliferation.

A TOXIC CONJUGATE BETWEEN EGF AND THE A-CHAIN OF RICIN

The variants described in Table 3 were all isolated by the colchicine procedure, which depends on an intact mitogenic response for its selective effectiveness. We have recently developed another selective approach with the intention of isolating variants altered in receptor synthesis, ligand binding, or ligand-induced internalization.

Ricin is a toxic glycoprotein found in castor beans. It is composed of two subunits joined through a single disulfide bond. One of the subunits, the B chain, binds to galactose-containing glycoproteins and glycolipids on the cell surface. The other subunit, the A chain, is a potent catalytic inactivator of the larger ribosomal subunit in cell free systems (34–36). Neither subunit alone is toxic to cells; both the binding moiety (the B chain) and the catalytic subunit (the A chain) are necessary for intoxication of intact cells by ricin. We have isolated the A chain of ricin and coupled it to the amino terminal residue of EGF (11). EGF was first derivatized with N-succinimidyl 3(2-pyridyldithio) propionate (SPDP) to make an N-terminal pyridine dithiopropionate derivative, EGF-PDP. (Murine EGF has only a single primary amino group, at the amino terminus.) The EGF-PDP conjugate was then reacted in a thiol-disulfide exchange with reduced ricin A chain. The conjugate, EGF-ricin A, was separated from the reactants by gel filtration. Reduction of the conjugate with dithiothreitol demonstrated that the conjugate was composed of native A chain and EGF (Fig. 5). The toxicity of the EGF conjugate for 3T3 cells was within an order of magnitude of ricin (Fig. 6), while both ricin A chain and unconjugated mixtures of EGF and ricin A chain were several orders of magnitude less effective in reducing protein synthesis in 3T3 cells. The toxicity of the EGF-ricin A conjugate could be completely inhibited by excess unconjugated EGF, but was unaffected by antisera to the ricin B chain or by lactose, a sugar inhibitor of ricin binding (11). The specificity of the toxic effect for the EGF-ricin A conjugate thus resides in its EGF binding activity. Toxic chimeric conjugates of this type should be extremely valuable in isolating variants both in the synthesis of cell surface receptors and in the processing of ligand-receptor complexes. We are currently selecting for EGF-RTA resistant variants of 3T3 cells and of A431 cells, a human epidermoid carcinoma which has nearly 30 times the number of EGF receptors found on 3T3 cells (9,10).

ACKNOWLEDGMENTS

We thank David Brankow for technical assistance in some portions of these studies. This work was supported by NIH Grant GM 24797 and DOE Contract DE AM03 76 SF00012 to HRH. JMS is a postdoctoral trainee of the National Cancer Institute (CA 9030); ERB is a predoctoral trainee of the National Cancer Institute (CA 09056). DBC is the recipient of a National Research Service Award (GM 07489). We thank Dr. D. G. Gilliland and Dr. R. J. Collier for their collaboration in the construction and characterization of the toxic EGF-ricin A conjugate.

REFERENCES

1. Aharonov, A., Vlodavsky, I., Pruss, R. M., Fox, C. F., and Herschman, H. R. (1978): Epidermal growth factor induced membrane changes in 3T3 cells. *J. Cell. Physiol.*, 95:195–202.
2. Antoniades, H. N., and Scher, C. D. (1977): Radioimmunoassay of a human serum growth factor for Balb/c 3T3 cells: derivation from platelets. *Proc. Natl. Acad. Sci. U.S.A.*, 74:1973–1977.
3. Barnes, D., and Colowick, S. P. (1976): Stimulation of sugar uptake in cultured fibroblasts by epidermal growth factor (EGF) and EGF-binding arginine esterase. *J. Cell. Physiol.*, 89:633–640.
4. Berenblum, I. (1941): The cocarcinogenic action of croton resin. *Cancer Res.*, 1:44–48.

5. Brown, K. D., Dicker, P., and Rozengurt, E. (1979): Inhibition of epidermal growth factor binding to surface receptors by tumor promoters. *Biochem. Biophys. Res. Commun.*, 86:1037–1043.
6. Butler-Gralla, E., and Herschman, H. R. (1981): Variants of 3T3 cells lacking mitogenic response to the tumor promoter tetradecanoyl-phorbol-acetate. *J. Cell Physiol.*, 107:59–68.
7. Carpenter, G., and Cohen, S. (1976): ^{125}I-labeled human epidermal growth factor: binding, internalization and degradation in human fibroblasts. *J. Cell Biol.*, 71:159–171.
8. Carpenter, G., and Cohen, S. (1979): Epidermal growth factor. *Ann. Rev. Biochem.*, 48:193–216.
9. Carpenter, G., King, L., and Cohen, S. (1978): Epidermal growth factor stimulates phosphorylation in membrane preparations *in vitro*. *Nature*, 276:409–410.
10. Carpenter, G., King, L., and Cohen, S. (1979): Rapid enhancement of protein phosphorylation in A-431 cell membrane preparations by epidermal growth factor. *J. Biol. Chem.*, 254:4884–4891.
11. Cawley, D. B., Herschman, H. R., Gilliland, D. G., and Collier, R. J. (1980): Epidermal growth factor toxin A chain conjugates: EGF-ricin A is a potent toxin while EGF-diphtheria fragment A is non-toxic. *Cell*, 22:563–570.
12. Chandler, C., and Herschman, H. R. (1980): Tumor-promoter modulation of epidermal growth factor and nerve growth factor-induced adhesion and growth factor binding of PC-12 pheochromocytoma cells. *J. Cell. Physiol.*, 105:275–285.
13. Cohen, R., Pacifici, M., Rubenstein, N., Biehl, J., and Holtzer, H. (1977): Effect of a tumor promoter on myogenesis. *Nature*, 266:538–540.
14. Das, M., Miyakawa, T., Fox, C. F., Pruss, R. M., Aharonov, A., and Herschman, H. R. (1977): Specific radiolabeling of a cell surface receptor for epidermal growth factor. *Proc. Natl. Acad. Sci. U.S.A.*, 74:2790–2794.
15. DeLarco, J. E., and Todaro, G. J. (1980): Sarcoma derived growth factor (SGF): Specific binding to epidermal growth factor (EGF) membrane receptors. *J. Cell. Physiol.*, 102:267–277.
16. Diamond, L., O'Brien, S., Donaldson, C., and Shimizu, Y. (1974): Growth stimulation of human diploid fibroblasts by the tumor promoter 12-0-tetradecanoyl-phorbol-13-acetate. *Int. J. Cancer*, 13:721–730.
17. Diamond, L., O'Brien, T. L., and Rovera, G. (1977): Inhibition of adipose conversion of 3T3 fibroblasts by tumor promoters. *Nature*, 269:247–249.
18. Dreidger, P. E., and Blumberg, P. M. (1980): Specific binding of phorbol ester tumor promoters. *Proc. Natl. Acad. Sci. U.S.A.*, 77:567–571.
19. Gospodarowicz, D. (1974): Localization of a fibroblast growth factor and its effect alone and with hydrocortisone on 3T3 cell growth. *Nature*, 249:123–127.
20. Greenberg, D. B., Barsh, G. S., Ho, T-S., and Cunningham, D. D. (1977): Serum stimulated phosphate uptake and initiation of fibroblast proliferation. *J. Cell. Physiol.*, 90:193–210.
21. Hecker, E. (1971): Isolation and characterization of the cocarcinogenic principles from croton oil. *Methods Cancer Res.*, 6:439–484.
22. Herschman, H. R., Passovoy, D. S., Pruss, R. M., and Aharonov, A. (1978): Mitogens for murine embryo cell lines. *J. Supramol. Struct.*, 8:41–46.
23. Hershko, A., Mamont, P., Shields, R., and Tompkins, G. (1971): Pleiotypic response. *Nature New Biol.*, 232:206.
24. Holley, R. W. (1975): Control of growth of mammalian cells in cell culture. *Nature*, 258:487–490.
25. Holley, R. W., and Kiernan, J. A. (1968): Contact inhibition of cell division in 3T3 cells. *Proc. Natl. Acad. Sci. U.S.A.*, 60:300–304.
26. Huberman, E., and Callaham, M. F. (1979): Induction of terminal differentiation in human promyelocytic leukemia cells by tumor promoting agents. *Proc. Natl. Acad. Sci. U.S.A.*, 76:1293–1297.
27. Huberman, E., Heckman, C., and Langenbach, R. (1979): Stimulation of differentiated functions in human melanoma cells by tumor promoting agents and dimethylsulfoxide. *Cancer Res.*, 39:2618–2624.
28. Jiminez de Asua, L., Clingan, L. D., and Rudland, P. S. (1975): Initiation of cell proliferation in cultured mouse fibroblasts by prostaglandin F2α. *Proc. Natl. Acad. Sci. U.S.A.*, 72:2724–2728.
29. Lee, L., and Weinstein, I. B. (1978): Tumor promoting phorbol esters inhibit binding of epidermal growth factor to cellular receptors. *Science*, 202:313–315.

30. Moehring, T. J., and Moehring, J. M. (1977): Selection and characterization of cells resistant to Diphtheria toxin and Pseudomonas exotoxin A: presumptive translational mutants. *Cell*, 11:447–464.

31. Mufson, R. A., Fisher, P. B., and Weinstein, I. B. (1979): Effect of phorbol ester tumor promoters on the expression of melanogenesis in B16 melanoma cells. *Cancer Res.*, 39:3915–3919.

32. Nissley, S. P., Passamani, J., and Short, P. (1976): Stimulation of DNA synthesis, cell multiplication and ornithine decarboxylase in 3T3 cells by multiplication stimulating activity (MSA). *J. Cell. Physiol.*, 89:393–402.

33. O'Brien, T. B., and Diamond, L. (1977): Ornithine decarboxylase induction and DNA synthesis in hamster embryo cell cultures treated in the tumor promoting phorbol diesters. *Cancer Res.*, 37:3895–3900.

34. Olsnes, S., Fernandez-Puentes, C., Carrasco, L., and Vazquez, D. (1975): Ribosome inactivation by the toxic lectins abrin and ricin. Kinetics of the enzymatic activity of the toxin A-chains. *Eur. J. Biochem.*, 60:281–288.

35. Olsnes, S., Refsnes, K., Christensen, T. B., and Pihl, A. (1975): Studies on the structure and properties of the lectins from Abrus precatorius and Ricinus communis. *Biochim. Biophys. Acta*, 405:1–10.

36. Olsnes, S., Saltvedt, E., and Pihl, A. (1974): Isolation and comparison of galactose binding lectins from Abrus precatorius and Ricinus communis. *J. Biol. Chem.*, 249:803–810.

37. Pardee, A. B., Dubrow, R., Hamlin, J. L., and Kletzien, R. F. (1978): Animal cell cycle. *Ann. Rev. Biochem.*, 47:715–750.

38. Pledger, W. J., Stiles, C. D., Antoniades, H. N., and Scher, C. D. (1977): Induction of DNA synthesis in Balb/c 3T3 cells by serum components: reevaluation of the commitment process. *Proc. Natl. Acad. Sci. U.S.A.*, 74:4481–4485.

39. Pruss, R. M., and Herschman, H. R. (1977): Variants of 3T3 cells lacking mitogenic response to epidermal growth factor. *Proc. Natl. Acad. Sci. U.S.A*, 74:3918–3921.

40. Pruss, R. M., and Herschman, H. R. (1979): Cholera toxin stimulates division of 3T3 cells. *J. Cell. Physiol.*, 98:469–474.

41. Pruss, R. M., and Herschman, H. R. (1979): Mitogenic effects of murine serum and fibroblast growth factor on EGF non-proliferative variants of 3T3. *J. Supramol. Struct.*, 12:467–470.

42. Pruss, R. M., Herschman, H. R., and Klement, V. (1978): 3T3 variants lacking receptors for epidermal growth factor are susceptible to transformation by Kirsten sarcoma virus. *Nature*, 274:272–274.

43. Rose, S. P., Pruss, R. M., and Herschman, H. R. (1975): Initiation of 3T3 fibroblast cell division by epidermal growth factor. *J. Cell. Physiol.*, 86:593–598.

44. Rovera, G., O'Brien, T. G., and Diamond, L. (1977): Tumor promoters inhibit spontaneous differentiation of Friend erythroleukemia cells in culture. *Proc. Natl. Acad. Sci. U.S.A.*, 74:2894–2898.

45. Rovera, G., O'Brien, T. G., and Diamond, L. (1979): Induction of differentiation in human promyelocytic leukemia cells by tumor promoters. *Science*, 204:868–870.

46. Rozengurt, E., and Heppel, L. A. (1975): Serum rapidly stimulates ouabain-sensitive [86]Rb[+] influx in quiescent 3T3 cells. *Proc. Natl. Acad. Sci. U.S.A.*, 72:4992–4995.

47. Rozengurt, E., Legg, A., and Peltican, P. (1979): Vasopressin stimulation of mouse 3T3 cell growth. *Proc. Natl. Acad. Sci. U.S.A.*, 76:1284–1287.

48. Rozengurt, E., Mierzejewski, K., and Wigglesworth, N. (1978): Uridine transport and phosphorylation in mouse cells in culture: effect of growth-promoting factors, cell cycle transit and oncogenic transformation. *J. Cell. Physiol.*, 97:241–252.

49. Savage, C. R., and Cohen, S. (1972): Epidermal growth factor and a new derivative: rapid isolation procedures and biological and chemical characterization. *J. Biol. Chem.*, 247:7609–7611.

50. Scatchard, G. (1949): The attraction of proteins for small molecules and ions. *Ann. N.Y. Acad. Sci.*, 51:660–672.

51. Schneider, J. A., Diamond, I., and Rozengurt, E. (1978): Glycolysis in quiescent cultures of 3T3 cells. *J. Biol. Chem.*, 253:872–877.

52. Seiffert, W. E., and Rudland, P. S. (1974): Possible involvement of cyclic GMP in growth control of cultured mouse cells. *Nature*, 248:138–140.

53. Shier, T. (1979): Activation of high levels of endogenous phospholipase A₂ in cultured cells. *Proc. Natl. Acad. Sci. U.S.A.*, 76:195–199.

54. Shoyab, M., DeLarco, J. E., and Todaro, G. J. (1979): Biologically active phorbol esters specifically alter affinity of epidermal growth factor membrane receptors. *Nature*, 279:387–391.

55. Sivak, A. (1972): Induction of cell division: role of cell membrane sites. *J. Cell. Physiol.*, 80:167–174.
56. Smith, J. A., and Martin, L. (1973): Do cells cycle? *Proc. Natl. Acad. Sci. U.S.A.*, 70:1263–1267.
57. Smith, J. B., and Rozengurt, E. (1978): Lithium transport by fibroblastic mouse cells: characterization and stimulation by serum and growth factors in quiescent cultures. *J. Cell. Physiol.*, 97:441–450.
58. Stiles, C. D., Capone, G. T., Scher, C. D., Antoniades, H. N., Van Wyk, J. J., and Pledger, W. J. (1979): Dual control of cell growth by somatomedins and platelet-derived growth factor. *Proc. Natl. Acad. Sci. U.S.A.*, 76:1279–1283.
59. Stuart, R. K., and Hamilton, J. A. (1980): Tumor-promoting phorbol esters stimulate hematopoietic colony formation *in vitro*. *Science*, 208:402–404.
60. Taylor, J. M., Mitchell, W. M., and Cohen, S. (1972): Epidermal growth factor: physical and chemical properties. *J. Biol. Chem.*, 247:5928–5934.
61. Todaro, G. J., and Green, H. (1963): Quantitative studies of the growth of mouse embryo cells in culture and their development into established cell lines. *J. Cell. Biol.*, 17:299–313.
62. Vogel, A., Risser, R., and Pollack, R. (1973): Isolation and characterization of relevant cell lines. II. Isolation of density-revertants of SV-40 transformed 3T3 cells using colchicine. *J. Cell. Physiol.*, 82:181–188.
63. Wigler, M., and Weinstein, I. B. (1976): Tumor promoter induces plasminogen activator. *Nature*, 259:232–233.

Maturation Factors and Cancer,
edited by Malcolm A. S. Moore.
Raven Press, © New York 1982.

Control of Cell Growth by Somatomedins and the Platelet-Derived Growth Factor

*Charles D. Scher, *Kathryn L. Locatell, **Jay Lilliquist, and **Charles D. Stiles

*Department of Pediatric Hematology-Oncology, Sidney Farber Cancer Institute, and Children's Hospital Medical Center, Harvard Medical School, Boston, Massachusetts 02115; **Laboratory of Tumor Biology, Sidney Farber Cancer Institute and Laboratory of Microbiology and Molecular Genetics, Harvard Medical School, Boston, Massachusetts 02115*

Serum is used to supplement tissue culture medium and allow the growth of cells *in vitro*. It contains agents which are needed in a nutritional sense, such as selenium or the iron transport protein transferrin (6,9,16), and proteins used for attachment, such as fibronectin (17). In addition, serum contains newly described polypeptide hormones which regulate the growth of fibroblasts (27,33). These hormones act synergistically in a sequential fashion to modulate "events" in the G_0/G_1 phase of the cell cycle which control the entry of cells into the S phase. The oncogenic virus SV40 overrides the requirement for these hormones, suggesting that the loss of the need for these regulatory factors causes cellular transformation.

PDGF

Tissue culture medium supplemented with serum supports the growth of fibroblasts, while that supplemented with plasma does not (15,22,26). Serum and plasma are similar body fluids: serum is the liquid portion of clotted blood, and plasma is the liquid portion of unclotted blood. Serum differs from plasma in lacking fibrinogen and in containing proteins liberated from platelets. Platelets are anucleate blood cells that have an important role in maintaining vascular integrity and preventing hemorrhage. Their α-granules contain several proteins, including the platelet-derived growth factor (PDGF), which are released during clotting (14). PDGF is an essential hormone required for the growth of fibroblasts and other connective tissue cells.

PDGF has recently been purified to homogeneity (1,10). It is a heat (100°C) stable cationic protein with an isoelectric point of 9.8 and a molecular weight of 35 k daltons on SDS-polyacrylamide gels. Disulfide bonds are required for activity because reduction with 2-mercaptoethanol destroys the activity of the protein, as does treatment with trypsin. The protein is active at about 10^{-10} M, a concentration typical for polypeptide hormones.

BALB/c-3T3 cells have proven useful for studying the action of PDGF. Their rate of replication and their saturation density are controlled by the concentration of serum in the medium. Under typical tissue culture conditions, in which the medium is replenished twice weekly, these cells become growth-arrested at confluence with a G_1 content of DNA. Addition of fresh serum stimulates DNA synthesis and cell replication, demonstrating that the "old" serum-supplemented medium overlying the density-arrested cells lacks an essential growth factor (11,24,34). These cells appear to deplete serum of an essential growth factor while they grow and thus become arrested when they reach a critical cell density (34). This growth factor appears to be PDGF. Addition of an electrophoretically homogeneous preparation of PDGF (1) to density-inhibited cells maintained in depleted medium induced DNA synthesis, while addition of plasma did not (Table 1). Thus the PDGF component of serum is a limiting factor for the growth of BALB/c-3T3 cells in tissue culture.

COMPETENCE

Although PDGF is an essential growth factor required for the replication of BALB/c-3T3 cells, it alone does not efficiently stimulate DNA synthesis. Pledger et al. (19) demonstrated that plasma contains growth factors which act synergistically with PDGF to induce cells to enter the S phase (Fig. 1). Density arrested BALB/c-3T3 cells were treated with partially purified PDGF in the presence of medium supplemented with various concentrations of plasma. The percentage of cells that entered the S phase, as determined by autoradiography, was regulated by both the concentration of plasma and the concentration of PDGF. Jimenez De Asua et al. (12,13) have also shown that growth factors act synergistically to promote DNA synthesis. The induction of DNA synthesis by PDGF can be plotted on linear graph paper as the percentage of cells that have entered S as a function of time (Fig. 2A), or on semilogarithmic paper as the percentage of cells remaining in G_0/G_1 versus time (Fig. 2B) (30). The latter method has some advantages and will be used for the remainder of this discussion.

TABLE 1. *The PDGF component of serum is limiting for BALB/c-3T3 cell growth*

Addition to cell depleted medium[a]	% DNA synthesis[b]	Cultures changed to[c]	% DNA synthesis[b]
Pure PDGF (0.3 ng)	62	PDGF (0.3 ng) and plasma (5%)	67
Plasma (5%)	<3	Plasma (5%)	<3
None	<3	No change	<3

[a]Additions were made to density-arrested cells that were in medium containing 10% bovine serum. This serum was depleted (24,34) of growth factors because the cells were not synthesizing DNA.
[b]The cells were fixed 30 hr after adding the growth factors, and the percentage synthesizing DNA was determined using (^{3}H)dThd uptake into nuclei with radioautography.
[c]Cultures were changed to fresh medium supplemented as shown.

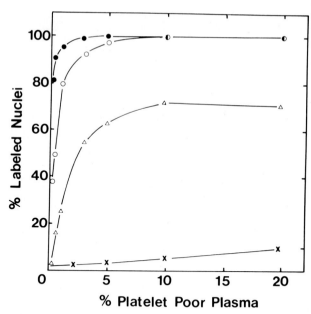

FIG. 1. Effect of concentration of platelet-poor plasma on platelet extract-induced DNA synthesis. Platelet extract (●, 100 μg; ○, 10 μg; △, 5 μg; or x, 0 μg) was added to cultures in 0.2 ml medium containing {³H} dThd and various concentrations of platelet-poor plasma. Cultures were fixed 36 hr later and processed for autoradiography. (Adapted from Pledger et al., ref. 19.)

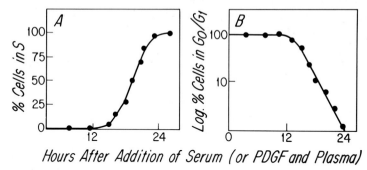

FIG. 2. Schematic illustration of the rate at which density-arrested BALB/c-3T3 cells enter the S phase following the addition of fresh culture medium containing serum (or PDGF and plasma). **A:** The data are plotted as percent cells that have entered S phase versus time. **B:** The same data are replotted on a semilogarithmic scale after the fashion of Smith and Martin (30).

PDGF does not have to be present continuously to initiate cellular entry into the S phase. A brief treatment with PDGF renders cells "competent" to synthesize DNA. These competent cells will synthesize DNA after transfer to medium supplemented with an optimal concentration of plasma. The rate that PDGF treated cells enter the S phase is regulated by the plasma concentration (Fig.3) (19). Plasma does not have to be added immediately after the PDGF is removed for cells to enter the S phase. The addition of plasma can be delayed as long as 13 hr, and the

CELL GROWTH, SOMATOMEDINS, AND PDGF

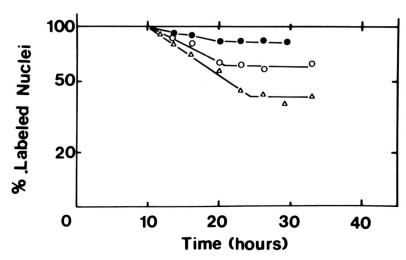

FIG. 3. Effect of concentration of platelet-poor plasma on the rate of cell entry into the S phase. Cultures were treated with 50 μg platelet extract at 37°C in 0.2 ml medium supplemented with {³H} dThd and platelet-poor plasma (●, 0.25%; ○, 2.5%; Δ, 5%). Cultures were fixed at the times indicated and processed for autoradiography. (Adapted from Pledger et al., ref. 19.)

majority of the PDGF treated cells enter the S phase. These cells begin to enter the S phase 12 hr after the addition of plasma, whether plasma is added immediately after PDGF is removed or 13 hr later (Fig. 4) (19).

Thus the cellular events modulated by PDGF can be separated from those controlled by plasma growth factors. PDGF primes cells to respond to growth factors present in plasma by inducing them to become competent to synthesize DNA. Plasma stimulates competent (but not incompetent) cells to progress through G_0/G_1 phase and synthesize DNA. Furthermore, treatment of cells with plasma before the addition of PDGF does not shorten the lag phase until DNA synthesis, indicating that PDGF initiates the growth response (20).

The ability of plasma to regulate the percentage of PDGF treated cells that enter the S phase has allowed complementation analysis to be used to define the growth factors that act like PDGF (31,33). Pituitary fibroblast growth factor (FGF) (8) precipitates of calcium phosphate (2,23) or wounding of the monolayer (34) act like PDGF and induce competence, because plasma acts synergistically with these

FIG. 4. The stability of the platelet extract-induced competent state. **A:** Cultures were treated with 50 μg platelet extract at 37°C in 0.2 ml medium containing 5% platelet-poor plasma and {³H} dThd. At the indicated times, cultures were fixed and processed for autoradiography. **B–E:** Cultures were treated with 50 μg platelet extract in 0.2 ml medium for 5 hr (↓) at 37°C, washed, and returned to 0.2 ml medium containing {³H} dThd but lacking platelet-poor plasma. At the times indicated (↑), the medium was supplemented with platelet-poor plasma (●, 5%, ○, 0.25%). The cultures were fixed and processed for autoradiography at timed intervals. (Adapted from Pledger et al., ref. 19).

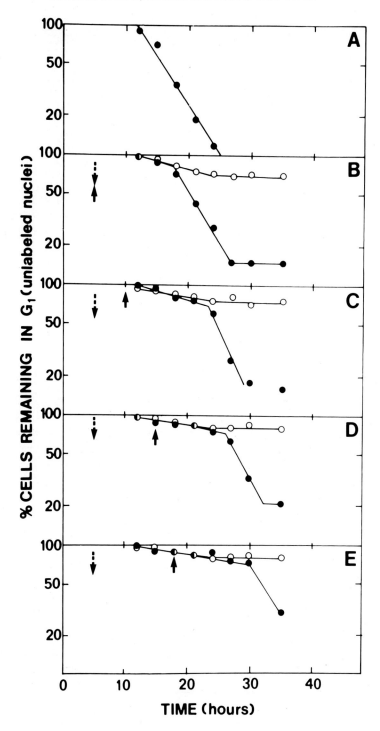

TABLE 2. Identification of progression factors and competence factors[a]

Factor or treatment	Progression activity	Competence activity
Somatomedin A (partially pure)	Potent: 1 unit = 20 ng	Weak: some activity at 330 ng
Somatomedin C	Potent: 1 unit = 2 ng	None: tested to 200 ng
MSA	Potent: 1 unit = 2 ng	None: tested to 200 ng
Insulin	Weak: 1 unit = 160 ng	None: tested to 120 µg
Hydrocortisone	Weak: 1 unit = 724 ng (10^{-5} M)	None: tested to 724 ng (10^{-5} M)
Growth hormone (50% pure)	None: was tested to 200 ng	None: tested to 200 ng
Tri-iodothyromine	None: was tested to 132 ng	Not tested
EGF	Partial: see text	None: tested to 200 ng
FGF	None: tested to 200 ng	Potent: 2 ng
PDGF (partially pure)	None: tested to 50 µg	Potent: 5 ng is active
$Ca_3(PO_4)_2$	None: tested to 18 mM	Potent: 3 mM is active
Wounding	None	Potent
Normal human serum	Potent: 1 unit = 2 µl	Potent: 5% serum is active
Normal human platelet-poor plasma	Potent: 1 unit = 2 µl	None: tested to 100%
SV40	Potent: 1 PFU/cell is active	Potent: 1 PFU/cell is active

[a] Growth factors were tested for progression factor activity according to the protocol outlined in refs. (31,33); a unit of progression factor is defined as the quantity of material which must be added to 3% hypophysectomized rat plasma to give progression activity comparable to that of 3% normal rat plasma. For competence testing, quiescent density-arrested microtiter cultures of BALB/c-3T3 cells were exposed for 3 hr to various quantities of growth factor; control cultures were exposed for 3 hr to 5% normal human plasma. The culture medium was then aspirated. Cell monolayers were washed once with saline containing 28 mM β-mercaptoethanol and once with saline only. The treated cultures were then incubated for 36 hr with DME containing 5% normal human plasma and [³H] dThd (5 µCi/ml). After 36 hr, the cells were fixed and processed for autoradiography. Under these conditions, less than 5% of cells from control cultures were stimulated to synthesize DNA; those factors with competence activity stimulated 60 to 95% of the cells to become labeled. Final concentrations of all growth factors can be derived by multiplying the quantities indicated × 5 ml⁻¹. Pure PDGF also acts as a competence agent (unpublished data). PFU = plaque forming units.

agents to promote DNA synthesis (Table 2) (31,33). A schematic view of the activity of these agents is shown in Fig. 5.

EXPONENTIAL GROWTH

The studies outlined above were performed by adding PDGF to density inhibited cells arrested in the G_0 phase of the growth cycle. Vogel et al. (38) demonstrated that 3T3 cells treated with an optimal concentration of both PDGF and plasma grew exponentially. Like all exponentially growing populations, these cells had a short interval between M and the next S phase, and did not appear to enter G_0.

We reasoned that cells may not enter G_0 if they are treated with PDGF during the preceding S phase (28). Confluent G_0-arrested BALB/c-3T3 cells were treated with PDGF and plasma in the presence of methotrexate, an inhibitor of dihydrofolate reductase, an enzyme needed for *de novo* purine and thymidine synthesis. Because the cells could not synthesize DNA, they become growth-arrested in an early part of the S phase. Removal of the methotrexate and addition of an optimal concentration of plasma allowed these cells to complete the cell cycle, but they did not enter the S phase of the subsequent cell cycle. Addition of PDGF and plasma to these cells after M allowed them to enter the S phase of the second cycle, with a lag of 12 hr, demonstrating that cells that lack PDGF are incompetent and become arrested at G_0 (Fig. 6) (28).

Methotrexate-blocked cells were released from methotrexate and treated with a short pulse of partially purified PDGF while traversing the S phase; the cells were then returned to 5% plasma and allowed to undergo mitosis. The daughter cells, which remained in plasma, entered a second S phase, with a lag period of 6 to 7 hr from the time of mitosis (Fig. 6). Thus the daughter cells "remembered" that their parents had been treated with PDGF during the S phase of the preceding cell cycle. Because the parent had been treated with PDGF, the daughters did not enter G_0, but synthesized DNA after a 6 to 7 hr lag period from the preceding M. Treatment of the parent cells with PDGF during S phase prevented the daughter cells from

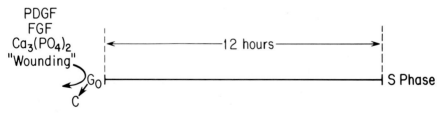

FIG. 5. Schematic illustration of the effects of competence factors, PDGF, FGF, $Ca_3(PO_4)_2$, or wounding, on density-arrested BALB/c-3T3 cells. Transient treatment with any of these agents renders density-arrested cells to become competent to synthesize DNA. However, competent cells do not enter the S phase until at least 12 hr following the transfer of cultures to plasma supplemented tissue culture medium. Unlike competence factors, which are required only transiently, the hormonal growth factors in plasma are required continuously for cellular entry into the S phase.

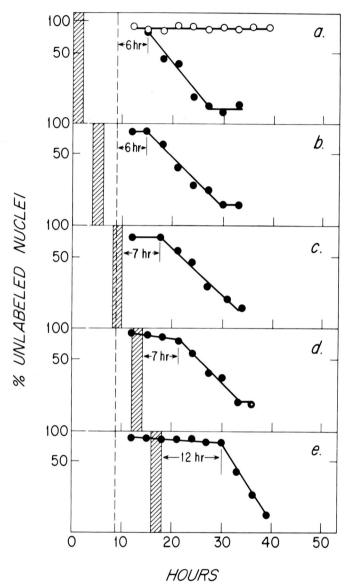

FIG. 6. Treatment with PDGF during S, G_2, or M phases, or immediately after mitosis, prevents replicating BALB/c-3T3 cells from becoming growth-arrested at G_0. Density-inhibited BALB/c-3T3 cells were treated with partially purified PDGF and transferred to 5% plasma-supplemented medium containing methotrexate. After 18 hr, the medium was removed from all cultures; some cultures were transferred to medium containing 5% plasma, hypoxanthine, and {³H} dThd (5 μCi/ml; 0.3 Ci/mmol) and fixed 8 hr later. Autoradiography demonstrated that 91% of the PDGF-stimulated parent cells entered the S phase. Duplicate cultures were transferred to 5% platelet-poor plasma containing hypoxanthine and thymidine. Some cultures (●) were treated with platelet extract (150 μg/ml) containing partially purified PDGF and hypoxanthine and thymidine for 2 hr periods at the times indicated by the shaded bars or were left untreated (○). {³H} dThd (5 μCi/ml; final concentration, 0.3 Ci/mmol) was added to these cultures 10 hr after the removal of the methotrexate. The cells were fixed at the indicated times and processed for autoradiography. The data are plotted according to the method of Smith and Martin (30). The dashed line is shown to mark the beginning of mitosis. (Adapted from Scher et al., ref. 28.)

becoming arrested at G_0. Thus PDGF has a dual function. It stimulates growth-arrested cells to leave G_0 and prevents replicating cells from entering G_0.

PROGRESSION

An optimal concentration of plasma (usually 5–10%) must be present continuously for PDGF-treated competent cells to enter the S phase. Withdrawal of plasma shortly before the onset of DNA synthesis causes cells to become growth arrested at one of two growth arrest points either 6 hr (V point) or immediately (W point) before the G_1/S phase boundary (20,33). Treatment of competent cells with a suboptimal concentration of plasma causes cells to become arrested at the same growth arrest points (20). Thus an optimal concentration of plasma is needed continuously to stimulate DNA synthesis.

Nutrients such as the essential amino acids are also required for serum stimulated cells to enter the S phase (18). However, deprivation of amino acids does not prevent PDGF from inducing density-arrested cells to become competent to replicate. Amino acid deprivation interferes with the plasma mediated progression sequence (32). In the presence of an optimal concentration of plasma these cells become arrested at the V or W growth arrest points (32). Thus nutrients are required for plasma mediated progression of cells into the S phase.

SOMATOMEDINS

The somatomedins are a group of polypeptide hormones with insulin-like activity and structural homology to proinsulin (21) that appear to be synthesized by the liver in response to pituitary growth hormone (37). The somatomedins have been shown to stimulate the growth of cartilage cells in organ culture. In contrast, growth hormone does not stimulate cartilage growth directly. Thus it appears that the growth stimulating activity of growth hormone *in vivo* is mediated through the somatomedins (5,37).

Although the somatomedins stimulate cartilage growth within organ explants, they have only a minimal effect in tissue culture. They stimulate suboptimal DNA synthesis in growth arrested chick embryo fibroblasts (21), but do not stimulate DNA synthesis in density arrested BALB/c-3T3 cells (25). This discrepancy was resolved by the realization that the treatment of fibroblasts in tissue culture with PDGF is required for an optimal response to the somatomedins (31).

PDGF-treated, competent BALB/c-3T3 cells were placed in medium supplemented with plasma from hypophysectomized animal donors. Relative to the plasma obtained from control animals, this plasma was deficient in progression activity. Only a small percentage of the PDGF treated cells that were transferred to the hypophysectomized animal plasma entered the S phase (Fig. 7A). The addition of 3 ng per ml (10^{-9} M) of pure somatomedin C to these cultures allowed the cells to synthesize DNA (Fig. 7B). In addition to the somatomedin, growth factors in the hypophysectomized animal plasma were needed because the addition of somatomedin alone to PDGF treated cells did not stimulate DNA synthesis (Fig. 7B).

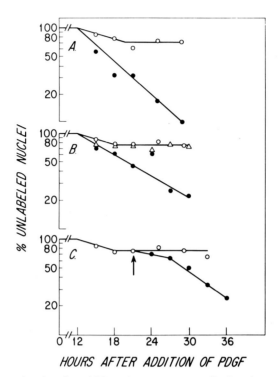

FIG. 7. Demonstration that the addition of pure somatomedin C to hypophysectomized rat plasma restores progression factor activity. Density-arrested BALB/c-3T3 cells were treated for 3 hr with 57 μg of partially purified PDGF. After the PDGF was removed, the cells were washed and returned to medium containing {³H} dThd. **A:** The medium was supplemented with 3% plasma from either normal (●) or hypophysectomized (○) rats. **B:** The medium was supplemented with 3% plasma from hypophysectomized animals (○), 3% plasma from hypophysectomized animals plus 3 ng/ml of pure somatomedin C (●), or 3 ng/ml of pure somatomedin C only (Δ). **C:** The medium was supplemented with 3% plasma from hypophysectomized rats. At the time indicated (↑), somatomedin C (30 ng/ml) was added to some cultures (●), while others (○) received an equivalent volume of 0.15 M NaCl. At periodic intervals, the cells were fixed and processed for autoradiography. (Adapted from Stiles et al., ref. 31.)

In a temporal analysis of S phase entry, PDGF treated competent cells were transferred to medium supplemented with hypophysectomized animal plasma; 21 hr later, somatomedin C was added to some cultures. The cells entered the S phase in a biphasic fashion. A small but significant increase in the entry of cells into the S phase was noted immediately, and at 6 hr, a major increase was noted (Fig. 7C) (33). It appears that somatomedin C is needed for cells to leave the V or W growth arrest points and synthesize DNA (33).

Other growth factors can substitute for somatomedin C to promote the progression through G_0/G_1 of cells maintained in hypophysectomized animal plasma (31). These growth factors, which include other somatomedins such as somatomedin A and multiplication stimulating activity (MSA), are listed in Table 2. High concentrations of insulin (10^{-6} M or greater) were found to have progression activity (31), presumably because of binding to the somatomedin receptor (37).

Of interest is the finding that competence factors do not promote progression and vice versa (31). Some factors, such as the epidermal growth factor (EGF) (3,4), have neither activity and may represent the activity present in hypophysectomized animal plasma. Serum has both competence and progression activities (Table 2) because it contains both PDGF and somatomedins.

CENTRIOLES

As proliferating cells replicate their DNA and proceed through mitosis, the centriole must also duplicate so that chromosomes can be distributed to the daughter cells. Tucker et al. (35) demonstrated that density-arrested BALB/c-3T3 cells contain one pair of centrioles which form a primary cilium; upon serum stimulation, such cells undergo early (1–2 hr) transient deciliation, followed by another deciliation which is associated with centriole duplication and DNA synthesis. The initial centriole deciliation, observed very rapidly after serum stimulation, is controlled by the PDGF component of serum (36). In dose-response studies, only doses of PDGF which produced centriole deciliation were capable of inducing competence for DNA synthesis. Other agents that induce competence, such as pituitary FGF or microprecipitates of calcium phosphate, also induce the initial transient deciliation of the centriole (36). In contrast, plasma or somatomedin, which do not induce competence, do not cause the transient centriole deciliation (36). These agents were required for the optimal progression of cells into the S phase and for the second centriole deciliation, which was associated with DNA synthesis.

SV40

The oncogenic virus SV40 stimulates quiescent BALB/c-3T3 cells to synthesize DNA. It was useful to analyze the replicative response of cells to SV40 in the context of competence and progression. The activity of SV40 in stimulating cellular DNA synthesis was complemented by neither PDGF nor plasma (Fig. 8) but was solely controlled by the viral multiplicity of infection. Thus an SV40 gene function(s) overrides the requirement for both the PDGF and plasma components of serum. Furthermore, unlike growth factor induced DNA synthesis, infection with SV40 stimulates cells to enter the S phase in nutrient deficient medium (32). The mitogenic response to SV40 differed from that induced by growth factors in another way. Unlike competence factors, SV40 did not induce an initial transient deciliation of the centriole (36).

TUMOR PROMOTER

The active ingredient of croton oil, 12-0-tetradecanoyl-phorbol-13-acetate (TPA), has been shown to stimulate the proliferation of BALB/c-3T3 cells in culture (29).

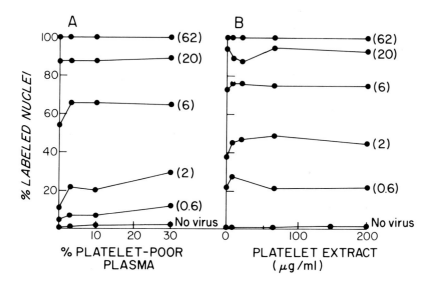

FIG. 8. Demonstration that SV40 overrides both competence and progression. Gradient-purified SV40 was added to density-arrested BALB/c-3T3 cells at the multiplicity of infection indicated in parentheses. **A:** After 3 hr, the medium was removed and the cells were washed. Fresh medium containing {³H} dThd and normal human plasma as indicated (●) was added to the cultures. **B:** Density-arrested cultures of BALB/c-3T3 cells were treated for 3 hr with partially purified PDGF as indicated (●). After 3 hr, the medium was removed and the cells were washed. Fresh medium containing {³H} dThd and 0.25% normal human plasma was added together with SV40. After 36 hr, all cultures were fixed and processed for autoradiography. (Adapted from Stiles et al., ref. 31.)

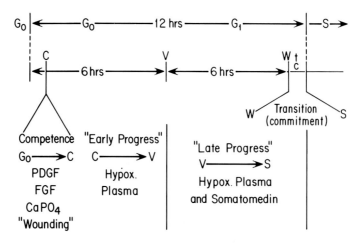

FIG. 9. Hormonal control of early events in the mitogenic response of BALB/c-3T3 cells to serum growth factors. (Adapted from Stiles et al., ref. 33.)

TPA is also a widely used model compound in studies on tumor promotion; for this reason, we analyzed the mitogenic action of TPA in the context of competence and progression (7). TPA functions in a fashion which differs from that of growth factors and also differs from SV40. Growth factors modulate either the competence or the progression events but never both. SV40 overrides both competence and progression activity. TPA functions as a competence factor, since it enhances the growth stimulatory activity of progression factors. TPA also functions as a progression factor, since it enhances the growth stimulatory activity of competence factors. TPA alone, however, does not stimulate cell replication, thus distinguishing this compound from SV40.

CONCLUSIONS

Temporal analysis of the mitogenic response of BALB/c-3T3 cells to serum growth factors indicates that PDGF and somatomedins regulate separate and sequential events in the cell cycle (Fig. 9). These data provide a useful context in which to study the molecular action of serum growth factors and nutrients in promoting DNA synthesis. Moreover, by examining the cellular growth response to tumor viruses and chemical tumor promoters in the context of competence and progression, it may be possible to establish functional analogies between these agents and specific polypeptide growth factors found in serum.

ACKNOWLEDGMENTS

We thank Dr. W. J. Pledger for helpful discussions. Portions of the work summarized within were supported by Grants CA 18662, CA 27113, CA 22042, and CA 22427. C. D. Scher is a Scholar of the Leukemia Society of America.

REFERENCES

1. Antoniades, H. N., Scher, C. D., and Stiles, C. D. (1979): Purification of human platelet-derived growth factor. *Proc. Natl. Acad. Sci. U.S.A.*, 76:1809–1813.
2. Barnes, D. W., and Colowick, S. P. (1977): Stimulation of sugar uptake and thymidine incorporation in mouse 3T3 cells by calcium phosphate and other extra-cellular particles. *Proc. Natl. Acad. Sci. U.S.A.*, 74:5593–5597.
3. Carpenter, G., Lembach, K. J., Morrison, M. M., and Cohen, S. (1975): Characterization of the binding of ^{125}I-labeled epidermal growth factor to human fibroblasts. *J. Biol. Chem.*, 250:4297–4304.
4. Das, M., Miyakawa, T., Fox, C. F., Pruss, R. M., Aharonov, A., and Hershman, H. R. (1977): Specific radiolabeling of a cell surface receptor for epidermal growth factor. *Proc. Natl. Acad. Sci. U.S.A.*, 74:2790–2794.
5. Daughaday, W. H., Hall, K., Raben, M. S., Salmon, Jr., W. D., Van Den Brande, J. L., and Van Wyk, J. J. (1972): Somatomedin: proposed designation for sulphation factor. *Nature*, 235:107.
6. Eagle, H. (1955): Nutrition needs of mammalian cells in culture. *Science*, 122:501–504.
7. Frantz, C. F., Stiles, C. D., and Scher, C. D. (1979): The tumor promoter 12-0-tetradecanoyl-phorbol-13-acetate enhances the proliferative response of BALB/c-3T3 cells to hormonal growth factors. *J. Cell. Physiol.*, 100:413–424.
8. Gospodarowicz, D. (1975): Purification of a fibroblast growth factor from bovine pituitary. *J. Biol. Chem.*, 250:2515–2520.
9. Hazashi, I., and Sato, G. (1976): Replacement of serum by hormones permits growth of cells in defined medium. *Nature*, 259:132–134.

10. Heldin, C. H., Westermark, B., and Wasteson, A. (1979): Platelet-derived growth factor: Purification and partial characterization. *Proc. Nato. Acad. Sci. U.S.A.*, 76:3722–3726.

11. Holley, R. W., and Kiernan, J. A. (1968): Contact inhibition of cell division in 3T3 cells. *Proc. Natl. Acad. Sci. U.S.A.*, 60:300–304.

12. Jimenez De Asua, L., O'Farrell, M., Bennett, D., Clingan, D., and Rudland, P. (1977): Interaction of two hormones and their effect on observed rate of initiation of DNA synthesis in 3T3 cells. *Nature*, 265:151–153.

13. Jimenez De Asua, L., O'Farrell, M. K., Clingan, D., and Rudland, P. S. (1977): Temporal sequence of hormonal interactions during the prereplicative phase of quiescent cultured fibroblasts. *Proc. Natl. Acad. Sci. U.S.A.*, 74:3845–3849.

14. Kaplan, D. R., Chao, F. C., Stiles, C. S., Antoniades, H. N., and Scher, C. D. (1979): Platelet α-granules contain a growth factor for fibroblasts. *Blood*, 53:1043–1052.

15. Kohler, N., and Lipton, A. (1974): Platelets as a source of fibroblast growth-promoting activity. *Exp. Cell Res.*, 87:297–301.

16. McKeehan, W., Hamilton, W. G., and Ham, R. G. (1976): Selenium is an essential trace nutrient for growth of WI-38 diploid human fibroblasts. *Proc. Natl. Acad. Sci. U.S.A.*, 73:2023–2027.

17. Only, J., and Sato, G. (1979): Fibronectin mediates cytokinesis and growth of rat follicular ceils in serum-free medium. *Cell*, 17:295–305.

18. Pardee, A. B. (1974): A restriction point for control of normal animal cell proliferation. *Proc. Natl. Acad. Sci. U.S.A.*, 71:1286–1290.

19. Pledger, W. J., Stiles, C. D., Antoniades, H. N., and Scher, C. D. (1977): Induction of DNA synthesis in BALB/c-3T3 cells by serum components: reevaluation of the commitment process. *Proc. Natl. Acad. Sci. U.S.A.*, 74:4481–4485.

20. Pledger, W. J., Stiles, C. D., Antoniades, H. N., and Scher, C. D. (1978): An ordered sequence of events is required before BALB/c-3T3 cells become committed to DNA. *Proc. Natl. Acad. Sci. U.S.A.*, 75:2839–2843.

21. Rinderknecht, E., and Humbel, R. E. (1976): Amino-terminal sequences of two polypeptides from human serum with nonsuppressible insulin-like and cell-growth-promoting activities: evidence for structural homology with insulin B chain. *Proc. Natl. Acad. Sci. U.S.A.*, 73:4379–4381.

22. Ross, R., Glomset, J., Kariya, B., and Harker, L. (1974): A platelet dependent serum factor that stimulates the proliferation of arterial smooth muscle cells. *Proc. Natl. Acad. Sci. U.S.A.*, 71:1207–1210.

23. Rubin, H., and Sanui, H. (1977): Complexes of inorganic pyrophosphate, orthophosphate, and calcium as stimulants of 3T3 cell multiplication. *Proc. Natl. Acad. Sci. U.S.A.*, 74:5026–5030.

24. Scher, C. D. (1971): SV40-induced DNA synthesis and the fixation of the transformed state. *Virology*, 46:956–957.

25. Scher, C. D., Stathakos, D., and Antoniades, H. N. (1974): Dissociation of cell division stimulating capacity for BALB/c-3T3 from the insulin-like activity in human serum. *Nature*, 247:279–281.

26. Scher, C. D., Pledger, W. J., Martin, P., Antoniades, H., and Stiles, C. D. (1978): Transforming viruses directly reduce the cellular growth requirement for a platelet-derived growth factor. *J. Cell. Physiol.*, 97:371–380.

27. Scher, C. D., Shepard, R. C., Antoniades, H. N., and Stiles, C. D. (1979): Platelet-derived growth factor and the regulation of the mammalian fibroblast cell cycle. *Biochim. Biophys. Acta*, 560:217–241.

28. Scher, C. D., Stone, M. E., and Stiles, C. D. (1979): Platelet-derived growth factor prevents G_0 growth arrest. *Nature*, 281:390–392.

29. Sivak, A. (1977): Induction of Cell division in BALB/c-3T3 cells by phorbol myristate acetate or bovine serum: effect of inhibitors of cyclic AMP phosphodiesterase and Na^+-K^+ ATPase. *In Vitro*, 13:1263–1266.

30. Smith, J. A., and Martin, L. (1973): Do cells cycle? *Proc. Natl. Acad. Sci. U.S.A.*, 70:1263–1267.

31. Stiles, C. D., Capone, G. T., Scher, C. D., Antoniades, H. N., Van Wyk, J. J., and Pledger, W. J. (1979): Dual control of cell growth by somatomedins and platelet-derived growth factor. *Proc. Natl. Acad. Sci. U.S.A.*, 76:1279–1283.

32. Stiles, C. D., Isberg, R. R., Pledger, W. J., Antoniades, H. N., and Scher, C. D. (1979): Control of the BALB/c-3T3 cell cycle by nutrients and serum factors: analysis using platelet-derived growth factor and platelet-poor plasma. *J. Cell. Physiol.*, 99:395–406.

33. Stiles, C. D., Pledger, W. J., Van Wyk, J. J., Antoniades, H., and Scher, C. D. (1979): Hormonal control of early events in the BALB/c-3T3 cell cycle: commitment to DNA synthesis. In: *Hormones and Cell Culture, Cold Spring Harbor Conferences on Cell Proliferation*, Vol. 6, edited by G. Sato and R. Ross, pp. 425–439. Cold Spring Harbor Laboratory Press, Cold Spring Harbor, N.Y.
34. Todaro, G. J., Maysuya, Y., Bloom, S., Robbins, A., and Green, H. (1967): Stimulation of RNA synthesis and cell division in resting cell by a factor present in serum. In: *Growth Regulating Substances for Animal Cells in Culture*, edited by V. Defendi and M. Stoker, pp. 87–101. Wistar Inst. Press, Philadelphia.
35. Tucker, R. W., Pardee, A. B., and Fujiwara, K. (1979): Centriole ciliation is related to quiescence and DNA synthesis in 3T3 cells. *Cell*, 17:527–535.
36. Tucker, R. W., Scher, C. D., and Stiles, C. D. (1979): Centriole deciliation associated with the early response of 3T3 cells to growth factors but not to SV40. *Cell*, 18:1065–1072.
37. Van Wyk, J. J., and Underwood, L. E. (1978): The somatomedins and their actions. In: *Biochemical Actions of Hormones*, Vol. 5, edited by G. Litwack, pp. 101–147. Academic Press, New York.
38. Vogel, A., Raines, E., Kariya, B., Rivest, M. J., and Ross, R. (1978): Coordinate control of 3T3 cell proliferation by platelet-derived growth factor and plasma components. *Proc. Natl. Acad. Sci. U.S.A.*, 76:2810–2814.

Maturation Factors and Cancer,
edited by Malcolm A. S. Moore.
Raven Press, © New York 1982.

The Role of the Extracellular Matrix and Growth Factors in the Control of Proliferation of Anchorage-Dependent Cells

D. Gospodarowicz and I. Vlodavsky

Cancer Research Institute and the Department of Medicine, University of California Medical Center, San Francisco, California 94143

Cell migration and growth *in vivo* are the result of a complex balance between cell-cell and cell-substrate interactions. Those forces which combine to modulate the cell shape may either permit or prevent cell proliferation and differentiation (13,19,50,71). Following its original proposal by Grobstein (35), a role for cell-substrate interactions in the control of cell proliferation and morphogenesis has been demonstrated (for reviews, see refs. 36,37,46,81,82). In the case of epithelial tissues with a high rate of cell turnover, such as the epidermis or the corneal epithelium, active cell proliferation is only localized to the basal layer, composed of tall and columnar cells. These cells are in close contact with a basal lamina or extracellular matrix (ECM). In contrast, cells in the upper layers, which have lost their ability to proliferate and gradually adopt a flattened configuration, are no longer in contact with the ECM. Thus contact between the cells and their substrate rather than contact between cells could have a permissive influence on cell proliferation. The ECM with which various tissues are closely associated has also been shown to modulate gene expression and cytodifferentiation (5,66,80). A major limitation of conventional tissue culture techniques has been that cells, in contrast to the *in vivo* situation, proliferate *in vitro* as a collection of individual cells resting on plastic rather than on an ECM. A number of *in vitro* studies demonstrate that the substrate upon which cells are cultured can alter both the cellular shape and proliferative response to various mitogens in an interrelated manner (4,19,32,50). In the present chapter, we describe the use of the ECM produced by cultured corneal endothelial cells as a substrate on which to culture both normal and transformed cells of various origins.

EXTRACELLULAR MATRIX: COMPOSITION

Although the exact nature and composition of ECM produced by various tissues are still to be elucidated, they are composed for the most part of collagen, glyco-saminoglycans, and glycoproteins. Collagen, a major component of the ECM, is a family of closely related proteins, each a different gene product. Three types of interstitial collagen (I, II, and III), as well as, tentatively, two types of basement membrane collagens (IV and V), are currently recognized (53). Glycosaminoglycans (GAGs) are sugar polymers of high molecular weight composed of repeating dimers of amino sugars, which tend to be linked to proteins to form the proteoglycans (54). Some GAGs are sulfated and, because they contain abundant free carboxyl groups, are the major anionic substance of the intracellular spaces. By variation of the types and distribution of GAGs associated with proteins, a fantastic diversity of proteoglycans can be generated. Glycoproteins such as fibronectin (39) and laminin (72) are also associated with the extracellular matrix and are considered to be involved mainly in cell-substrate adhesion.

The effect of the ECM on the proliferation of cells maintained in cultures has not been studied. This is mostly due to the fact that, with the exception of lens capsule, it is difficult *in vivo* to isolate such material from neighboring tissues. *In vitro*, the reconstitution of an ECM from its separate elements (collagens, proteoglycans, glycosaminoglycans, and glycoproteins) may be difficult, if not impossible. Not only must the correct ratio of components constituting the ECM be respected, but they must also be linked in such a way that the resulting tridimensional structure will be like that of the extracellular scaffolding *in vivo*. The problem in reconstituting an ECM *in vitro* is made even more difficult by the fact that collagen types IV and V, which *in vivo* are the main components of basement membrane collagens, are most often extracted from tissue following limited proteolysis. This could result in structural alterations and prevent their proper polymerization *in vitro*. One must also consider that our knowledge of the components of the ECM is limited and that components such as laminin (72) have only recently been isolated. The number of components which remain to be isolated can only be guessed.

CULTURED CORNEAL AND VASCULAR ENDOTHELIAL CELLS AND THE PRODUCTION OF AN ECM *IN VITRO*

As pointed out earlier, in order to test whether or not the ECM can affect cell proliferation and differentiation, one has to reconstitute it *in vitro*. The *in vitro* reconstitution of the ECM from its isolated and purified components is a formidable, if not impossible task. One can, however, take advantage of the fact that cell types such as corneal endothelial cells, when maintained in tissue culture, still retain their ability to synthesize and secrete an ECM found underneath, but not on top of the cells (21). As shown in Fig. 1A, corneal endothelial cells form, upon reaching

FIG. 1. Scanning electron microscopy of a monolayer of bovine corneal endothelial cells before and after exposure to Triton X-100. A monolayer composed of polygonal, highly flattened, and closely apposed cells can be seen in (**A** (×600). After the monolayer has been treated with Triton X-100, it is composed of nuclei and cytoskeletons, which no longer attach firmly to the extracellular matrix. In some areas, the extracellular matrix has been exposed (**B**, ×600). Washing the dishes with PBS removed the cytoskeleton and exposed the extracellular matrix present underneath the cells (**C**, ×200). The plate has been scratched with a needle to expose the plastic (p) to which the extracellular matrix (em) strongly adheres. In some areas, heavy deposits of extracellular matrix material form hexagonal ridges (**D**, ×600) on top of an amorphous material covering the whole dish.

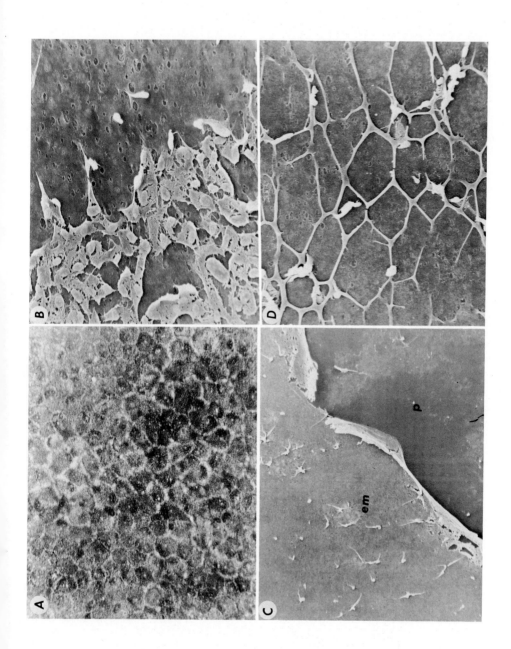

confluence, a monolayer of small, highly flattened, tightly packed (1,300 cells per mm^2) and nonoverlapping cells. Secretion of an ECM takes place only underneath the cell layer (21,31), and the underlying matrix is revealed after exposing the cell layer to 0.5% Triton X-100 and subsequent washing with PBS to remove remaining nuclei and cytoskeletons (17) (Fig. 1B,C). The matrix then appears as a uniform layer of amorphous material coating the entire area of the dish (Fig. 1C,D).

The collagen composition of the ECM produced by corneal endothelial cells *in vitro* has been analyzed. Type III collagen is the major component found in the ECM. Basement membrane collagen types IV and V were also found, and the ratio of type III : IV + V collagen synthesized by corneal endothelial cells is 16 to 1 (73). Fibronectin, as well as laminin, which codistributed with collagen type IV, are also present in large quantities (20) (Fig. 2). Likewise, vascular endothelial cells, which at confluence adopt all the morphological and functional characteristics of their *in vivo* counterparts, retain their ability to secrete underneath the cell layer an extensive ECM composed of laminin, fibronectin (20) (Fig. 2), and collagen type III, as well as of types IV and V, present at a ratio of 3 to 1 (74).

These ECMs, whose appearance has been shown to correlate with the acquisition by cultured corneal and vascular endothelial cells of their normal "in vivo" morphology, cell surface polarity, and function (31), could substitute for the ECM produced by other cell types (Fig. 3. The ability of endothelial cells in tissue culture to produce an extensive ECM could therefore provide us with a tailor-made ECM with which to test the proliferative response of other cell types to growth factors. We have therefore compared the rates of attachment and proliferation of various cell types maintained on plastic versus dishes coated with an ECM produced by corneal endothelial cell cultures.

TUMOR CELLS

A central issue in tumor biology is the understanding of the interactions between tumor cells and their environment. It is of interest in this regard to study the tumor cells' interaction with extracellular matrices, since this could throw light on the need for stromal and fibroblastic support for tumor cell growth (1,48), on the ability of tumor cells to reorganize their local environment in order to grow and invade (49,60), and on the mechanisms through which various artificial substrates that are introduced *in vivo* into the animal result in the production of malignant mesothelioma and fibrosarcoma (70). We have therefore studied the use of the ECM produced by cultured corneal endothelial cells as a substrate on which to culture human cells originating from solid tumors (colon carcinoma and Ewing's sarcoma). These were chosen primarily because, although they were derived from "solid tumors," they showed a poor ability to attach to tissue culture dishes and grow either as loosely attached aggregates or in suspension. In this respect, the Ewing's cells were of particular interest, because the cellular origin of this tumor, which is the most common primary malignant bone tumor in children (56), has been controversial.

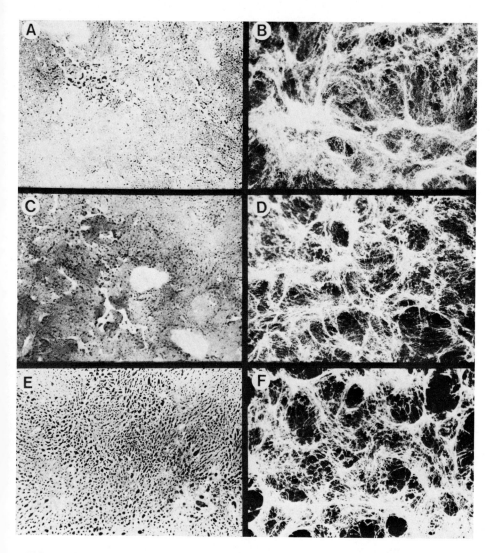

FIG. 2. Distribution of laminin **(A,B)**, type IV collagen **(C,D)**, and fibronectin **(E,F)** in the ECM of corneal endothelial **(A,C,E)** and vascular endothelial **(B,D,F)** cell cultures. ECMs were prepared and stained by indirect immunofluorescent microscopy as described in ref. 20.

In vivo they appeared as small and closely apposed cells growing between partitions of connective tissue. Because of this morphology, they were regarded by Ewing (9) as a myeloma derived from the endothelium. When grown on plastic, the cells appeared different from the original tumor cells and resembled fibroblastic cells when viewed by electron microscopy (41). Since the environmental requirements

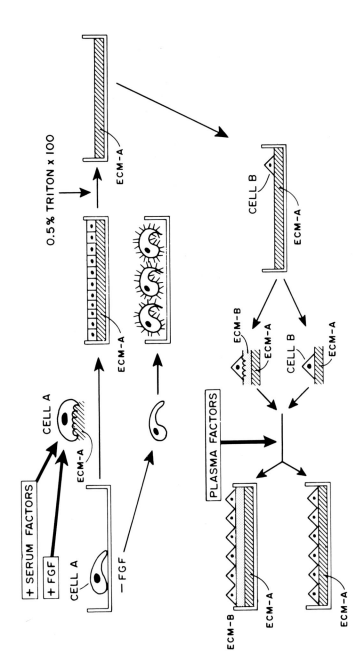

FIG. 3. The extracellular matrix (ECM) and cell proliferation. Cells maintained in the absence of FGF at very low cell density cannot produce a normal ECM. They therefore produce an aberrant ECM and cannot proliferate in response to serum or plasma factors (porcupine cells). In the presence of FGF (cell A), the cells make an ECM with a given polarity and with the correct composition. Cells resting on the ECM can respond to serum or plasma factors and will form a cell monolayer. That cell monolayer can then be exposed to Triton X. After washing, the ECM produced by the cell is exposed (ECM-A). If a cell type such as that represented by cell B, which does not have the ability to produce an ECM when maintained on plastic, is provided with an ECM, it will now proliferate in response to plasma factors and escape the restrictive influence of the plastic substrate. Alternatively, cell B, which cannot produce an ECM when maintained on plastic, will produce its own ECM (ECM-B) when maintained on ECM-A. This will in turn make the cells sensitive to plasma factors, and cells, because they are now making their own ECM, will divide rapidly.

for long-term cultures of human cancer cells, particularly for those of epithelial morphology, are currently poorly defined (58), we have limited ourselves to tumor cells of human origin in hope of improving their growth.

Cell Morphology and Organization of Colon Carcinoma and Ewing's Sarcoma Cells when Maintained on ECM-Coated Dishes Versus Plastic Dishes

Colon carcinoma cells seeded on plastic attach poorly to it and form tightly packed, ball-like cell aggregates (Fig. 4A–C). In contrast, cells seeded on an ECM (Fig. 4D) adopt within 1 to 2 hr after seeding a flattened morphology, spreading out and showing no signs of cell aggregation. At confluence, a monolayer composed of small and tightly packed cells that cover the entire area of the dish was observed

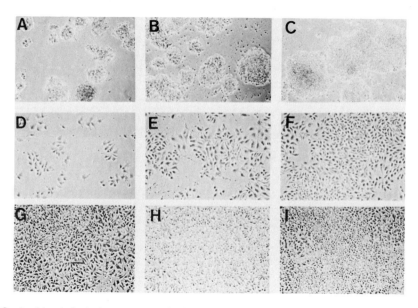

FIG. 4. Morphological appearance of colon carcinoma cells maintained on plastic versus extracellular matrix. Stock cultures maintained on plastic tissue culture dishes were dissociated with STV and the cells seeded into plastic **(A–C)** or extracellular matrix-coated **(D–I)** dishes in DMEM (H-21) containing 10% fetal calf serum. Photographs were taken (phase contrast, × 100) starting on day 1 **(A,D)** and up to 10 days **(C,I)** after seeding in order to demonstrate the culture's morphological appearance at various cell densities. **A–C:** Cells seeded on plastic. The cells form aggregates composed of small and spheroidal cells and proliferate as such to form large, multiple layered aggregates. Most of these aggregates are firmly attached to the tissue culture dish, but the percentage of floating cells (aggregates and single cells) increases when the cells reach confluence. **D–I:** Cells seeded on extracellular matrix. Cell spreading and flattening with no signs of cell aggregation and overlapping can be seen at either a low **(D–E)** or high cell density **(F,G)**. A layer of cuboidal and tightly packed cells is formed at confluence **(H,I)**, but as the cells continue to proliferate, areas of cell overlapping, and particularly shedding of single cells into the culture medium, are observed.

(Fig. 4F–I). Although the cells did grow on top of one another late at confluence (Fig. 4F–I), the overgrowing cells rounded up and floated free into the medium, probably because, unlike the cells underneath, they were prevented from attaching to the ECM. Upon dissociation of the cell layer and reseeding on plastic, the cells reaggregate, pile up, and proliferate to form large, multilayered clumps that may eventually cover the surface of the dish or float in the medium (78).

Similar morphological differences were observed with the Ewing's sarcoma cells grown on plastic versus an ECM (78) (Fig. 5). Cell aggregates that are seeded on plastic adopt at either low (Fig. 5A,B) or high cell density (Fig. 5C) the configuration of loosely attached aggregates of cells. In contrast, if the same cells are seeded either singly or as aggregates on dishes coated with an ECM, they spread and adopt a flattened morphology (Fig. 5C). This could be observed both at a sparse density prior to the formation of cell-cell contacts (Fig. 5D), as well as at confluence, when

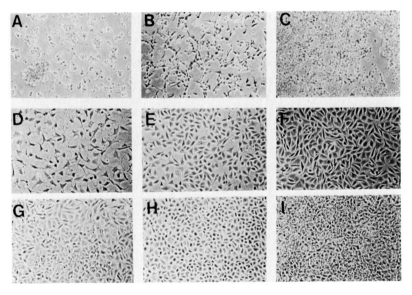

FIG. 5. Morphological appearance of Ewing's sarcoma cells maintained on plastic versus extracellular matrix. Stock cultures maintained in plastic dishes were dissociated with STV and the cells seeded into plastic **(A–C)** or extracellular matrix-coated **(D–I)** dishes in DMEM (H-12) containing 1% calf serum. Photographs (phase contrast, × 100) were taken starting on day 1 **(A,D)** and up to 9 days **(C,I)** after seeding in order to demonstrate the culture's morphological appearance at both high and low cell densities. Loosely attached aggregates **(A)**, as well as single spherical or elongated cells **(B)** that hardly contact each other can be seen at a sparse density 1 to 3 days after seeding. The elongated and firmly attached configuration was seldom or not observed in medium containing fibronectin-depleted rather than untreated calf serum. Cell aggregation and overgrowth is most prominent at higher cell densities **(C)**, with a large proportion of cells floating in the medium. In contrast, cells on extracellular matrix are highly flattened and spread at either a sparse **(D,E)** or confluent **(F–H)** cell density, showing no signs of cell aggregation and overlapping, and in some areas adopt the configuration of a highly organized and contact inhibited cell monolayer **(H)**. Late at confluence (7–9 days after seeding), cells start to grow on top of one another and become less spread **(I)**.

an organized, nonoverlapping cell monolayer is formed (Fig. 5F-H). The morphological configuration of confluent cultures was similar to that of a confluent vascular
endothelial cell monolayer, thereby corroborating the initial impression of Ewing
(9) with regard to the source of the disease.

Preliminary studies with human choroidal melanoma cells also demonstrate a
striking morphological response to seeding on dishes coated with an ECM (78).
On plastic, the cells appear as aggregates composed of spheroidal cells densely
packed with dark melanin granules. In contrast, when the same cell aggregates are
in contact with an ECM, extensive cell migration is observed, the cells adopt a
flattened and spindly morphology characteristic of melanoma cells and show numerous and distinct cytoplasmic granules.

Time Course of Tumor Cell Attachment to Plastic Dishes Versus Dishes Coated with an ECM

In the case of either colon carcinoma cells (Fig. 6A) or Ewing's cells (Fig. 6B),
as many as 50 to 80% of the cells seeded on ECM attached firmly within 30 min,
as compared to only about 5 to 10% of the cells on plastic. After 24 hr, no more
than 35% of the seeded cells attached to plastic. In contrast, 70 to 90% of them
attached firmly within the first hour of incubation to dishes coated with an ECM.
The looser attachment of either the hepatocarcinoma or Ewing's cells to plastic
then to ECM was easily demonstrated by subjecting the cultures to a gentle pipetting.
This released up to 95% of the cells grown on plastic, while no more than 5% of
the cells cultured on the ECM were released. An even looser attachment of the
Ewing cells could be observed at confluence, since in this case only a gentle shaking
of cultures maintained on plastic was required to release the cells from the dish.
Coating of plastic culture dishes with fibronectin (20 μg/ml) induced cell attachment
in the case of Ewing's cells (albeit to a lesser extent than on ECM) (Fig. 6B), but
had no effect on the colon carcinoma cells. These results demonstrate that cells
seeded on ECM adhere tenaciously to this substrate. In particular terms, this unique
adhesive interaction may be advantageous for the culture of anchorage-dependent
cells that fail to attach properly to currently available substrates and are not capable
of producing an ECM *in vitro*.

The Respective Involvement of Laminin and Fibronectin in the Adhesion of Human Carcinoma and Sarcoma Cells

Since colon carcinoma cells show a strict requirement for ECM and do not adhere
to dishes coated with fibronectin, while Ewing's sarcoma cells adhere and flatten
almost equally well when seeded on ECM or dishes coated with purified fibronectin,
it is possible that different adhesive proteins may mediate the attachment of sarcoma-
and carcinoma-derived cells to extracellular matrices. The most likely candidates
for mediating cell attachment are fibronectin (43,49,79) and laminin (12,72). Fibronectin has been shown to stimulate the adhesion of fibroblasts, but not of
epidermal cells, to collagen type IV (55). It could therefore mediate the attachment

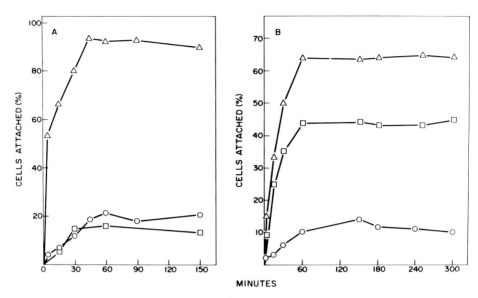

FIG. 6. Attachment of tumor cells as a function of time to plastic dishes versus dishes coated with an extracellular matrix or fibronectin. **A,B:** Stock cultures of the colon carcinoma cells **(A)** and Ewing's sarcoma **(B)** cells were dissociated with STV and seeded (10^5 cells per 35 mm dish) in DMEM containing 10% fetal calf serum or 2.5% fibronectin-depleted calf serum, respectively, into plastic tissue culture dishes ($\bigcirc$), dishes coated with fibronectin (20 μg fibronectin per dish) ($\square$), and dishes coated with extracellular matrix ($\triangle$). Nonattached cells were removed at various times by a gentle pipetting and rinsing of the dishes (twice) with PBS. In the absence of such a treatment, some of the cells remained on the culture dish without showing signs of spreading or any firm attachment. These represent cells which were either left over after aspiration of the medium or which settled down on the tissue culture dish without changing their spherical morphology. The remaining attached cells were dissociated with STV and triplicate cultures counted with a Coulter counter.

of sarcoma cells to their substrate. Studies on the *in vivo* distribution of laminin have shown that it was confined to the lamina lucida region of basement membranes (12,79) and was localized to cellular adhesion sites (2). Recent studies on the attachment of epidermal cells *in vitro* (V. P. Terranova, personal communication) suggest that laminin is an adhesive factor for epithelial cells. It could therefore play the same role for carcinoma cells as that played by fibronectin for sarcoma cells.

Vascular endothelial cells maintained in culture secrete large amounts of fibronectin (6,42,77) and laminin (20), which can be found in both the extracellular matrix lying beneath the cell layer and the tissue culture medium. This medium can therefore provide a convenient source of soluble fibronectin as well as of laminin with which to study their respective involvements in promoting the attachment and flattening of carcinoma and sarcoma cells. We have therefore explored the effect of precoating plastic dishes with culture medium conditioned by bovine aortic vascular endothelial cells on the attachment and flattening of both human colon carcinoma (Fig. 6C) and Ewing's sarcoma cell lines.

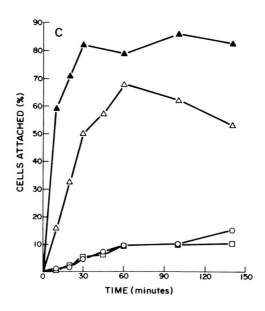

FIG. 6C.   Colon carcinoma cell stock cultures grown on ECM-coated dishes were dissociated into single cells by treatment with STV (0.5% trypsin, 0.02% EDTA). Two $\times 10^5$ cells were then seeded on plastic tissue culture dishes (□), dishes coated with 10 μg per dish of affinity purified bovine plasma fibronectin (○), dishes coated with an ECM (▲), or dishes coated with vascular endothelial cell conditioned medium (△). To coat dishes with conditioned medium, plastic dishes were exposed to a medium (DMEM, H-16 supplemented with 10% calf serum) taken from vascular endothelial cells maintained for 8 days in culture (from the day of seeding until 3–4 days after reaching confluence). This medium was centrifuged (1,500 g for 5 min), incubated (14 hr, 37°C) with the dishes, and replaced with fresh medium prior to seeding the tumor cells. When a serum-free conditioned medium was used, it was collected 7–9 days after replacing the medium of subconfluent endothelial cultures with DMEM (H-16) containing no serum. Because the production and secretion of laminin by endothelial cells is greatly reduced when they reach confluence (25), medium conditioned by confluent cultures was not as active as medium conditioned by actively growing vascular endothelial cells. At various times after seeding carcinoma cells, unattached cells were removed by a gentle pipetting and rinsing of the dishes (twice) with phosphate-buffered saline (PBS). The remaining firmly attached cells were dissociated with STV and duplicate cultures counted with a Coulter counter. The variations of different determinations did not exceed ± 10% of the mean.

When the time course of attachment of carcinoma cells to plastic or fibronectin-coated dishes was compared to that observed with dishes coated with ECM or preexposed to vascular endothelial cell conditioned medium, less than 30% of the cells seeded on plastic or fibronectin-coated dishes attached to these substrates and no cell flattening was observed, regardless of the time in culture (up to 10 days) and regardless of whether or not serum (10%) was present. In contrast, 70 and 80% of the seeded cells firmly attached and flattened within the first hour of incubation on dishes preexposed to endothelial conditioned medium or coated with ECM, respectively (Fig. 6C).

Preexposure of dishes to the endothelial cell conditioned medium (either serum-free or containing fibronectin-depleted calf serum) also induced the attachment of the Ewing's sarcoma cells. However, in this case and in contrast to carcinoma cells, coating of dishes with purified fibronectin was either more or as effective in promoting cell attachment and subsequent flattening (78).

The nature of the agents which mediate the attachment and flattening of the human carcinoma and Ewing's sarcoma cells to dishes preexposed to conditioned medium was analyzed by subjecting the endothelial cell conditioned medium to specific double immunoprecipitation with either rabbit antilaminin (12) or antifibronectin antisera (6), followed by goat antirabbit IgG antiserum (77), and coating the dishes with either fibronectin-depleted or laminin-depleted conditioned medium (76). As seen in Fig. 7B, carcinoma cells no longer attached to dishes preexposed to conditioned medium from which laminin was removed by immunoprecipitation. On the other hand, immunoprecipitation of fibronectin (Fig. 7A) or collagen type IV (76) by specific antibodies did not have any effect on the induction of attachment and flattening of carcinoma cells. In contrast, when the same immunoprecipitated fibronectin-free conditioned medium was used to coat dishes, a complete loss of attachment-promoting activity for Ewing's sarcoma cells was observed (Fig. 7D). The induced attachment and flattening of Ewing's cells was not affected by subjecting the conditioned medium to immunoprecipitation with antilaminin (Fig. 7E), anticollagen type IV, or nonimmune rabbit serum (Fig. 7F), followed by coating the dishes. These results demonstrate that the human carcinoma- and sarcoma-derived cells show a specific response to different adhesive glycoproteins, such as laminin and fibronectin, respectively (76).

Since both laminin and fibronectin have been shown to be secreted underneath the endothelial cell layer and to be part of the ECM produced by these cells, they may function as conditioned medium does and may promote the tenacious attachment to the underlying extracellular matrix and rapid spreading of carcinoma- and sarcoma-derived cells (78). The production of both laminin and fibronectin by vascular endothelial cells may therefore facilitate the arrest of blood-born metastatic cells (45) that produce little or no such adhesive glycoproteins (64).

FIG. 7. Induction of tumor cell attachment promoted by coating dishes with vascular endothelial cell conditioned medium from which fibronectin or laminin had been removed by double immunoprecipitation. One ml of vascular endothelial cell conditioned medium was princubated (1 hr, 37°C) with 10 μl of rabbit antisera against fibronectin **(A,D)**, laminin **(B,E)**, or with 10μl of nonimmune rabbit serum **(C,F)**. Antibodies to laminin and to bovine plasma fibronectin were the same as those previously used in studies already reported (20,21,31). The specificities of the antisera and lack of cross-reactivity between the various antigens have been established in these previous reports. The conditioned media were then incubated (2 hr, 37°C, followed by 14 hr at 4°C) with 30 μl of goat anti-rabbit IgG antiserum (35% ammonium sulphate cut), centrifuged (12,000 g for 5 min), and the supernatant incubated in 35 mm tissue culture dishes for 12 hr at 37°C. The conditioned media were then removed and 2 ml of DMEM supplemented with 5% fibronectin-depleted calf serum and containing either 2×10^5 colon carcinoma cells **(A–C)** or Ewing's sarcoma cells **(D–F)** was then added to the dishes. Phase micrographs of cell attachment and spreading were taken 3 hr after seeding.

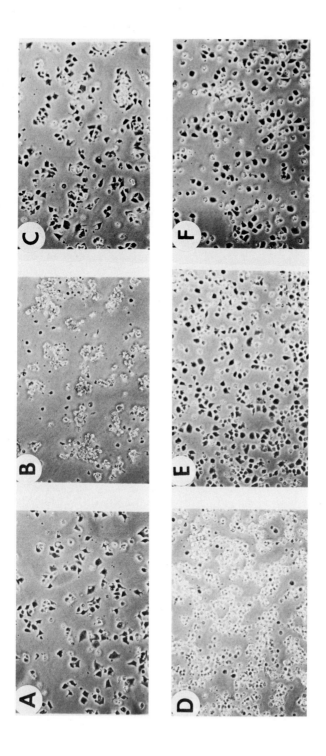

Tumor Cell Migration on ECM-Coated Dishes

Cell migration was studied quantitatively by seeding cell aggregates rather than single cells on plastic or ECM and observing the extent of cell migration out of the aggregates. Cell migration was studied in most cases during the first 4 hr after seeding in order to minimize any possible effect of cell proliferation. Cell aggregates that were seeded into plastic dishes retained their previous morphology (78). The Ewing sarcoma cells remained mostly in the form of floating and loosely packed cell aggregates, while the colon carcinoma cells remained as tightly packed aggregates, mostly attached to the substrate. In neither case and even after 10 days in culture, did cells migrate out of the cell aggregates (78). In contrast, seeding of the same cell aggregates on dishes coated with ECM was associated with spreading and migration of cells that could be observed within 5 to 15 min after seeding. Migratory activity was best observed in the cells located at the periphery of the aggregates (78). Small aggregates flattened out in less than 1 hr, leading to the formation of colonies composed of flat and nonoverlapping cells. Depending on the size of the initial aggregate, cell overlapping could be seen in the center of some of these colonies, but as time proceeded, the cells reorganized and adopted a monolayer configuration (78). Since cell migration is observed prior to cell proliferation, it can be regarded as a specific cellular response to the mere contact between cells and the ECM. This may reflect the preferential adhesion of the cells to the ECM components, whose force can overcome the adhesive forces between cells themselves and is much stronger than the adhesive forces between cells and plastic.

Effect of the ECM on Tumor Cell Growth

Normal human epithelial cells are difficult to grow using conventional culture techniques. This applies even to malignant cells of epithelial origin (57,58), some of which, when maintained in culture, have an extremely long doubling-time (10–20 days). Since cell shape has been shown to be a major factor in regulating cell growth (14,50,52), we have compared the growth rate of cells plated on plastic (spherical configuration) to that of cells plated on ECM, which adopt a flattened morphology. Although differences in growth rate were observed, both the Ewing's and colon carcinoma cells proliferated in either configuration (Fig. 8A–B). This observation therefore demonstrated that cell adhesion to the ECM and their subsequent flattening imposed no restriction on their proliferation. On the contrary, when cells flattened out, a stimulation of cell growth, which depended on the cell type and culture conditions, was observed. This stimulation was particularly evident with the colon carcinoma cells (Fig. 8A) which, when seeded on plastic, showed a lag period of 3 to 4 days before resuming a logarthmic growth rate (16 hr doubling time). In contrast, seeding of the same cells on ECM resulted in an active cell migration concomitant with a rapid resumption of proliferation, so that after 3 to

4 days, the cell density of cultures maintained on an ECM was 4- to 10-fold higher than that of cultures maintained on plastic (78) (Fig. 8A).

Specific binding of EGF (2×10^4 receptor sites per cell) to colon carcinoma cells grown on either plastic or ECM was observed. When the effect of EGF on cell proliferation was studied, it was found to stimulate cell growth on plastic but had little or no effect with cells maintained on an ECM (Fig. 8A). This demonstrates that binding of a mitogen to a given cell type can, depending on the substrate, be followed not by a mitogenic response. The likely explanation for such a difference in the response to EGF by cells maintained on plastic versus ECM is that cells in contact with the ECM are already induced, possibly via a change in cell shape, to express their full proliferative potential in response to serum components, thereby no longer requiring other stimuli. In contrast, cells on plastic, because they are free of such an extracellular dependent modulation, require an additional mitogenic stimulus in order to express fully their proliferative potential.

An increased growth rate of cells maintained on ECM was also observed with the Ewing's cells (Fig. 8B,C). Since these cells showed a very loose attachment to plastic, both attached and floating cells had to be counted in order to reach a meaningful conclusion regarding an effect on the total number of cells. When the cultures were maintained on ECM, the number of firmly attached and floating cells exceeded by two- to fourfold that of cultures maintained on plastic. This difference was only observed at low serum concentrations (0.5–1%) (Fig. 8B). In the case of Ewing's cells, therefore, the effect of the ECM on the rate of cell proliferation was mainly reflected in a lowering of the serum requirement of the cells and not so much in an imposition of a faster growth rate. The final cell density late at confluence was similar on plastic and ECM. If only the number of firmly attached cells was compared while the floating cells were ignored, activity proliferation of the attached cells was observed only in dishes coated with an ECM. This resulted in a 10- to 50-fold higher final density of attached cells in cultures maintained on an ECM than on plastic (Fig. 8C). Although detachment of cells from the ECM was observed 3 to 5 days after they reached confluence, it could be prevented or delayed by changing the growth medium every other day. Similar studies with human choroidal melanoma cells have also demonstrated that cells maintained on an ECM proliferate rapidly (78). This contrasts with a very slow rate of proliferation of these cells (12 to 18 days average doubling time) when maintained on plastic. Effects similar to those of the ECM as far as cell attachment and proliferation are concerned were not observed when tumor cells were seeded on plastic dishes coated with purified preparations of collagen types I, III, or IV (78).

The above results therefore demonstrate that cultured tumor cells can proliferate when they are highly flattened and firmly attached to the substrate, as well as when they are either loosely attached or in suspension. Cell attachment to the ECM results in a stimulation of cell growth, which is best observed at a low cell density and with cells maintained in low serum concentrations.

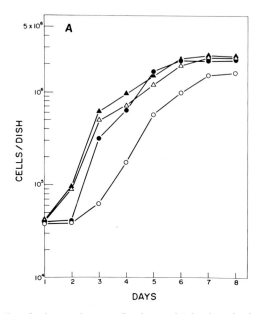

FIG. 8A: Proliferation of colon carcinoma cells when maintained on plastic versus extracellular matrix and exposed or not to EGF. Four $\times 10^4$ cells in 2 ml DMEM containing 10% fetal calf serum, were seeded into each plastic (○) or extracellular matrix-coated (△) 35 mm dishes. EGF (10 ng/ml) was added every day to half of the uncoated (●) and extracellular matrix-coated (▲) dishes, and duplicate cultures were counted every day for both floating cells present in the tissue culture medium and attached cells dissociated with STV. The percentage of floating cells increased with time but did not exceed 20% of the total cell number. The curves represent the total number of cells (attached plus floating).

NORMAL CELLS

Vascular Endothelial Cells

Previous studies (18,28,29) have shown that vascular endothelial cell cultures maintained on plastic and propagated in the presence of fibroblast growth factor (FGF) divide with an average doubling time of 18 hr when seeded at either a high (up to 1 : 1,000) or low split ratio. Upon reaching confluence, the cells adopt a morphological configuration similar to that of the confluent culture from which they originated. In contrast, seeding of the same cells at a high split ratio in the absence of FGF results in a much longer doubling time (60 to 78 hr), and within a few passages, cultures maintained in the absence of FGF exhibit, in addition to a much slower growth rate, morphological as well as structural alterations, which mostly involve changes in the composition and distribution of the extrecellular matrix (ECM) (53,54). This raises the possibility that the ECM produced by these cells could have an effect on their ability to proliferate and to express their normal phenotype once confluent.

This is what was in fact observed when the growth of bovine vascular endothelial cells seeded at low density on plastic versus ECM was compared. Cells maintained

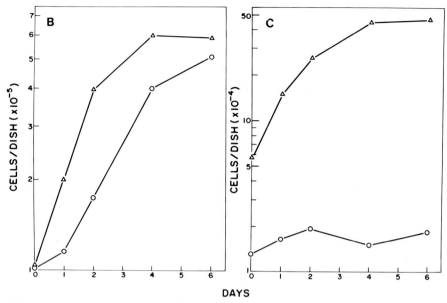

FIGS. 8B and C: Proliferation of Ewing's sarcoma cells when maintained on plastic versus extracellular matrix. Cells, 10^5 in 2 ml DMEM containing 0.5% calf serum, were seeded into each plastic (○) or extracellular matrix-coated (Δ) 35 mm dishes. Duplicate cultures were counted every day to determine the number of floating cells (present in the tissue culture medium) and of cells that are firmly attached (dissociated with STV). (**B**) Total cell number (floating plus attached). (**C**) Firmly attached cells. The number of firmly attached cells was higher than 80% of the total cell number found in dishes coated with extracellular matrix and lower than 10% of the total cell number obtained on plastic.

on an ECM produced by either confluent corneal or vascular endothelial cells divided extremely rapidly, regardless of whether they were exposed or not to FGF (Fig. 9) and regardless of the initial cell density (sparse culture, 10 cells/mm², or clonal density, 1 cell/cm²). Addition of FGF to cultures maintained on an ECM did not decrease their mean doubling time, which was already at a minimum (18 to 20 hr), nor did it result in a higher final cell density, which was already at a maximum (900–1,000 cells/mm²). One can therefore conclude that, while low density cell cultures maintained on plastic proliferate poorly and therefore require FGF in order to become confluent within a few days, when the cultures are maintained on ECM, they proliferate actively and no longer require FGF in order to become confluent. In both cases (either maintained on plastic and exposed to FGF or maintained on an extracellular matrix), the rate of proliferation is a direct function of the serum or plasma concentration to which cultures are exposed. It is therefore likely that the effect of the ECM is more a permissive than a direct mitogenic effect, since cells still required serum or plasma in order to proliferate (24). It was also observed that, while cultures maintained on plastic and passaged at low cell density rapidly lose their phenotypic expression, cultures maintained on ECM retain it. ECM can therefore stabilize the phenotypic expression of vascular endothelial cells.

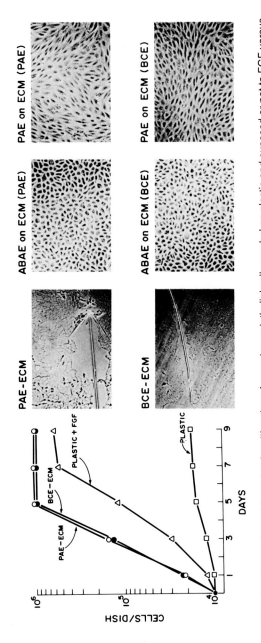

FIG. 9. Comparison of the rate of proliferation of vascular endothelial cells seeded on plastic and exposed or not to FGF versus that of cultures seeded on an ECM produced by either bovine corneal endothelial cells or porcine aortic endothelial cells. One × 10⁴ bovine (ABAE) or porcine aortic endcthelial cells (PAE) were seeded on either plastic dishes or dishes coated with an ECM produced by porcine aortic endotheliɑ cells (PAE) or bovine corneal endothelial cells (BCE). Cultures on plastic were exposed or not to FGF. The rate of proliferation of the various cultures was analyzed as a function of time, and photographs were taken once cultures became confluent. The morphology of the ECM produced by confluent cultures of either BCE (BCE-ECM) or PAE (PAE-ECM) is shown. The dishes were scratched with a needle to expose the underlying plastic and demonstrate the degree of coating. Maintenance of ABAE cultures on either an ECM produced by PAE or BCE cultures did not affect their morphology once cells became confluent. The same is true of PAE cultures.

The present results also raise the possibility that, although the final effect of FGF is that of a mitogen (18,26,27), its action could be indirect. It could either replace the cellular requirement for a substratum such as the ECM and thereby make the cells fully responsive to growth factors present in serum and plasma even when the cells are maintained on plastic, or alternatively, it could induce the synthesis and secretion of the ECM produced by the cells. Such induction could in turn make the cells sensitive to factors present in serum or plasma. That the latter alternative could occur finds support in previous observations that FGF can control the production by vascular endothelial cells of extracellular and cell surface components such as fibronectin and various collagen types (33,77). Since sparse cultures of endothelial cells proliferate poorly when maintained on plastic but not when maintained on an ECM, it may be that at very low cell density, cultures maintained on plastic are unable to produce enough extracellular material to support further growth. The mitogenic effect of FGF on these cells could be the result of an increased synthesis of the ECM by vascular endothelial cells.

These results emphasize how drastically one can modify the proliferative response of a given cell type to serum factors depending on the substrate upon which the cells are maintained. It is possible that the lack of response of different cell types maintained under tissue culture conditions to agents responsible *in vivo* for their proliferation and differentiation could be attributed to the artificial substrate, whether plastic or glass, upon which the cells rest and which limits their ability to produce an ECM.

Among the plasma factors which could be held directly or indirectly responsible for the active proliferation of vascular endothelial cells are the high density lipoproteins (HDL), as well as the low density lipoproteins (LDL). Earlier studies have shown that both LDL and HDL can interact specifically with vascular endothelial cells (10,59,65,68,69,75), and others have shown that LDL could be mitogenic for vascular smooth muscle cells and dermal fibroblasts when added to lipoprotein-deficient serum (LPDS) (7,11,61) or to serum from abetalipoproteinemic subjects (47). Likewise, in the case of cells which have a limited ability to make cholesterol *de novo* or in the case of cells maintained in the presence of compounds such as compactin, which totally inhibits their ability to make cholesterol, addition of LDL to the medium leads to resumption of cell proliferation (16). In that case, LDL could act by providing an exogenous source of cholesterol to the cells, thereby obviating the block in cholesterol synthesis resulting from the presence of the inhibitor in the medium (16). We have therefore compared the respective mitogenic activities of HDL and LDL on vascular endothelial cell cultures exposed to LPDS or to serum-free medium.

Vascular endothelial cells maintained in the presence of medium supplemented with LPDS grow poorly (67). Such cultures therefore require the presence of lipoproteins in order to proliferate optimally. Of the two classes of lipoproteins (HDL and LDL) which have been studied, HDL seems to be the major factor involved in the proliferation of vascular endothelial cells. This is mostly due to its lack of toxicity when added at high concentration, as well as to its lack of dependence on LPDS in order to exhibit its mitogenic properties (Fig. 10).

LDL, unlike HDL, has a biphasic effect (67). Although mitogenic for vascular endothelial cells when added at low concentration, once physiological concentrations are reached, it becomes toxic for the cells. Moreover, and in contrast with HDL, the mitogenic effect of LDL was found to be a function of the LPDS concentration to which cultures were exposed (Fig. 10). LDL at concentration of 200 μg protein/ml did not stimulate cells to proliferate at an optimal growth rate unless cultures were maintained in high (5 to 10%) LPDS concentration (Fig. 10). This mitogenic effect on the part of HDL, as opposed to the cytotoxic effect of LDL, was observed regardless of the density at which cultures were seeded (clonal or high density cultures) (Fig. 11). Therefore, HDL at physiological concentrations can fully replace serum or plasma. This is best exemplified by our observation that

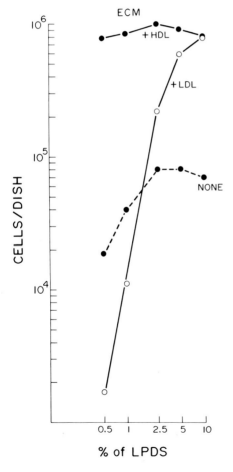

FIG. 10. Effect of increasing concentrations of lipoprotein-deficient serum (LPDS) on the proliferative response of bovine vascular endothelial cells exposed to constant concentrations of LDL or HDL. Vascular endothelial cells were seeded at 2×10^4 cells per 35 mm dish on ECM-coated dishes and exposed to DMEM supplemented with increasing concentrations, ranging from 0.5 (0.3 mg/ml) to 10% (6 mg/ml), of LPDS (●---●), increasing concentrations of LPDS plus 500 μg protein/ml of HDL (●——●), or increasing concentrations of LPDS plus 200 μg protein/ml of LDL (○———○). After 6 days, cultures were trypsinized and counted.

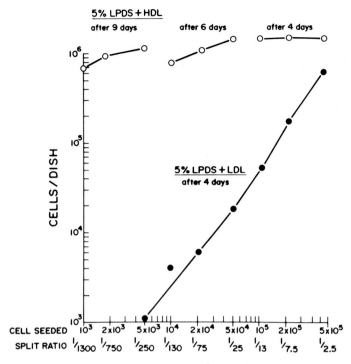

FIG. 11. Proliferation of bovine vascular endothelial cells seeded at various cell densities on ECM-coated dishes and exposed to serum supplemented with 5% LPDS and HDL (500 μg protein/ml) or LDL (500 μg protein/ml). Vascular endothelial cells were seeded at a split ratio ranging from 1/1,300 (1,000 cells per 35 mm dish) to 1/2.5 (5 × 10^5 cells per 35 mm dish) and maintained in 5% LPDS supplemented with either HDL or LDL (500 μg protein/ml). Cultures maintained with HDL were counted, depending on the split ratio to which they were seeded, after 4, 6, and 9 days. In all cases, and even when cultures were seeded at a split ratio as low as 1/1,300, cultures exposed to HDL became confluent. In contrast, when exposed to LDL, cultures seeded at high density did not proliferate, while those seeded at low density died. All cultures exposed to LDL had therefore to be counted on day 3. Cell death became evident upon comparing the seeding density of cultures exposed to LDL with their density at day 4.

cells maintained in serum-free medium will proliferate at an optimal rate if HDL is added to the medium. In contrast, in the absence of LPDS, LDL concentrations as low as 80 μg protein/ml resulted in cell death and at 30 μg protein/ml had a small mitogenic effect when compared to that of HDL (Fig. 12).

The substrate upon which cultures are maintained has been found to be important if a mitogenic effect on the part of either HDL or LDL is to be observed. When maintained on plastic, cells exposed to LPDS did not survive and therefore could not respond to either lipoprotein (67). In contrast, when maintained on ECM they survived quite well, thereby making it possible to observe the mitogenic effect of either HDL or LDL. This suggests that, *in vivo*, the integrity of the basement membrane upon which endothelial cells rest and migrate is an important factor in determining the cells' response to lipoproteins present in plasma (67).

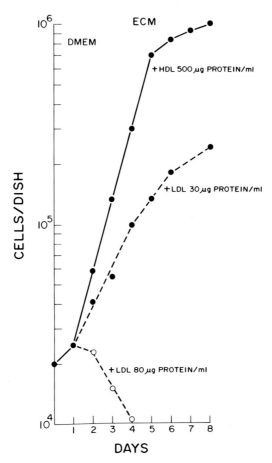

FIG. 12. Proliferative rae of bovine vascular endothelial cells maintained on ECM-coated dishes and exposed to DMEM supplemented with either HDL or LDL. Vascular endothelial cells were seeded at 2 × 10⁴ cells per 35 mm dish on ECM-coated dishes and exposed to medium supplemented with 10% calf serum. Six hours later, the medium was removed and cultures were washed twice. Medium supplemented with 500 μg protein/ml of HDL (●————●), 30 μg protein/ml of LDL (●–––●), or 80 μg protein/ml of LDL (○–––○) was then added. Triplicate plates representing each condition were trypsinized and counted every day.

Plasma Versus Serum: Is There a Difference in their Abilities to Promote Cell Growth?

Culture of most cells *in vitro* requires the presence of serum (8). Consequently, investigators have spent much effort in a search to identify the various factors in serum that stimulate cell growth *in vitro*. An important step in the search for serum growth factors has been the finding that one of the most potent mitogenic factors present in serum is derived from platelets (3,4). While plasma was unable to support the growth of aortic smooth muscle cells (62) or that of BALB/c 3T3 cells (44), serum made from the same pool of blood stimulated their proliferation. Addition of a platelet extract to cell-free plasma-derived serum restored the growth-promoting activity (44,62,63). One could therefore conclude that one of the principal mitogens responsible for the induction of DNA synthesis present in whole blood serum is derived from platelets (44,63). The difference in the proliferative ability of cells exposed to plasma versus serum results from the absence of the platelet factor in the former. However, all studies have thus far used cells maintained on plastic rather than an ECM. This difference in the substrate upon which the cells are maintained could have prevented their response to factors present in plasma, thereby creating the difference in mitogenic activity between plasma and serum. To explore the possibility that the serum factors to which cells maintained on ECM become sensitive are also present in plasma, we have compared the mitogenic activity of plasma versus serum, using as target cells vascular smooth muscle cells maintained on either plastic or an ECM (23).

Vascular smooth muscle cells maintained on plastic and exposed to plasma (10%) proliferate poorly, while when exposed to serum (10%) instead of plasma, the cells proliferate actively (23,63) (Fig. 13). In contrast to the above results, when cells were maintained on an ECM and exposed to plasma, they proliferated actively, and plasma was observed to be even more mitogenic for cells maintained on an ECM than was serum for cells maintained on plastic (Fig. 13). When the growth rate and the final cell density of cultures maintained on an ECM and exposed to either plasma or serum were compared, they were found to be the same. When the final cell density of cultures maintained on an ECM and exposed to either plasma or serum was analyzed as a function of the serum or plasma concentration to which they were exposed, it was found to be a direct function of the serum or plasma concentration. It is therefore likely that the proliferation of vascular smooth muscle cells, like that of vascular endothelial cells maintained on an ECM, is controlled by factor(s) present in plasma and that the ECM has only a permissive role (23).

If in the case of vascular smooth muscle cells one were to extrapolate to the *in vivo* situation, maintaining them on an ECM and plasma is clearly a closer approximation to physiological conditions than exposing them to plastic and serum. Since vascular smooth muscle cells proliferate at a maximal rate when maintained on an ECM and exposed to plasma, it is likely that they are responding to mitogen(s) already present in plasma rather than to FGF or to mitogen(s) generated during the coagulation process.

Factors in Plasma Which Control the Proliferation of Vascular Smooth Muscle Cells

Among the plasma components which could affect the proliferation of VSM cells are the high (HDL) and low density lipoproteins (LDL). As already pointed out, both of these components have already been shown to be mitogenic for that cell type when cultures are exposed to lipoprotein-deficient serum (LPDS) (7,11,61) or to serum from abetalipoproteinemic subjects (47). Transferrin, somatomedin C, insulin, epidermal growth factor (EGF), and FGF are also likely to affect VSM

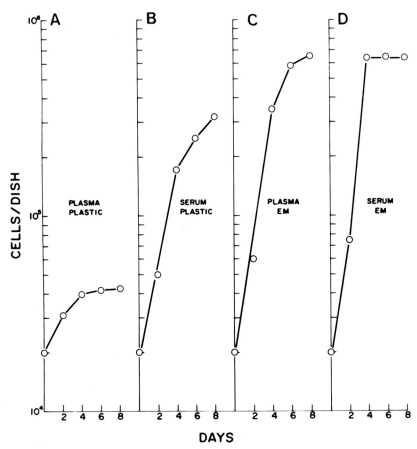

FIG. 13. Proliferation of bovine vascular smooth muscle cells when maintained on plastic versus extracellular matrix (ECM) and exposed to either plasma or serum. Vascular smooth muscle cells were seeded at 2 × 10⁴ cells per 35 mm dish and maintained in the presence of DMEM supplemented with either 10% plasma **(A,C)** or serum **(B,D)**. The cells were maintained on either plastic **(A,B)** or ECM **(C,D)**.

cell proliferation, since those agents have been shown to be mitogenic for a wide variety of cell types maintained under serum-free conditions (52) as well as for VSM cell cultures exposed to plasma (26,28).

We have therefore compared the effects of the substrate (either ECM or plastic) on the proliferative response of low density VSM cell cultures exposed to a synthetic medium supplemented with these various factors. We were further encouraged to take this approach by previous observations which indicated that VSM cells maintained on ECM-coated dishes had a much lower requirement for either serum or plasma in order to proliferate actively than when they were maintained on plastic. It is therefore possible that VSM cells, when maintained on ECM-coated dishes, could survive and still be responsive to plasma factors even when maintained in a well-defined synthetic medium unsupplemented with either plasma or serum (22).

Preliminary studies demonstrated that transferrin, which is the main iron-carrying protein in the bloodstream, must be present if any mitogenic response to plasma factors on the part of VSM cells seeded and maintained in total absence of serum is to be observed. It is likely that this absolute requirement for transferrin either reflects its role in delivering iron to the cells or its ability to detoxify the medium by removing toxic traces of metals.

When low density VSM cell cultures were maintained on ECM-coated dishes and exposed to a synthetic medium supplemented with transferrin (10 µg/ml), HDL (250 µg protein/ml), insulin (2 µg protein/ml), and FGF (100 ng/ml), cells proliferated as actively as when they were exposed to optimal serum concentration. The single omission of HDL, insulin, or FGF resulted in a lower growth rate of the cultures, as well as in a lower final cell density (Fig. 14A). This indicates that all of these factors have an additive effect upon one another and must be present simultaneously in order to induce optimal cell growth. Neither FGF nor insulin, either singly or in combination, had a significant effect on cell growth (Fig. 14A). When the ability of EGF (50 ng/ml) to substitute for FGF was tested, it was found to be as potent as FGF. Likewise, somatomedin C at low concentration (10 ng/ml) can fully substitute for insulin (22).

Since HDL, insulin, and EGF are all normally present in plasma, these factors may reflect the plasma constituents involved in the control of the proliferation of VSM cells when such cells are maintained on ECM-coated dishes and exposed to plasma (22).

The concentrations at which insulin was mitogenic are clearly pharmacological. However, since insulin can be replaced by somatomedin C, and since it is known to have a low affinity for somatomedin binding sites, it may be that the high concentrations of insulin required are due to its weak interaction with the somatomedin binding sites. If this is the case, the mitogenic activity of insulin on VSM cells is not directly mediated through its interaction with high affinity insulin binding sites. In contrast, the effect of EGF, which was further documented by the presence on the cell surface of EGF receptor sites, is probably due to a direct interaction of EGF with the cells (22).

The mitogenic effect of HDL over a wide range of concentrations and its lack of toxicity for VSM cells are in accord with previous observations with vascular endothelial cells. However, in the case of vascular endothelial cells exposed to a synthetic medium, the addition of HDL alone is capable of insuring an optimal growth rate similar to that observed with optimal concentration of serum or plasma. In the case of VSM cells, addition of HDL alone, even at high concentration, does not fully replace plasma or serum, as reflected by the growth rate of the cultures, which is suboptimal. In contrast to HDL, concentrations of LDL higher than 50 µg protein/ml were cytotoxic. This observation agrees with earlier reports of Hessler et al (40) who, using human aortic medial smooth muscle cells maintained in the

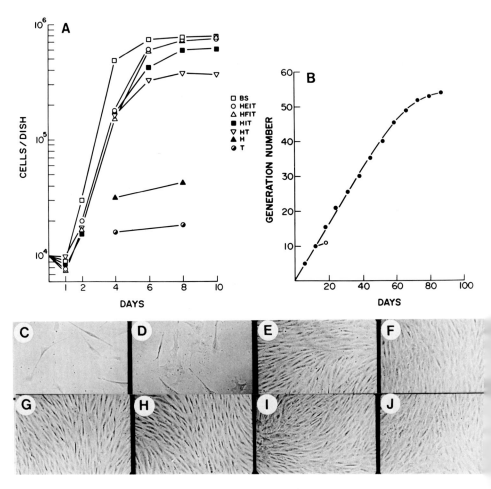

FIG. 14. Growth rate, life span, and morphological appearance of low density VSM cell cultures seeded on ECM-coated dishes and passaged in the total absence of serum. **(A)** VSM cells were seeded at 1 × 10⁴ cells per 35 mm dish coated with ECM (22). Cells were exposed to 10% bovine serum (BS□); transferrin (10 μg/ml, T, ◑); HDL (250 μg/ml, H ▲); HDL and transferrin (HT ▽); HDL, insulin (2.5 μg/ml), and transferrin (HIT ■); HDL, FGF (100 ng/ml), insulin, and transferrin (HFIT △); or HDL, EGF (50 ng/ml), insulin, and transferrin (HEIT ○). **(B)** Life span of VSM cell cultures seeded in the absence of serum and passaged repeatedly at low cell density. Cultures were passaged at 10⁴ cells per 35 mm dish (○). Cultures were exposed to DMEM supplemented with HDL (250 μg/ml), insulin (2.5 μg/ml), FGF (100 ng/ml), and transferrin (10 μg/ml). Similar life spans were observed when cultures were passaged in the presence of EGF (50 ng/ml) instead of FGF (22). As soon as transferrin was omitted from the medium, cells no longer proliferated (○) and cultures therefore could no longer be passaged. **(C–J)** Morphological appearance of bovine VSM cells seeded as described above on ECM-coated dishes and exposed to **(C)** transferrin (10 μg/ml); **(D)** HDL (250 μg protein/ml); **(E)** HDL and transferrin (10 μg/ml); **(F)** HDL, transferrin, and insulin (2.5 μg/ml); **(G)** HDL, transferrin, and EGF (50 ng/ml); **(H)** HDL, transferrin, and FGF (100 ng/ml); **(I)** HDL, transferrin, insulin, and FGF; or **(J)** HDL, transferrin, insulin, and EGF (22).

presence of medium supplemented with LPDS, have reported a cytotoxic effect of LDL at concentrations as low as 80 μg cholesterol/ml of medium, a concentration to which cultured cells would be exposed if whole serum from a normalipemic human donor were added as 10% of the culture medium.

The use of a synthetic medium supplemented with transferrin, HDL, insulin, and EGF has allowed VSM cells not only to proliferate actively but also to be passaged repeatedly (Fig. 14B). This therefore makes realization of the goal of serial passage in a totally defined medium possible.

The substrate upon which VSM cells are maintained is an important factor in their response to the various factors to which they are exposed. When cells are maintained on plastic and exposed to a synthetic medium, they will not proliferate. The addition of FGF, which in previous studies has been shown to replace the requirement for an ECM, will allow the cells to proliferate and to respond to either HDL or LDL. Yet, the lifespans of the cultures are far from impressive, since even when exposed to HDL and FGF cells senesce after undergoing 23 generations. In contrast, when cells are maintained on ECM-coated dishes, even when exposed to a synthetic medium unsupplemented with any factor, cells can undergo 15 generations before senescing and, while the addition of FGF to the medium no longer has any effect on the lifespan of the cultures, that of HDL, insulin, and FGF or EGF will allow the cells to undergo 46 generations before senescing. The effect of the ECM in delaying cell senescence is even more impressive if one considers the case of cells exposed to synthetic medium supplemented with an optimal concentration of serum (Fig. 15). While cultures maintained on plastic can be maintained at best for 16 generations, cultures maintained on ECM and exposed to serum can undergo 80 to 90 generations before senescing (Fig. 15). It may therefore be concluded that the ECM upon which VSM cells were maintained not only made cells sensitive to factors present in plasma but also delayed to a considerable extent the ultimate senescence of the cells when they were exposed to a synthetic medium supplemented with either well-defined factor or with serum. Furthermore, since the lifespan of the cultures exposed to serum is longer than that of cultures exposed to HDL, insulin, it is likely that there are other factor(s) present in serum which could protect them from senescing.

Our observation that the close contact of the VSM cells with the ECM increases the longevity of the culture raises the possibility that it could also stabilize the phenotypic expression of VSM cell cultures with respect to their enzyme contents and ultrastructural properties. Previous studies done by Fowler et al. (15) have shown that, when calf aortic smooth muscle cells are grown *in vitro* under various conditions, striking alterations in enzyme contents, physical properties, and morphological appearances of lysosomes, endoplasmic reticulum, plasma membranes, and to a lesser extent, mitochondria were observed. Their results therefore demonstrate significant differences in specific cellular characteristics and functions of aortic smooth muscle cells grown *in vitro* compared to aortic cells *in situ*. Whether such differences would be observed if cells were maintained on an ECM rather than on plastic remains a question.

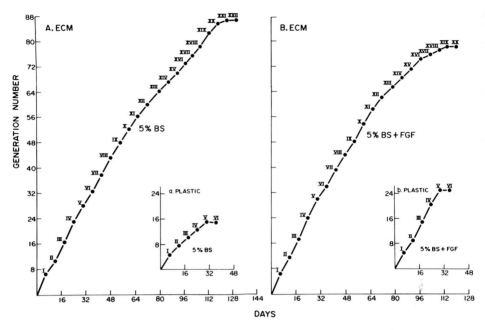

FIG. 15. Comparison of the effect of the substrate (ECM versus plastic) upon which VSM cells are maintained on the lifespan of the culture. VSM cells were maintained and passaged on plastic dishes **(a, b)** or on dishes coated with an ECM **(A, B)**. Cultures were exposed to DMEM supplemented with 5% bovine serum (BS) and in the presence (B, b) or absence (A, a) of FGF (100 ng/ml) added every other day. The cultures were seeded at 1×10^4 cells per 35 mm dish and passaged every 6 or 7 days. The number of generations was determined from the initial cell density 8 hours after seeding and the number of cells harvested at each transfer. Each point represents a single transfer. Roman numerals indicate the passage number.

OTHER CELL TYPES FOR WHICH THE PERMISSIVE EFFECT OF THE ECM CAN BE OBSERVED

The permissive effect of the ECM produced by corneal endothelial cells on cell proliferation has also been observed in the case of fibroblasts, granulosa cells, and adrenal cortex cells (7), as well as corneal endothelial cells and corneal and lens epithelial cells (25,34). Although these various cell types, when maintained on plastic, required either serum and/or growth factor in order to proliferate, when maintained on an ECM, they no longer required FGF, and the addition of plasma alone was sufficient to make them proliferate at an optimal rate. It is therefore likely that, when maintained on ECM, cells respond to plasma growth factors. In fact, one of the disadvantages to using the ECM as a natural substrate for growing cells is that too often, cells which do not grow on plastic and do not respond to FGF grow readily when maintained on an ECM. Among these are capillary endothelial cells, which now represent one of the main cellular contaminants in primary culture derived from various tissues (30).

CONCLUSIONS

Soluble factors that control the production of the ECM have not previously been reported. Until now, production of ECM was thought to be an automatic process that was mostly a function of the substrate upon which cells rest and of cell density. Although it is quite possible that *in vivo* the production of an ECM is not under any control other than that provided by the substrate upon which cells migrate during the early embryological phase, our results suggest that, at least *in vitro*, factors such as FGF could influence the formation of an ECM scaffolding. We do not yet know the extent of this influence.

The observations presented above emphasize how drastically one can modify the proliferative response of a given cell type to serum factors by modifying the substrate upon which the cells are maintained. It is possible that the lack of response of various cell types maintained under tissue culture conditions to agents responsible *in vivo* for their proliferation and differentiation could be directly attributed to the artificial substrate, whether plastic or glass, upon which the cells rest and which limits their ability to produce an ECM. It is likely that the study of cell cultures, which for past the 50 years, in Wilt's words, has been "almost a history of the adequacy of media," will become a history of the inadequacy of substrates.

ACKNOWLEDGMENTS

This work was supported by grants EY 02196, HL 20197, and 23678 from the National Institutes of Health. The authors wish to thank Mr. Harvey Scodel for his invaluable help in the preparation of this manuscript.

REFERENCES

1. Aaronson, S. A., Todaro, G. J., and Freeman, A. E. (1970): Human sarcoma cells in culture. *Exp. Cell Res.*, 61:1–5.
2. Alitalo, K., Kurkinen, M., Vaheri, A., Krieg, T., and Timpl, R. (1980): Extracellular matrix components synthesized by human amniotic epithelial cells in culture. *Cell*, 19:1053–1062.
3. Balk, S. D., (1971): Calcium as a regulator of the proliferation of normal, but not of transformed, chicken fibroblasts in a plasma-containing medium. *Proc. Natl. Acad. Sci. U.S.A.*, 68:271–275.
4. Balk, S. D., Whitefield, J. F., Youdale, T., and Braun, A. C. (1973): Roles of calcium, serum, plasma, and folic acid in the control of proliferation of normal and Rous sarcoma. *Proc. Natl. Acad. Sci. U.S.A.*, 70:675–679.
5. Bernfield, M. R. (1978): The cell periphery in morphogenesis. In: *Birth Defects, Excerpta Medica, Int. Congress Series 432*, edited by J. W. Littlefield and J. de Grouchy, pp. 111–125. Elsevier North-Holland, New York.
6. Birdwell, C. R., Gospodarowicz, D., and Nicolson, G. (1978): Identification, localization, and role of fibronectin in cultured bovine endothelial cells. *Proc. Natl. Acad. Sci. U.S.A.*, 75:3272–3277.
7. Brown, G., Mahley, R., and Assmann, G. (1976): Swine aortic smooth muscle in tissue culture—some effects of purified swine lipoproteins on cell growth and morphology. *Circ. Res.*, 39:415–424.
8. Carrel, A. J. (1912): On the permanent life of tissue outside of the organism. *Exp. Med.*, 15:516–536.
9. Ewing, J. (1921): Diffuse endothelioma of bone. *Proc. N.Y. Pathol. Soc.*, 21:17–24.

10. Fielding, P. E., Vlodavsky, I., Gospodarowicz, D., and Fielding, C. J. (1979): Effect of contact inhibition on the regulation of cholesterol metabolism in cultured vascular endothelial cells. *J. Biol. Chem.*, 254:749–755.

11. Fischer-Dzoga, K., Fraser, R., and Wissler, R. W. (1976): Aortic smooth muscle cells: 1. Effect of lipoprotein fractions of hyperlipemic serum and lymph. *Exp. Mol. Pathol.*, 24:346–359.

12. Foidart, J. M., Bere, E. W., Yaar, M., Beenard, S. I., Gullino, M., Martin, G. R., and Katz, S. I. (1980): Distribution and immunoelectron microscopic localization of laminin, a noncollageneous basement membrane glycoprotein. *Lab. Invest.*, 42:336–341.

13. Folkman, J. (1977): In: *Recent Advances in Cancer Research: Cell Biology, Molecular Biology, and Tumor Virology*, Vol. 1, edited by R. C. Gallo, pp. 119–130. CRC, Cleveland.

14. Folkman, J., and Moscona, A. (1978): Role of cell shape in growth control. *Nature*, 273:345.

15. Fowler, S., Shio, H., and Wolinsky, H. (1977): Subcellular fractionation and morphology of calf aortic smooth muscle cells. *J. Cell Biol.*, 75:166–184.

16. Goldstein, J. L., Helgeson, J. A. S., and Brown, M. S. (1979): Inhibition of cholesterol synthesis with compactin renders growth of cultured cells dependent on the low density lipoprotein receptor. *J. Biol. Chem.*, 254:5403–5409.

17. Gospodarowicz, D., Delgado, D., and Vlodavsky, I. (1980): Permissive effect of the extracellular matrix on cell proliferation in vitro. *Proc. Natl. Acad. Sci. U.S.A.*, 77:4094–4098.

18. Gospodarowicz, D., Greenburg, G., Bialecki, H., and Zetter, B. (1978): Factors involved in the modulation of cell proliferation in vivo and in vitro: the role of fibroblast and epidermal growth factors in the proliferative response of mammalian cells. *In Vitro*, 14:85–118.

19. Gospodarowicz, D., Greenburg, G., and Birdwell, C. (1978): Determination of cellular shape by the extracellular matrix and its correlation with the control of cellular growth. *Cancer Res.*, 38:4155–4171.

20. Gospodarowicz, D., Greenburg, G., Foidart, J.-M., and Savion, N. (1981): The production and localization of laminin in cultured vascular and corneal endothelial cells. *J. Cell Physiol.*, 107:173–183.

21. Gospodarowicz, D., Greenburg, G., Vlodavsky, I., Alvardo, J., and Johnson, L. K. (1979): The identification and localization of fibronectin in cultured corneal endothelial cells: cell surface polarity and physiological implications. *Exp. Eye Res.*, 29:485–509.

22. Gospodarowicz, D., Hirabayashi, K., Giguere, L., and Tauber, J.-P. (1980): Control of proliferation of vascular smooth muscle cells by high and low density lipoproteins, insulin, and by fibroblast and epidermal growth factors. *J. Cell Biol.*, 89:568–578.

23. Gospodarowicz, D., and Ill, C. R. (1980): Do plasma and serum have different abilities to promote cell growth? *Proc. Natl. Acad. Sci. U.S.A.*, 77:2726–2730.

24. Gospodarowicz, D., and Ill, C. R. (1980): The extracellular matrix and the control of proliferation of vascular endothelial cells. *J. Clin. Invest.*, 65:1351–1364.

25. Gospodarowicz, D., and Ill, C. R. (1980): The extracellular matrix and the control of proliferation of corneal endothelial and lens epithelial cells. *Exp. Eye Res.*, 31:181–199.

26. Gospodarowicz, D., Mescher, A. L., and Birdwell, C. R. (1978): Control of cellular proliferation by the fibroblast and epidermal growth factors. In: *Gene Expression and Regulation in Cultured Cells, Third Decennial Review Conference, National Cancer Institute Monographs, no. 48*, pp. 109–130.

27. Gospodarowicz, D., Mescher, A. L., and Moran, J. (1978): Cellular specificities of fibroblast growth factor and epidermal growth factor. In: *Molecular Control of Proliferation and Cytodifferentiation. 35th Symposium of the Society for Developmental Biology*, edited by J. Papaconstantinou and W. J. Rutter, pp. 33–61. Academic Press, New York.

28. Gospodarowicz, D., Moran, J. S., and Braun, D. (1977): Control of proliferation of bovine vascular endothelial cells. *J. Cell Physiol.*, 91:377–385.

29. Gospodarowicz, D., Moran, J. S., Braun, D., and Birdwell, C. R. (1976): Clonal growth of bovine endothelial cells in tissue culture: fibroblast growth factor as a survival agent. *Proc. Natl. Acad. Sci. U.S.A.*, 73:4120–4124.

30. Gospodarowicz, D., and Tauber, J.-P. (1980): Growth factors and extracellular matrix. *Endocrine Rev.*, 1:201–227.

31. Gospodarowicz, D., Vlodavsky, I., Greenburg, G., Alvarado, J., Johnson, L. K., and Moran, J. (1979): Studies on atherogenesis and corneal transplantation using cultured vascular and corneal endothelia. *Rec. Prog. Hormone Res.*, 35:375–448.

32. Gospodarowicz, D., Vlodavsky, I., Greenburg, G., and Johnson, L. K. (1979): Cellular shape is determined by the extracellular matrix and is responsible for the control of cellular growth and

function. In: *Cold Spring Harbor Conferences on Cell Proliferation, Vol. 6: Hormones and Cell Culture*, edited by R. Ross and G. Sato, pp. 561–592. Cold Spring Harbor, N.Y.

33. Greenburg, G., Vlodavsky, I., Foidart, J.-M., and Gospodarowicz, D. (1980): Conditioned medium from endothelial cell cultures can restore the normal phenotypic expression of vascular endothelium maintained *in vitro* in the absence of fibroblast growth factor. *J. Cell Physiol.*, 103:333–347.

34. Gospodarowicz, D., Vlodavsky, I., and Savion, N. (1980): The role of fibroblast growth factor and the extracellular matrix in the control of proliferation and differentiation of corneal endothelial cells. *Vision Res.*, 21:87–103.

35. Grobstein, C. J. (1955): Inductive interaction in the development of the mouse metanephros. *J. Exp. Zool.*, 130:319–340.

36. Grobstein, C. (1967): Mechanisms of organogenetic tissue interaction. *Cancer Inst. Monograph*, 26:279–299.

37. Grobstein, C. (1975): Developmental role of intercellular matrix: retrospective and prospective. In: *Extracellular Matrix Influences on Gene Expression*, edited by H. C. Slavkin and R. C. Grenlich, pp. 9–16, 804–814. Academic Press, New York.

38. Hay, E. D. (1977): Interaction between the cell surface and extracellular matrix in corneal development. In: *Cell and Tissue Interaction*, edited by J. W. Lash and M. M. Burger, pp. 115–137. Raven Press, New York.

39. Hedman, K., Vaheri, A., and Wartiovaara, J. (1978): External fibronectin of cultured human fibroblasts is predominantly a matrix protein. *J. Cell Biol.*, 76:748–762.

40. Hessler, J. R., Lazzarini, A., Robertson, A. L., and Chisolm, G. M. (1979): LDL-induced cytotoxicity and its inhibition by HDL in human vascular smooth muscle and endothelial cells in culture. *Atherosclerosis*, 32:213–231.

41. Howe-Jensen, K., Priori, E., and Dmochowoki, L. (1972): Studies on ultrastructure of Ewing's sarcoma and bone. *Cancer*, 29:280–286.

42. Jaffe, E. A., and Mosher, D. F. (1978): Synthesis of fibronectin by cultured human endothelial cells. *J. Exp. Med.*, 147:1779–1791.

43. Klebe, R. J. (1974): Isolation of a collagen-dependent cell attachment factor. *Nature*, 250:248–251.

44. Kohler, N., and Lipton, A. (1974): Platelets as a source of fibroblast growth-promoting activity. *Exp. Cell Res.*, 87:297–301.

45. Kramer, R. H., and Nicolson, G. L. (1979): Interactions of tumor cells with vascular endothelial cell monolayers: a model for metastatic invasion. *Proc. Natl. Acad. Sci. U.S.A.*, 76:5704–5708.

46. Kratochwil, K. (1972): In: *General Properties in Tissue Interaction in Carcinogenesis*, edited by D. Tarin, pp. 1–48. Academic Press, New York.

47. Layman, D. L., Jele, B. J., and Illingworth, D. R. (1980): Inability of serum from abetalipoproteinemic subjects to stimulate proliferation of human smooth muscle cells and dermal fibroblasts in vitro. *Proc. Natl. Acad. Sci. U.S.A.*, 77:1511–1515.

48. Leighton, J. (1957): Contributions of tissue culture studies to an understanding of the biology of cancer: a review. *Cancer Res.*, 17:929–935.

49. Liotta, L. A., Abe, S., Robey, P. G., and Martin, G. R. (1979): Preferential digestion of basement membrane collagen by an enzyme derived from a metastatic murine tumor. *Proc. Natl. Acad. Sci. U.S.A.*, 76:2268–2272.

50. Maroudas, N. G. (1973): Chemical and mechanical requirements for fibroblast adhesion. *Nature*, 244:353–354.

51. Maroudas, N. G., O'Neill, C. H., and Stanton, M. F. (1973): Fibroblast anchorage in carcinogenesis by fibres. *Lancet*, 1:807–809.

52. Mather, J. P., and Sato, G. H. (1979): The use of hormone-supplemented serum-free media in primary cultures. *Exp. Cell Res.*, 124:215–221.

53. Miller, E. J. (1977): The collagens of the extracellular matrix. In: *Cell and Tissue Interactions, Society of General Physiologists Series*, Vol. 32, edited by J. W. Lash and M. M. Burger. pp. 71–86. Raven Press, New York.

54. Muir, H. (1977): Structure and function of proteoglycans of cartilage and cell-matrix interaction. In: *Cell and Tissue Interactions, Society of General Physiologists Series*, Vol. 32, edited by J. W. Lash and M. M. Burger, pp. 87–88. Raven Press, New York.

55. Murray, J. C., Stingl, G., Kleinman, H. K., Martin, G. R., and Kidwell, W. R. (1979): Epidermal cells adhere preferentially to type IV (basement membrane) collagen. *J. Cell Biol.*, 80:197–202.

56. Nesbit, M. E. (1976): CA, 26:174–183.
57. Owens, R. B. (1976): Selective cultivation of mammalian epithelial cells. In: *Methods Cell Biol.*, 14:341–373.
58. Rafferty, K. A. (1975): Epithelial cells: growth in culture of normal and neoplastic forms. *Adv. Cancer Res.*, 21:249–272.
59. Reckless, J. P. D., Weinstein, D. B., and Steinberg, D. (1978): Lipoprotein and cholesterol metabolism in rabbit arterial endothelial cells in culture. *Biochim. Biophys. Acta*, 529:475–487.
60. Rifkin, D. B., Loeb, J. N., Moore, G., and Reich, E. (1974): Properties of plasminogen activators formed by neoplastic human cell cultures. *J. Exp. Med.*, 139:1317–1328.
61. Ross, R., and Glomset, J. A. (1973): Atherosclerosis and the arterial smooth muscle cell. *Science*, 180:1332–1339.
62. Ross, R., Glomset, J., Kariya, B., and Harker, L. (1974): A platelet dependent serum factor that stimulates the proliferation of arterial smooth muscle cells in vitro. *Proc. Natl. Acad. Sci. U.S.A.*, 71:1207–1210.
63. Ross, R., and Vogel, A. (1978): The platelet-derived growth factor. *Cell*, 14:203–301.
64. Smith, H. S., Riggs, J. L., and Mosesson, M. W. (1979): Production of fibronectin by human epithelial cells in culture. *Cancer Res.*, 39:4138–4142.
65. Stein, O., and Stein, Y. (1976): High density lipoproteins reduce the uptake of low density lipoproteins by human endothelial cells in culture. *Biochim. Biophys. Acta*, 23:563–568.
66. Sun, T. T., and Green, H. (1977): Cultured epithelial cells of cornea, conjunctiva and skin: absence of marked intrinsic divergence of their differentiated states. *Nature*, 269:489–493.
67. Tauber, J.-P., Cheng, J., and Gospodarowicz, D. (1980): The effect of high and low density lipoproteins on the proliferation of vascular endothelial cells. *J. Clin. Invest.*, 66:696–708.
68. Tauber, J.-P., Goldminz, D., Vlodavsky, I., and Gospodarowicz, D. (1980): The interactions of the high density lipoproteins with cultured vascular endothelial cells. *J. Clin. Invest. (in press).*
69. Tauber, J.-P., Vlodavsky, I., Goldminz, D., and Gospodarowicz, D. (1980): Up regulation in vascular endothelial cells of high density lipoprotein receptor sites induced by 25 hydroxycholesterol. *J. Cell Physiol. (in press).*
70. Thomassen, M. J., Buoen, L. C., and Brand, K. G. (1975): Foreign-body tumorigenesis: number distribution, and cell density of preneoplastic clones. *J. Natl. Cancer Inst.*, 54:203–207.
71. Thompson, D. (1961): In: *On Growth and Form*, edited by J. T. Bonner. Cambridge University Press, Cambridge.
72. Timpl, R., Rohde, H., Gehran-Robey, P., Rennard, S. I., Foidart, J.-M., and Martin, G. R. (1979): Laminin—a glycoprotein from basement membrane. *J. Biol. Chem.*, 254:9933–9937.
73. Tseng, S. C., Savion, N., Gospodarowicz, D., and Stern, R. (1981): Characterization of collagens synthesized by bovine corneal endothelial cell cultures. *J. Biol. Chem.*, 256:3361–3365.
74. Tseng, S., Savion, N., Stern, R., and Gospodarowicz, D. (1982): Fibroblast growth factor maintains the phenotypic expression of collagen synthesis in cultured bovine vascular endothelial cells. *Eur. J. Biochem. (in press.)*
75. Vlodavsky, I., Fielding, P. E., Fielding, C. J., and Gospodarowicz, D. (1978): Role of contact inhibition in the regulation of receptor mediated uptake of low density lipoprotein in cultured vascular endothelial cells. *Proc. Natl. Acad. Sci. U.S.A.*, 75:356–360.
76. Vlodavsky, I., and Gospodarowicz, D. (1980): Respective involvement of laminin and fibronectin in the adhesion of human carcinoma and sarcoma cells. *Nature* 289:304–306.
77. Vlodavsky, I., Johnson, L. K., Greenburg, G., and Gospodarowicz, D. (1979): Vascular endothelial cells maintained in the absence of fibroblast growth factor undergo structural and functional alterations that are incompatible with their in vivo differentiated properties. *J. Cell Biol.*, 83:468–486.
78. Vlodavsky, I., Lui, G.-M., and Gospodarowicz, D. (1980): Morphological appearance, growth behavior and migratory activity of human tumor cells maintained on extracellular matrix versus plastic. *Cell*, 19:607–616.
79. Yamada, K. M., and Olden, K. (1978): Fibronectins— adhesive glycoproteins of cell surface and blood. *Nature*, 275:179–184.
80. Yang, J., Richards, J., Bowman, P., Guzman, R., Eham, J., McCormick, K., Hamamoto, S., Pitelka, D., and Nandi, S. (1979): Substained growth and three-dimensional organization of primary mammary tumor. *Proc. Natl. Acad. Sci. U.S.A.*, 76:3401–3405.
81. Wessels, N. K. (1964): Substrate and nutrient effects upon epidermal basal cell orientation and proliferation. *Proc. Natl. Acad. Sci. U.S.A.*, 52:252–259.
82. Wessels, N. K. (1977): In: *Tissue Interaction and Development*, pp. 213–229. W. A. Benjamin, London.

Maturation Factors and Cancer,
edited by Malcolm A. S. Moore.
Raven Press, © New York 1982.

N,N-Dimethylformamide-Induced Modulation of Responses of Tumor Cells to Conventional Anticancer Treatment Modalities

*Daniel L. Dexter, **John T. Leith, †Gerald W. Crabtree, †Robert E. Parks, Jr., **Arvin S. Glicksman, and *Paul Calabresi

*Department of Medicine, Roger Williams General Hospital, and Section of Medicine, Division of Biology and Medicine, Brown University, Providence, Rhode Island 02912; **Department of Radiation Oncology, Rhode Island Hospital, and Section of Radiation Medicine, Division of Biology and Medicine, Brown University, Providence, Rhode Island 02912; †Section of Biochemical Pharmacology, Division of Biology and Medicine, Brown University, Providence, Rhode Island 02912*

Cancer has been defined as a disease of differentiation (28), and the past two decades have seen the implementation of various approaches designed to influence or direct the maturation of neoplastic cells. Much of the original impetus for this work was derived from studies with spontaneously differentiating tumors. Reports from the laboratories of L. C. Stevens (35) and G. B. Pierce, Jr. (22) have elegantly described the differentiation of murine teratomas to benign cell types. Pierce (30) has also described the differentiation of a chondrosarcoma in the hamster, and a squamous cell carcinoma in the rat. Maturation of human neuroblastomas to ganglioneuromas or ganglioneuroblastomas has been reported (11). Thus the spontaneous differentiation of animal and human tumors, although uncommon, is well documented.

Investigators have used two basic approaches, or strategies, in an attempt to trigger the differentiation of tumor cells. One approach uses naturally occurring metabolites produced by cell lines or tissues, which can be shown to play a role in the maturation of target cancer cells. The work done in the laboratory of L. Sachs (12,26) provides a good example of this method. Sachs and co-workers have reported extensively on the ability of the naturally produced protein MGI to induce the differentiation of both normal and neoplastic hematopoietic cells. The second strategy utilizes synthetic chemicals to effect the differentiation of tumor cells. The term "biological modifier" can be applied to both naturally produced and chemically synthesized inducers.

Polar solvents, principally dimethylsulfoxide (DMSO) and N,N-dimethylformamide (DMF), have been used as chemical inducers in many systems. The prototype of this work has been the DMSO induction of the erythroid program of differentiation in Friend virus-transformed murine erythroleukemia (MEL) cells (13). DMF and other polar solvents are also effective inducers in this system (36). DMSO has induced morphological and bioelectrical differentiation of murine neuroblastoma cells (21) and has effected cilia formation in human lung adenocarcinoma cells (38). DMSO and DMF have caused the differentiation of human myelocytic leukemia cells to cells resembling human granulocytes in their morphological and phagocytic properties (4). Both polar solvents have been shown to induce morphological differentiation in murine fibrosarcoma cells, and DMF or DMSO has caused an alteration in the membrane glycoprotein profile of these cells (1). It has also been reported that DMF induces a marked reduction in the tumorigenicity of a murine rhabdomyosarcoma cell line as well as pronounced morphological changes in these cells (6).

Our laboratory has focused on human colon cancer cells as targets for differentiation induction. Pierce (30) has advocated for some time that many tumors are stem cell tumors, and that a strategy for treating such cancers would be to enable them to differentiate to more benign end cell types; Potter (31) has advanced a similar hypothesis. Human colon carcinoma would appear to be a likely candidate for such an approach because of the population of rapidly turning over stem cells in the crypts of the colon. One can ask the question whether there is any connection between the facts that neoplasms occur so frequently in the colon, and that colonic epithelial cells divide every 24 hr and are completely replaced every 3 to 4 days (25). We therefore selected colon cancer as one tumor type that might be appropriate for an induction study, and we used DMF as the inducing chemical.

RESULTS AND DISCUSSION

The Effects of Polar Solvents on Cultured Human Colon Cancer Cells

We initially studied the effect of DMF on the growth properties of a series of human colon carcinoma cell lines and clones established in our laboratory (7). That work can be summarized as follows: DMF at a concentration of 0.8% in the tissue culture medium causes alterations in the growth characteristics of four colon cancer cell lines. Treatment with DMF caused the doubling times of these cells to be increased from about 20 to almost 50 hr, the saturation densities of the cultures to be significantly decreased, and the clonogenicity of the cells in soft agar to be totally abolished. When DLD-1 human colon cancer cells were pretreated in culture with DMF, and then injected into nude mice, their tumorigenicity was greatly reduced compared to their untreated counterparts. An inoculum of 1×10^6 DMF-treated cells produced a tumor in only 1 of 10 recipient mice, whereas 10 of 10 mice injected with 1×10^6 untreated cells developed carcinomas. Such alterations in the malignant properties of the colon carcinoma cells subsequent to DMF exposure are consistent with changes expected in cells that have acquired a more benign phenotype (23,34). Kim and co-workers have shown similar changes in doubling times and clonogenicity in agar for two other human colon cancer cell lines treated with DMSO (20).

The effect of DMF on specific cell surface markers was also examined (18). DMF caused an increased expression of carcinoembryonic antigen (CEA) in our colon cancer lines. As increased CEA expression correlates with a higher degree of differentiation in human colon carcinomas and derivative cell lines (2,5), this result indicates that DMF caused the differentiation of several colon cancer cell types with respect to this marker. The modulation of the expression of the colonic mucoprotein antigen (CMA), described by Gold and Miller (15), was also studied. Our group was able to show, with DMF-treated colon cancer cells, an increased expression of the CMA molecule found on the plasma membrane of normal colonic mucosal cells (NCMA), with a concomitant decrease in the colon tumor-specific CMA (TCMA) molecule. These data provide further evidence that DMF causes the maturation of the cultured colon carcinoma cells. Our study also showed that DMF causes a decrease in the amount of detectable O blood group substance (H gene– determined product) on the surface of treated cells. This has also been interpreted as a maturational event (18).

The alteration of the malignant phenotype of colon cancer cells concomitant with corresponding maturational events can thus be effected by treatment with DMF. We have presented this system as a suitable model to investigate the relationship between colon cancer and differentiation and have suggested that this approach might be extended to other human carcinomas as well (8).

Rationale for the Combination of Biological Modifiers with Conventional Cancer Treatment Modalities

We, as well as other groups, are continuing to study the possibility that differentiation-inducing agents might be employed in the maturational therapy of experimental animal cancers. Success with human tumor xenograft maturation would suggest the use of these agents in a clinical setting. However, the possibility certainly exists that differentiation-inducing compounds might also cause the sensitization of cancer cells to conventional therapies. Therefore, we have begun extensive studies with combinations of DMF and anticancer drugs, X-irradiation, hyperthermia, and hormone or immunotherapy. The feasibility of this strategy is supported by results from many laboratories, including our own, on maturation induction with polar solvents as single agents. A careful analysis of the data has led us to the following working hypotheses, shown schematically in Fig. 1.

First, polar solvents induce alterations in cell surface components of cancer cells (1,18,21,27,38), and DMSO has been shown to cause decreased membrane fluidity (27). Therefore, pretreatment with polar solvents might result in the appearance of increased numbers of cell surface antigens or hormone receptors. This could result from an increased synthesis of such macromolecules, or from the exposure of masked or cryptic components, or both. Induced cells with new, or newly revealed, antigens or hormone receptors on their surface could then become more sensitive to the appropriate hormone or immunotherapy. Also, polar solvents might facilitate the transport of chemotherapeutic drugs into tumor cells. This could be important

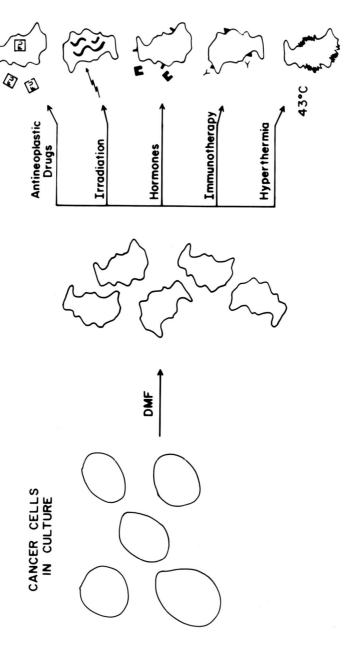

FIG. 1. Schematic diagram of DMF-induced sensitization of cancer cells to conventional treatments. Cancer cells are exposed to the polar solvent and undergo morphological and biochemical differentiation; changes could occur in the plasma membrane, nucleus, and metabolic processes of treated cells. The DMF-exposed cells are rendered more sensitive to anticancer drugs, hyperthermia, irradiation, hormone therapy, or immunotherapy.

in cases where the drug is not well transported, or where the active form of the drug cannot be given because of transport problems. Finally, membrane changes might sensitize the cancer cell to hyperthermic treatment.

Second, polar solvents cause a wide range of effects on metabolic processes in tumor cells. The synthesis of a number of molecular species (heme, hemoglobin, spectrin, an erythrocyte antigen, heme mRNA) has been induced by polar solvent treatment of MEL cells (for a review, see ref. 32). It is reasonable to hypothesize that DMF-induced alterations in the levels of key enzymes in the purine and pyrimidine pathways, for example, would significantly affect the cytotoxic action of antimetabolites such as fluorouracil, 6-thioguanine, or methotrexate in cancer cells. A therapeutic-enhancing effect could be achieved either through an increase in the activity in a drug-activating enzyme, or through a decrease in the activity of a drug-inactivating enzyme following exposure of target cells to DMF.

Third, DMSO causes an increase in the number of single strand breaks in the DNA of MEL cells (33,37). The scissions might result from increased nuclease attack on regions of DNA that have been exposed due to polar solvent-induced changes in the chromatin structure. Alternatively, the treated cells may not be able to repair the breaks as efficiently as their untreated counterparts. Regardless of the mechanism, the data suggest that cells pretreated with DMSO or DMF might be more sensitive to radiation or to alkylating agents for the following reasons. Both treatments cause DNA breaks, and any change in the microenvironment in the nucleus that facilitates increased nicks in the DNA might also facilitate increased DNA damage by irradiation or an alkylating agent. Furthermore, if cells pretreated with DMF cannot repair single strand breaks as well as their untreated counterparts, this could result in a far more effective cytotoxic effect than could be achieved by a given dose of X-rays or alkylating drug without polar solvent pretreatment.

Effect of DMF on Drug Metabolizing Enzymes

Our laboratory has taken the following approach to the problem of selecting combinations of inducers and conventional antineoplastic drugs for treatment of colon cancer cells. The activities of a spectrum of enzymes important in purine metabolism were determined in four human colon cancer cell lines. The activities of these enzymes were also determined in cells preexposed to 0.8% DMF or 3 mM sodium butyrate (another compound known to induce differentiation in tumor cells; refs. 4,14,24). The data were analyzed for changes in enzyme activities that could be exploited to increase the efficacy of a conventional anticancer drug against these cells.

Our results, recently presented in preliminary form (10), indicate that the activities of two enzymes, adenosine deaminase (ADA) and guanine deaminase, might be modulated to provide a potentiation of the appropriate drugs. DMF caused an 11-fold decrease in ADA activity in the clone A cells of the heterogeneous DLD-1 human colon carcinoma, and a fourfold decrease in ADA activity in clone D cells, also derived from the DLD-1 carcinoma. These data suggest that some human colon tumor cells pretreated with DMF could be more sensitive to adenosine analogs such as formycin and 8-azaadenosine, which are good substrates for ADA and are converted to chemotherapeutically inactive forms by this enzyme. DMF also causes a threefold decrease in guanine deaminase levels in clone D colon cancer cells. Thus one can speculate that the activity of an analog such as 8-azaguanine, which is a substrate for the enzyme, might be potentiated in clone D cells pretreated with DMF.

This approach provides a rational basis for selection of the appropriate inducer and antineoplastic drug to more efficaciously inhibit an enzyme catalyzing a key reaction in purine biosynthesis in tumor cells. The enzymes in the pyridimine pathway are also being examined for their sensitivity to modulation by biological modifiers. Information provided by these biochemical analyses will then allow testing of selected inducer-antimetabolite combinations against appropriate human colon carcinoma cell lines and xenograft tumors.

Effect of DMF on Sensitivity of Tumor Cells to X-Irradiation

We have recently begun to test the effect of DMF pretreatment on the sensitivity of tumor cells to X-irradiation. Initial studies have focused on two subpopulations (lines 66 and 67) isolated in our laboratory from a heterogeneous, spontaneously occurring mouse mammary tumor (9). These two lines were selected because one of them (line 66) was shown to be quite radioresistant. Line 66 or 67 cells were pretreated for 4 days with DMF (0.8% in the growth medium), and were then exposed to graded doses of X-rays. After irradiation, cells were trypsinized, counted, and plated in regular growth medium at the appropriate inocula. Control cultures (no DMF pretreatment) were irradiated and processed at the same time. Colonies were allowed to develop for 8 days, stained with crystal violet, and colonies with 50 or more cells were counted. Data were then fitted to the single-hit, multitarget equation (16).

The results (Fig. 2) showed that DMF had little effect on the response of the more radiosensitive 67 cells to X-ray treatment. In contrast, the more radioresistant 66 cells showed an increased sensitivity to X-irradiation subsequent to exposure to the polar solvent. The DMF modifying effect is seen in the shoulder region of the 66 cell survival curve, suggesting that repair function in these cells may be affected by DMF. Line 66 cells not exposed to DMF but irradiated had an extrapolation number *(n)* of 4.5 and a "shoulder" or quasi-threshold dose (D_q) of 2.8 Gy. In contrast, 66 cells pretreated with DMF and then irradiated had $n = 1.5$ and $D_q = 0.8$ Gy.

This finding, recently presented in a preliminary report (3), that DMF modifies the shoulder region of the survival curve of irradiated tumor cells, is important in terms of implications about repair of DNA damage and the potential use of biological modifiers in combination with radiation therapy. It is of course necessary to establish whether other tumor cell types, particularly human tumors, can respond in a similar manner. Experiments are currently being carried out to determine whether human

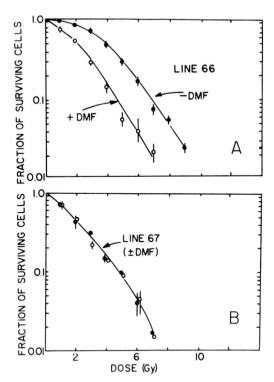

FIG. 2. Response of DMF-treated and untreated mouse mammary tumor cell subpopulations to *in vitro* X-irradiation. Mouse mammary tumor cells from sublines 66 and 67, isolated from a culture obtained from a mouse mammary adenocarcinoma, were grown either in the presence (+DMF) or in the absence (−DMF) of 0.8% DMF in the culture medium. Cells were plated in duplicate flasks, and exponentially growing cultures were treated with X-irradiation at graded doses. The cells were removed from the flasks and were plated at appropriate inocula in culture dishes. After 8 days, dishes were stained with crystal violet, and colonies of more than 50 cells were scored. Fractional cell survival is plotted against dose on semilogarithmic paper. (Reprinted with permission from Leith et al., *Int. J. Rad. Oncol. Biol. Phys.*, Vol. 7, 1981. Pergamon Press, Ltd.)

colon carcinoma cells or their xenograft tumors can be sensitized to X-irradiation by pretreatment with differentiation-inducing compounds.

Implications of DMF-Induced Cell Surface Changes For Hormone and Immunotherapy

A number of laboratories have described cell surface changes caused by exposure of cancer cells to differentiation-inducing chemicals. Several of these studies have already been referenced in this chapter (1,18,21,27,38). In addition, Tralka et al. (39) have described surface changes in butyrate-treated human lung cancer cells. DMSO has induced the appearance of an erythrocyte membrane antigen in MEL cells (19) and has caused changes in the ganglioside composition of human colon cancer cells (20). Morphological differentiation, obviously reflecting changes in membrane structure, has been reported in many tumor cell types treated with a variety of chemical inducers (1,4,6,7,20,23).

Work in our laboratory with DMF has provided the following evidence that carcinoma cells can have their antigenicity modified by exposure to the polar solvent. Two subpopulations isolated from an autochthonous mouse mammary tumor did not have the mouse mammary tumor virus (MMTV) antigen when assayed by the indirect immunofluorescence test. After pretreatment with DMF for several days, significant fluorescence could be assayed (17). Work with human colon cancer cell lines has shown that CEA, CMA, and H blood group substance levels can also be modulated by DMF treatment (18). Therefore, we have described four examples of the ability of DMF to change the antigenicity of cultured carcinoma cells. It would also be reasonable to hypothesize that DMF, DMSO, or butyrate might change the levels of estrogen receptor, for example, in the appropriate tumor cell type. The findings from many laboratories, taken together, certainly suggest that exposure of cancer cells to an inducer might sensitize the cell to antibody, immunocyte, or hormone attack.

CONCLUSIONS

In vitro studies using a variety of inducing chemicals against a spectrum of rodent and human tumor cell lines have clearly demonstrated that these agents can induce maturational changes in cancer cells and can alter the malignant phenotype to a phenotype characteristic of a more benign cell type. *In vivo* experiments with animal and human xenograft tumors will be carried out in increasing numbers by many investigators in the next several years to determine whether biological modifiers can effect a maturational change in solid tumors. Encouraging results would indicate that agents such as polar solvents, butyrate, retinoic acid (29), etc., should be considered for use in the clinic. However, the possibility remains that solid tumors will not be affected in any dramatic fashion by biological modifiers used as single agents in a treatment protocol. Another strategy would be to use the inducer in combination with conventional treatment modalities. This could result in a modulation of tumor cell growth, structure, or metabolism in a way that would sensitize the cancer cell to other forms of treatment. With such an approach, the host would benefit from whatever maturational or growth-inhibiting effects the inducer alone might achieve, as well as from any potentiation of the effects of chemotherapeutic drugs, irradiation, etc. Sensitization of tumor cells *in situ* might also permit the use of a lower dose of drug or irradiation to achieve the same response as a higher dose without inducer, thus reducing the toxicity for the host. Such *in vivo* experiments are feasible because very large doses of DMF or DMSO can be given without toxicity; many biological modifiers are quite innocuous to cultured cells or living tissue.

A number of model systems employed by various investigators to study maturational changes induced in tumor cells by chemicals would be appropriate for the combination treatment studies proposed here. In our laboratory, biochemical analyses of inducer-treated and untreated human colon cancer cells are being carried out to select rationally the appropriate companion antimetabolite for a combination protocol. We have detected significant antigenic changes effected by DMF in both human colon carcinoma cells and in mouse mammary tumor cells. These observations have implications for immunotherapy. An important finding of our group was that DMF induced an increase in radiosensitivity in a radioresistant mouse mammary tumor cell line. These results support the concept that a protocol combining an inducer with a conventional treatment modality might prove to be the most efficacious method of using biological modifiers in the treatment of neoplastic disease.

ACKNOWLEDGMENT

This work was partially supported by USPHS Grants CA20892, CA13943, and CA23225.

REFERENCES

1. Borenfreund, E., Steinglass, M., Karngold, G., and Bendich, A. (1975): Effect of dimethyl sulfoxide and dimethylformamide on the growth and morphology of tumor cells. *Ann. N.Y. Acad. Sci.*, 243:167–171.
2. Breborowicz, J., Easty, C. G., Birbeck, M., Robertson, D., Nery, R., and Neville, A. M. (1975): The monolayer and organ culture of human colorectal carcinomata and the associated "normal" colonic mucosa and their production of carcinoembryonic antigen. *Br. J. Cancer*, 31:559–569.
3. Brenner, H., Dexter, D., Glicksman, A., Calabresi, P., and Tefft, M. (1980): Alteration of intrinsic tumor cell radiosensitivity *in vitro* by N,N-dimethylformamide. *Proc. Am. Assoc. Cancer Res.*, 21:273.
4. Collins, S. J., Ruscetti, F. W., Gallagher, R. E., and Gallo, R. C. (1978): Terminal differentiation of human promyelocytic leukemia cells induced by dimethyl sulfoxide and other polar compounds. *Proc. Natl. Acad. Sci. U.S.A.*, 75:2458–2462.
5. Denk, H., Tappeiner, B., Davidovits, A., Eckerstorfer, R., and Holzner, J. H. (1972): Carcinoembryonic antigen (CEA) in gastrointestinal and extragastrointestinal tumors and its relationship to tumor-cell differentiation. *Int. J. Cancer*, 10:262–272.
6. Dexter, D. L. (1977): N,N-Dimethylformamide-induced morphological differentiation and reduction of tumorigenicity in cultured mouse rhabdomyosarcoma cells. *Cancer Res.*, 37:3136–3140.
7. Dexter, D. L., Barbosa, J. A., and Calabresi, P. (1979): N,N-Dimethylformamide-induced alteration of cell culture characteristics and loss of tumorigenicity in cultured human colon carcinoma cells. *Cancer Res.*, 39:1020–1025.
8. Dexter, D. L., and Hager, J. C. (1980): Maturation-induction of tumor cells using a human colon carcinoma model. *Cancer*, 45:1178–1184.
9. Dexter, D. L., Kowalski, H. M., Blazar, B. A., Fligiel, Z., Vogel, R., and Heppner, G. H. (1978): Heterogeneity of tumor cells from a single mouse mammary tumor. *Cancer Res.*, 38:3174–3181.
10. Dexter, D. L., Parks, R. E., Jr., and Calabresi, P. (1980): Sodium butyrate and N,N-dimethylformamide modulation of the activities of purine metabolizing enzymes in cultured human colon cancer cells. *Proc. Am. Assoc. Cancer Res.*, 21:30.
11. Dyke, P. C., and Mulkey, D. A. (1967): Maturation of ganglioneuroblastoma to ganglioneuroma. *Cancer*, 20:1343–1349.
12. Fibach, E., Landau, T., and Sachs, L. (1972): Normal differentiation of myeloid leukaemic cells induced by a differentiation-inducing protein. *Nature*, 237:276–278.
13. Friend, C. W., Scher, W., Holland, J. G., and Sato, T. (1971): Hemoglobin synthesis in murine virus-induced leukemic cells *in vitro*: stimulation of erythroid differentiation by dimethylsulfoxide. *Proc. Natl. Acad. Sci. U.S.A.*, 68:378–382.

14. Ghosh, N. K., Rukenstein, A., and Cox, P. (1977): Induction of human choriogonadotropin in HeLa-cell cultures by aliphatic monocarboxylates and inhibitors of deoxyribonucleic acid synthesis. *Biochem. J.*, 166:265–274.
15. Gold, D. V., and Miller, F. (1978): Comparison of human colonic mucoprotein antigen from normal and neoplastic mucosa. *Cancer Res.*, 38:3204–3211.
16. Goldstein, A. (1964): *Biostatistics: An Introductory Text.* MacMillan, New York.
17. Hager, J. C., Dexter, D. L., Calabresi, P., and Heppner, G. H. (1979): Heterogeneity of MMTV antigen expression and induction in mouse mammary tumor cells. *Proc. Am. Assoc. Cancer Res.*, 20:61.
18. Hager, J. C., Gold, D. V., Barbosa, J. A., Fligiel, Z., Miller, F., and Dexter, D. L. (1980): N,N-Dimethylformamide-induced modulation or organ- and tumor-associated markers in cultured human colon cancer cells. *J. Natl. Cancer Inst.*, 64:439–446.
19. Ikawa, Y., Furasawa, M., and Sugano, H. (1973): Erythrocyte membrane-specific antigens in Friend virus-induced leukemia cells. *Bibl. Haematol.*, 39:955–967.
20. Kim, Y. S., Tsao, D., Siddiqui, B., Whitehead, J. S., Arnstein, P., Bennett, J., and Hicks, J. (1980): Effects of sodium butyrate and dimethylsulfoxide on biochemical properties of human colon cancer cells. *Cancer*, 45:1185–1192.
21. Kimhi, Y., Palfrey, C., Spector, I., Barak, Y., and Littauer, V. F. (1976): Maturation of neuroblastoma cells in the presence of dimethylsulfoxide. *Proc. Natl. Acad. Sci. U.S.A.*, 73:462–466.
22. Kleinsmith, L. J., and Pierce, G. B. (1964): Multipotentiality of single embryonal carcinoma cells. *Cancer Res.*, 24:1544–1551.
23. Leavitt, J., Barrett, J. C., Crawford, B. D., and Ts'o, P. O. P. (1978): Butyric acid suppression of the *in vitro* neoplastic state of syrian hamster cells. *Nature*, 271:262–265.
24. Leder, A., and Leder, P. (1974): Butyric acid, a potent inducer of erythroid differentiation in cultured erythroleukemic cells. *Cell*, 5:319–322.
25. Lipkin, M., Bell, B., and Sherlock, P. (1963): Cell proliferation kinetics in the gastrointestinal tract of man. I. Cell renewal in colon and rectum. *J. Clin. Invest.*, 42:767–776.
26. Lotem, J., and Sachs, L. (1978): *In vivo* induction of normal differentiation in myeloid leukemia cells. *Proc. Natl. Acad. Sci. U.S.A.*, 75:3781–3785.
27. Lyman, G. H., Preisler, H. D., and Papahadjopoulos, D. (1976): Membrane action of DMSO and other chemical inducers of Friend leukemic cell differentiation. *Nature*, 262:360–363.
28. Markert, C. L. (1968): Neoplasia: a disease of cell differentiation. *Cancer Res.*, 28:1908–1914.
29. Meyskens, F. L., Jr., and Fuller, B. B. (1980): Characterization of the effects of different retinoids in the growth and differentiation of a human melanoma cell line and selected subclones. *Cancer Res.*, 40:2194–2196.
30. Pierce, G. B. (1974): The benign cells of malignant tumors. In: *Developmental Aspects of Carcinogenesis and Immunity*, edited by T. J. King, pp. 3–22. Academic Press, New York.
31. Potter, V. R. (1978): Phenotypic diversity in experimental hepatomas: the concept of partially blocked ontogeny. *Br. J. Cancer*, 38:1–23.
32. Rifkind, R. A., and Marks, P. A. (1978): Regulation of differentiation in transformed erythroid cells. *Blood Cells*, 4:189–206.
33. Scher, W., and Friend, C. (1978): Breakage of DNA and alterations in folded genomes by inducers of differentiation in Friend erythroleukemia cells. *Cancer Res.*, 38:841–849.
34. Shin, S., Freedman, V. H., Risser, R., and Pollack, R. (1975): Tumorigenicity of virus-transformed cells in nude mice is correlated specifically with anchorage independent growth *in vitro*. *Proc. Natl. Acad. Sci. U.S.A.*, 72:4435–4439.
35. Stevens, L. C. (1970): The development of transplantable teratocarcinomas from intratesticular grafts of pre- and postimplantation mouse embryos. *Dev. Biol.*, 21:364–382.
36. Tanaka, M., Levy, J., Terada, M., Breslow, R., Rifkind, R. A., and Marks, P. A. (1975): Induction of erythroid differentiation in murine virus infected erythroleukemia cells by highly polar compounds. *Proc. Natl. Acad. Sci. U.S.A.*, 72:1003–1006.
37. Terada, M., Nudel, V., Fibach, E., Rifkind, R. A., and Marks, P. A. (1978): Changes in DNA associated with induction of erythroid differentiation by dimethyl sulfoxide in murine erythroleukemia cells. *Cancer Res.*, 38:835–840.
38. Tralka, T. S., and Rabson, A. S. (1976): Cilia formation in cultures of human lung cancer cells treated with dimethyl sulfoxide. *J. Natl. Cancer Inst.*, 52:1101–1110.
39. Tralka, T. S., Rosen, S. W., Weintraub, B. D., Lieblich, J. M., Engel, L. W., Wetzel, B. K., Kingsbury, E. W., and Rabson, A. S. (1979): Ultrastructural concomitants of sodium butyrate-enhanced ectopic production of chorionic gonadotropin and its alpha subunit in human bronchogenic carcinoma (Cha Go) cells. *J. Natl. Cancer Inst.*, 62:45–61.

Maturation Factors and Cancer,
edited by Malcolm A. S. Moore.
Raven Press, © New York 1982.

Properties of Growth Factors Produced by Sarcoma Virus-Transformed Cells

George J. Todaro*

**Laboratory of Viral Carcinogenesis, National Cancer Institute,
Frederick, Maryland 21701*

The murine sarcoma virus (MSV) genome basically contains three genes that are required for replication (1): *env, gag,* and *pol.* Each is essential for replication of type C viruses, but they do not appear to be involved in the process of transforming normal fibroblasts into fibrosarcoma cells. There is also a fourth gene that is essential for transformation, but is not essential for virus growth. This has been called *sarc* or *onc* (18,20). Some of the properties that would be expected of a potential transforming gene are that (a) it is present in normal cellular DNA, (b) it is well conserved in evolution, (c) it codes for protein (maximum molecular weight of 60,000 daltons), (d) it is not essential for virus replication, and (e) its product acts as a regulator of cell growth. It is evident that one of the classes of proteins that could satisfy the requirements for transforming proteins would be normal or abnormal forms of the polypeptide growth hormones, such as epidermal growth factor (EGF), fibroblast growth factor, or the insulin-like growth factors (3,7,14). The discovery of the specific loss of EGF receptors from MSV-transformed cells was the first indication that there was, in fact, an association between viral transformation and the expression of available receptors for specific growth factors on these cells.

Mouse, rat, and mink cells transformed by murine sarcoma virus characteristically lose their cell surface receptors which bind EGF. The sarcoma virus-transformed cells show a dramatic decrease or total absence of cell surface EGF receptors. This, however, is not a general phenomenon of transformation, since neither the DNA virus-transformed cells nor the majority of chemically transformed cells showed this characteristic loss of available EGF receptors (23,24). Over the years, we have accumulated cells transformed by a variety of agents, including DNA viruses such as simian virus 40 (SV40) and polyoma, RNA viruses such as murine and avian sarcoma viruses, chemical carcinogens, and radiation, as well as cells which have become transformed spontaneously during passage in cell culture. These have been obtained from Swiss 3T3, BALB/3T3, and other mouse and rat cell systems. In collaboration with Stanley Cohen, these transformed cells were tested for their ability to bind ^{125}I-labeled EGF (23). Of 47 independently isolated, chemically transformed cells, 5 show a pattern like the MSV-transformed cells, i.e., almost complete loss of EGF receptors with normal levels of other receptors maintained. The chemically transformed cells without detectable EGF receptors have not yet been further characterized for the growth factors they may be producing. They represent a minority of chemically transformed cells that, with respect to this phenotype, behave like the MSV-transformed cells.

One explanation for the loss of available EGF receptors following sarcoma virus transformation is that the cells themselves produce a substance capable of interacting with these receptors. The possibility was suggested that a product of the MSV-transformed cells blocks the EGF receptors and might also serve as an endogenous growth stimulator that is either directly produced by the viral genomes or is a cellular gene product expressed in mammalian sarcoma virus-transformed cells (23,24). The hypothesis was presented which stated that tumor viruses produce their transforming action on cells, at least in part, by the production of endogenous polypeptide growth-stimulating factors. Subsequently, our laboratory isolated, purified, and characterized a family of growth factors called "sarcoma growth factors" (SGFs) from sarcoma virus-transformed cells (5). Sufficient quantities are released into serum-free medium of Moloney MSV-infected mouse 3T3 cells to allow for their partial purification and characterization (5).

The growth factors that are produced by the sarcoma virus-transformed cells are a family of heat- and acid-stable, trypsin-sensitive transforming polypeptides, which are destroyed by disulfide reducing agents. Addition of these SGFs to the culture medium of normal cells results in rapid and reversible changes. These factors have EGF-competing activity and growth-stimulating activity that coelute in gel filtration. SGFs not only stimulate normal fibroblasts to divide and overgrow in monolayer cultures, but they also produce a profound morphologic alteration in the cells, rapidly converting them to transformed cells that pile up and are virtually indistinguishable from those genetically transformed by sarcoma viruses. They cause normal rat fibroblasts to form progressively growing colonies in soft agar (induction of anchorage-independent cell growth), a property closely associated with the transformed phenotype. The morphological alterations produced in monolayer cultures and the ability to induce anchorage-independent growth are observable within a few days after treatment with nanogram quantities of partially purified SGFs and continue as long as the peptides are supplied. The phenotypic changes in cellular morphology seen in the presence of SGFs are illustrated in Fig. 1. The untreated fibroblastic cells were present as a flat monolayer containing a regular growth pattern, whereas the treated cells were refractile, displayed no discernible overall growth pattern, crisscrossed in an apparently random fashion, and grew in multiple layers. In soft agar, the untreated cells (Fig. 1C) were present as single cells.

SGF can bring about a phenotypic change in the growth pattern of epithelial cells as well as of fibroblasts (8). Mouse epithelial cells (MMC-E), in the presence of SGF, can be induced to form foci, grow in soft agar, can be stimulated to synthesize DNA, and grow to higher densities than untreated epithelial control cells. MMC-E cells can respond to SGFs produced by virus-transformed mouse 3T3 fibroblasts. Thus the effects of Moloney MSV-induced SGFs are not restricted to the cell type from which they were isolated.

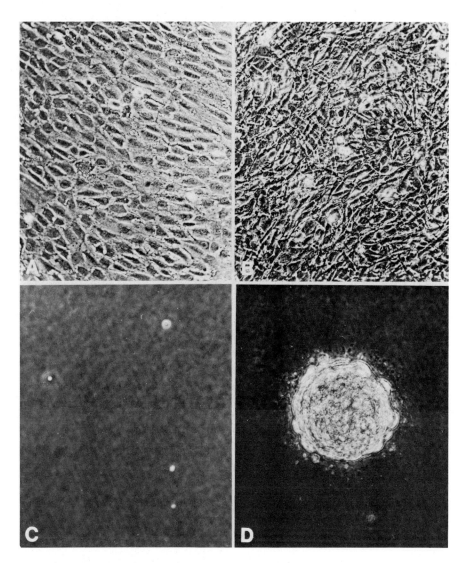

FIG. 1. **A:** Untreated NRK cells. **B:** NRK cells treated with an aliquot of SGF at 10 μg/ml and photographed 6 days later. The cells have grown to considerably higher cell density and display a morphology similar to that of virus-transformed cells. Magnification: **A** and **B**, ×69. **C:** Untreated NRK cells plated in 0.3% soft agar. **D:** NRK cells plated in 0.3% soft agar, treated with an aliquot of SGF at 10 μg/ml and photographed 2 weeks after treatment. The untreated cultures show primarily single cells with two or three cell colonies, but none of larger size. In the treated cultures, many colonies contained well over 500 cells. Magnification: **C** and **D**, ×137.

There is as yet no evidence that SGFs produce permanent genetic changes in the responding cells. Upon removal of SGFs from the medium, the cells resume their normal growth properties. These cells can be cycled back and forth between the untransformed and the transformed phenotype, without an apparent genetic change, by growing them in the absence or presence of the SGFs. It appears, therefore, that these peptides are able to act as effectors of cell transformation. The SGFs are specific for murine or feline sarcoma virus-transformed cells in that supernatants from untransformed cells or DNA tumor virus-transformed cells do not contain detectable quantities of these factors (5).

The factor(s) which has been characterized differs from mouse EGF purified from male salivary glands. First, each of the three fractions, even the smallest, appears to be significantly larger than EGF. Second, antiserum prepared against mouse EGF had no activity against the SGFs as measured in radioimmunoassays, in direct immunoprecipitation, or as an inhibitor of the growth-stimulating activity. Thus despite the fact that they can compete with the EGF receptor systems, SGFs and EGF are not closely related immunologically. Third, SGFs will permit fibro-blasts to grow progressively in agar, but EGF has no such effect. EGF, and other normal growth factors such as fibroblast growth factor and multiplication stimulating activity, will allow rat fibroblast cells to pass through one or two extra cell divisions in agar but will not produce progressively growing agar colonies. Although they are able to compete with EGF binding, SGFs may act through a separate receptor system that does not bind EGF.

One of the SGFs has been further purified and shown to specifically bind to EGF membrane receptors (6). The ability to bind to and be eluted from EGF receptors provides an important purification step in the isolation and characterization of EGF-like growth factors. SGF binding to EGF receptors can be completely blocked by mouse salivary gland EGF. The chemical properties of radiolabeled SGF that has been purified using this method give further support to the idea that SGF and EGF are distinctly different molecules. The SGFs have been shown to compete with EGF for available membrane receptors, yet they do not crossreact with antibodies to EGF, and their biological activity is distinct from that of EGF. Cells lacking EGF receptors are unable to respond to the growth stimulating effects of this partially purified SGF. We concluded, therefore, that SGF released by MSV-transformed cells elicits its biologic effects via specific interaction with EGF membrane recep-tors.

Polypeptides, which are characterized by their ability to confer a transformed phenotype on an untransformed indicator cell, have also been isolated directly from tumor cells growing both in culture and in the animal, rather than from conditioned medium, using an acid-ethanol extraction procedure (16). The properties of these intracellular polypeptides from both virally and chemically transformed cells are similar to those described for the SGFs isolated from the conditioned medium of sarcoma virus-transformed mouse 3T3 cells, suggesting the definition of a new class of transforming growth factors common to tumor cells of different origin. Thus the TGFs represent a new class of polypeptides common to cells transformed either by chemicals or by sarcoma viruses and possess biological activity distinct from that of EGF.

The conclusion which we have reached is that the sarcoma virus genome alters the cells in such a way that SGFs are produced which have at least some of the properties that one would expect of a cell transformation protein. There is no direct evidence at the moment that the SGFs are direct gene products of the sarcoma genome. The viruses could, rather, act by allowing the expression of cellular genes that normally are repressed. Given the rapidity of the change after MSV transformation and the observation that it is a general property of MSV-transformed cells, it would appear that the production of the SGFs is, at least in part, the mechanism by which sarcoma viruses transform cells. It has been suggested that one of the ways in which cells become transformed is by endogenous production of growth factors for which they have receptors and to which they are capable of responding. This internal production of growth polypeptides serves as a constant stimulus for cell division, thereby releasing these cells from some of their normal physiological controls. The MSVs, then, would have acquired either the structural or regulatory genes, which when expressed, allow the production of endogenous growth factors by cells such as fibroblasts, which are capable of responding to this product. Therefore, just as the genetic information for making whole virogenes resides in the cellular DNA of most species (25), so the capacity to make growth factors and/or transforming proteins also resides in the cellular DNA. Viral genes may contain this information or could recombine with it in such a way as to be able to transmit it from cell to cell.

Since it was established that mouse sarcoma virus-transformed cells produced transforming growth factors (TGFs), we decided to screen human tumor cells for similar endogenous factors related to EGF and SGF. The human tumor cells tested for production of factors analogous to SGF were chosen for study because they have no apparent EGF receptors and readily form colonies in soft agar. Normal embryonal lung fibroblasts, unable to grow in soft agar, and A431 epidermoid carcinoma cells, which have a very high number of EGF receptors and grow poorly in soft agar, were used as controls.

Figure 2 shows the results of experiments comparing five human cultures for their ability to form colonies in soft agar. The cells were grown in monolayer cultures, harvested, and seeded at varying densities into medium with 0.3% agar. Colonies were scored at 5 and 10 days. Colonies with more than 10 cells were counted as positive. The results shown in Fig. 2 were obtained at 5 days; the later reading showed no additional positive cells. The cell line 9812 (a bronchogenic carcinoma) formed progressively growing colonies even when relatively low numbers of cells were seeded. A431 cells only showed colony growth when high cell inocula were used. This suggests that a critical concentration of diffusible factors from these cells is required for anchorage-independent growth.

Cells which are potential producers of factors that stimulate growth in soft agar (e.g., human tumor cells) were seeded in one layer of agar at 1×10^6 cells per plate and overlaid with indicator cells (e.g., rat fibroblasts) at 1×10^4 cells per plate. The indicator cells formed colonies when certain human tumor cells were seeded in the other layer. A673 (human rhabdomyosarcoma), 9812 and A2058 (human metastatic melanoma) cells elicited the greatest response and released as much agar growth-stimulating activity as did a comparable number of MSV-transformed mouse 3T3 cells.

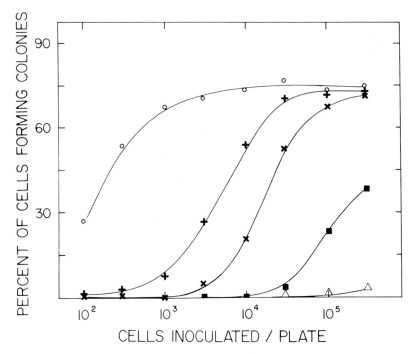

FIG. 2. Soft agar colony formation as a function of cell density. Soft agar assays were set up in 60-mm tissue culture dishes (Falcon #3002) by applying a base layer of 0.5% soft agar (Difco, Noble) and a 2-ml layer of 0.3% agar containing the appropriate cell number. HEL 299 (△), A431 (■), 9812 (○), A673 (+), A2058 (×).

Figure 3 shows the results of experiments in which serum-free supernates from A673 cells were collected, concentrated, and run over a Bio-Gel P-100 column in 1 M acetic acid. Individual fractions were tested for protein concentration, ability to stimulate cells to form colonies in soft agar, and ability to compete with ^{125}I-labeled EGF (4). The majority of the protein is in the void volume of the column. A major peak of soft agar growth-stimulating activity was found in the included volume with maximal activity in fraction 54. When the same fractions were tested for competition with ^{125}I-EGF binding, one major peak was again found, with maximal activity also in fraction 54. Aliquots were tested for stimulation of cell division in serum-depleted cultures of mouse 3T3 cells, rat NRK cells, and human skin fibroblasts; in all cases, the major growth-stimulating activity was found in fraction 54. Fractions 51 to 57 were pooled, concentrated by lyophilization, and used for further studies.

The identical procedure was used to test for growth-stimulating factors and EGF-competing peptides from the supernates of four other human cell cultures. Figure 4 shows that the two highly transformed tumor cell lines, 9812 and A2058, release a growth-stimulating and EGF-competing activity with an apparent molecular weight of 20,000 to 23,000 daltons (Fig. 4B and C). A2058 cells release a second factor

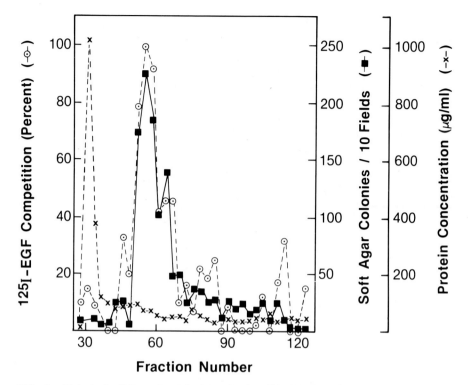

FIG. 3. Biological activity and protein determination of P-100 column fractions of concentrated conditioned media from A673 cells. EGF competition was performed as described. Nonspecific binding, determined by an addition of a 500-fold excess of unlabeled EGF, was approximately 200 counts per min (cpm). Specific binding was approximately 1,200 cpm. Percent competition was determined after correcting for nonspecific binding. Soft agar assays were performed as described. Protein concentration was determined by the method of Lowry et al. (9).

with an apparent molecular weight of 6,000 to 7,000 daltons. Figure 4A shows that the supernate from normal human fibroblast cells did not release a detectable growth-stimulating activity and had no significant EGF-competing activity. A431 cells showed a smaller peak of growth-stimulating activity with an apparent molecular weight of 21,000 daltons; no EGF-competing activity was found.

Figure 5A shows a dose response curve measuring soft agar growth as a function of protein concentration. The pooled, peak fractions from A673 cells are compared with those from normal human fibroblasts. There was a 50- to 100-fold difference in soft agar growth-stimulating activity.

The relative sensitivities of three different assays for growth-stimulating activity are compared in Fig. 5B. The data are presented as the percentage of the maximal response. Induction of DNA synthesis as tested with serum-depleted rat fibroblast monolayer cultures was slightly more sensitive than the soft agar growth assay; EGF-competing ability was the least sensitive. The latter two assays were used in

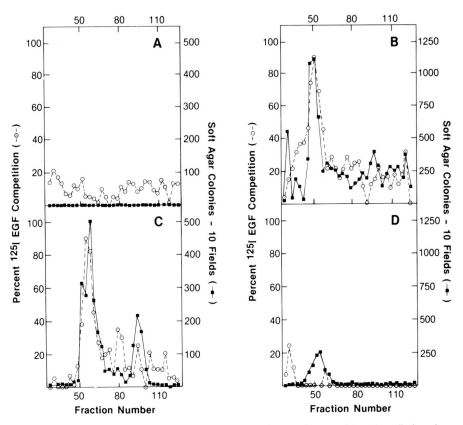

FIG. 4. Biological activity in P-100 column fractions of serum-free conditioned media from four human cells in culture. EGF competitions and soft agar assays were performed as described. **A**, HEL 299; **B**, 9812; **C**, A2058; **D**, A431.

further studies since they have greater specificity. Each of the TGF activities was destroyed by trypsin or dithiothreitol but was stable at 100°C for 2 min and to repeated lyophilization from 1 M acetic acid.

Table 1 shows that the growth-stimulatory factor(s) released by the human tumor cells induce anchorage-independent growth of normal human fibroblasts. Two cell strains were tested; passage 8 of HEL 299 (a human embryonic lung cell line) and the 14th passage of HsF (a skin strain from a normal human adult). A673 cells

FIG. 5. **A.** Soft agar colony formation as a function of protein concentration. Bio-Gel P-100 column fractions from the 20,000–23,000 dalton region were pooled and lyophilized. Aliquots in 0.1 M acetic acid were added with the cells in the soft agar overlay. A673 (○); HEL 299 (×). **B.** plot of the percent of the maximal effect as a function of protein. ³H-thymidine incorporation (×), EGF competition (▲), and soft agar growth assays (○) were performed as described. Maximal response was seen at 25–50 μg of protein; 73,500 cpm and 1,800 cpm, respectively, were incorporated for the ³H-thymidine assays and control plates; 430 colonies were counted per 10 fields, whereas there were no colonies in the control plates for the soft agar growth assay; inhibition of ¹²⁵I-EGF binding was 96%.

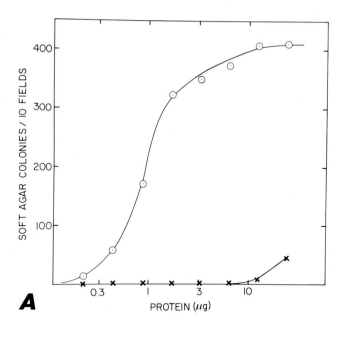

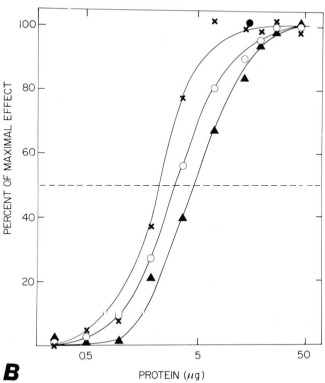

TABLE 1. *Stimulation of growth in agar of human diploid fibroblasts and human tumor cells by TGF*

| | | Colonies >10 cells/1,000 cells | | |
| | | Control | +TGF (10 µg/ml) | +TGF (1 µg/ml) |
Cell	Type			
HEL299	Embryonic lung fibroblast	1	42	3
HsF	Adult skin fibroblast	2	31	2
A431	Epidermoid carcinoma	3	31	8
TE85	Osteosarcoma	1	75	14
NRK (clone 49F)	Rat kidney fibroblasts	0	236	37

were tested at 10 and 1 µg/ml. One $\times$ 10^4 cells were seeded per plate and 1,000 single cells were followed for two weeks. Those that grew to colonies containing 10 cells were scored as positive. The percentages of HEL 299 and HsF single cells that gave rise to colonies were 4.2 and 3.1%, respectively, using 10 µg/ml of P-100 purified TGF. In contrast, 23.6% of the rat fibroblast cells showed a pronounced response even at 1 µg/ml. TGF also induced soft agar growth of the mouse epithelial cell line MMC-1 (8) (data not shown).

In order to test whether human tumor cell lines could also respond to TGFs, cells such as A431, that untreated could not form colonies in agar unless inoculated at high density, were used. Carcinoma cell growth in agar also depends on "conditioning" factors, such as TGFs, which partially replace the requirement for high cell density. The results were more striking when the human osteosarcoma line TE85, which can be further transformed by MSV and certain chemical carcinogens (2), was used as an indicator cell. These results demonstrate that normal and tumor cells respond to TGFs in the same manner as rat fibroblasts. The results, then, are not dependent on an unusual property of a particular indicator cell.

The active fractions from P-100 columns of A673 and A431 cells were pooled, concentrated, and applied to carboxymethyl cellulose columns. Two peaks of agar growth-stimulating activity were obtained from A673 cells; only the major activity was associated with the peak of EGF-competing activity. Dose response curves from each peak show an activity detectable when concentrations of 10 to 20 ng/ml are added to soft agar. The comparable fraction from supernates of the normal human fibroblast showed no activity. Fractions derived from A431 cells showed (Fig. 6) only the less active, earlier eluting peak, which is not associated with EGF-competing activity. We conclude that A431 cells, which grow poorly in agar and have a high level of EGF receptors, produce a factor capable of stimulating anchorage-independent growth of cells through a mechanism independent of the EGF receptor system. The highly transformed A673 cells, however, make at least two different factors. One interacts with the EGF receptor system and accounts for over 90% of the total activity in the fraction. The other is independent of the EGF receptor system and may be analogous to the factor produced by the A431 cells.

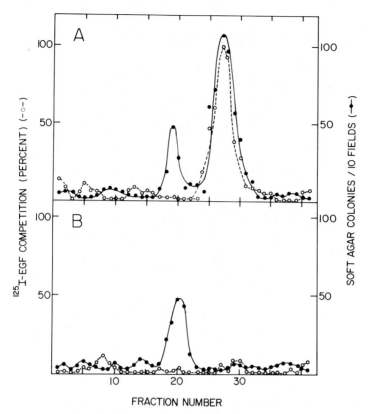

FIG. 6. Chromatography of biological activities in the peak region of Bio-Gel P-100 columns rechromatographed on a carboxymethyl cellulose column. **A**, A673; **B**, A431.

These results demonstrate that human tumor cells produce a growth factor (or factors) capable of inducing transformation in normal indicator cells. It has many properties in common with the factor from mouse and rat sarcoma virus-transformed cells. The major activity, although considerably larger than SGF, is closely associated with EGF-competing activity. We have found that a chemically transformed mouse 3T3 cell line produces growth-stimulating factor(s) active in the soft agar growth assay (unpublished experiments). Production of these factors, then, is not restricted to RNA tumor virus-transformed cells, sarcoma cells or rodent cells, but, rather, may be a more general expression of the transformed phenotype. In assays comparing growth stimulation of mouse, rat, and human fibroblasts in monolayer cultures, there is no evidence for species specificity of the factors produced by human cells. Conclusions as to whether the carcinoma, sarcoma, and melanoma cells are producing an identical factor (or factors) await further chemical purification. The present experiments show that anchorage-independent growth of tumor and normal cells is stimulated by these growth factors. Their production by transformed cells and the responses of their normal counterparts raise the possibility that cells "autostimulate" their growth by releasing factors that rebind at the cell surface (21). Experiments demonstrating that growth in soft agar of tumor cells depends on the number of cells seeded per unit area argue that diffusible substances released by cells stimulate neighboring cells. Those cells that grow best in soft agar are the most efficient producers of transforming peptides. Additional cell lines will have to be tested under different conditions before conclusions can be drawn as to the significance of this association.

Roberts et al. (16) described a procedure for purifying TGFs. The peptides are stable in acidic 70% alcohol. Intracellular growth factors have been extracted from cultured MSV-transformed mouse cells and from tumor cells in athymic mice. The major peptide with soft agar growth-stimulating activity has an apparent molecular weight of 6,700 daltons. The peak of EGF-competing activity is in the same fraction. A transplantable, transitional cell, mouse bladder carcinoma had agar growth-stimulating activity for rat fibroblasts. Ozanne et al. (13) described a transforming factor from Kirsten sarcoma virus-transformed rat fibroblasts with properties like SGF and TGFs and reported a similar activity in a spontaneously transformed rat cell line. The effect of the transforming factor on morphologic transformation can be blocked by actinomycin D early after treatment, suggesting that new RNA is produced prior to the change in phenotype of the indicator cells. Inhibitors of protein synthesis also produce a rapid reversion in the phenotype of the treated cells (13).

If release of the factor and rebinding to EGF receptors is essential for growth stimulation, tumor cell growth could be interrupted by exogenous agents, perhaps analogues that interact with the receptors but do not confer the ability to proliferate under anchorage-independent conditions (19). Anchorage-independent growth is a cell culture property closely associated with the transformed state *in vivo* (10,17). These peptides, then, are potent proximal effectors of cell transformation. Their continued production appears to play a role in maintaining the transformed phenotype. This can be directly demonstrated in temperature-sensitive mutant transformants of rodent cells (13,22) but has not yet been shown for factors produced by human tumor cells. The approach described here offers a sensitive assay for growth-stimulatory factors associated with maintaining the transformed state. Purification of such factors may lead to the development of specific immunologic assays for their production by tumor cells and their presence in body fluids. The factors may be analogous to peptide growth factors expressed early in normal embryonic development (22). This is supported by experiments by Nexo et al. (11). In the mouse embryo (days 11 to 18) there is 5 to 10 times more EGF-like material than mouse EGF. Why the factors produced by transformed cells are so potent in stimulating anchorage-independent growth while EGF is not effective is unclear but suggests the possibility that there may be more "transforming" variants of the normally expressed growth factors produced in adult life. We suggest that these factors, like SGFs, are EGF-related peptides as insulin and somatomedins are related (15), and they appear to have evolved from common ancestral proteins (12). Further purification of these and other growth factors from human tumor cells is needed to define their relationship to other biologically active peptides that cells produce. We are also testing the possibility that certain tumor cells may also produce factors related to the phorbol ester family of growth promoters.

ACKNOWLEDGMENT

The author acknowledges Patricia Ann Johnson for technical information support and editorial assistance in the preparation of this manuscript.

REFERENCES

1. Baltimore, D. (1974): Tumor viruses. *Cold Spring Harbor Symp. Quant. Biol.*, 39:1187–1200.
2. Cho, H. Y., and Rhim, J. S. (1979): Cycloheximide-dependent reversion of human cells transformed by MSV and chemical carcinogen. *Science*, 205:691–693.
3. Cohen, S., and Taylor, J. M. (1974): Epidermal growth factor: chemical and biological characterization. *Recent Prog. Hormone Res.*, 30:533–550.
4. De Larco, J. E., Reynolds, R., Carlberg, K., Engle, C., and Todaro, G. J. (1980): Sarcoma growth factor from mouse sarcoma virus-transformed cells: purification by binding and elution from epidermal growth factor receptor-rich cells. *J. Biol. Chem.*, 255:3685–3690.
5. De Larco, J. E., and Todaro, G. J. (1978): Growth factors from murine sarcoma virus-transformed cells. *Proc. Natl. Acad. Sci. U.S.A.*, 75:4001–4005.
6. De Larco, J. E., and Todaro, G. J. (1980): Sarcoma growth factor: specific binding to and elution from epidermal growth factor membrane receptors. *Cold Spring Harbor Symp. Quant. Biol.*, 44:643–649.
7. Gospodarowicz, D., and Moran, J. S. (1976): Growth factors in mammalian cell culture. *Ann. Rev. Biochem.*, 45:531–558.
8. Keski-Oja, J., De Larco, J. E., Rapp, U. R., and Todaro, G. J. (1980): Murine sarcoma growth factors affect the growth and morphology of cultured mouse epithelial cells. *J. Cell. Physiol.*, 104:41–46.
9. Lowry, O. H., Rosebrough, N. J., Farr, A. L., and Randall, R. J. (1951): Protein measurement with the folin phenol reagent. *J. Biol. Chem.*, 193:265–275.
10. Montesano, R., Drevon, C., Kuroki, T., Saint Vincent, L., Handelman, S., Sanford, K. K., DeFeo, D., and Weinstein, I. B. (1977): Test for malignant transformation of rat liver cells in culture: cytology, growth in soft agar, and production of plasminogen activator. *J. Natl. Cancer Inst.*, 59:1651–1658.
11. Nexo, E., Hollenberg, M. D., Figueroa, A., and Pratt, R. M. (1980): Detection of epidermal growth factor-urogastrone and its receptor during fetal mouse development. *Proc. Natl. Acad. Sci. U.S.A.*, 77:2782–2785.
12. Niall, H. D. (1977): Evolution of structure and function in natural peptides. In: *Peptides: Proceedings of the Fifth American Peptide Symposium,* edited by G. Goodman, and J. Meienhofer, pp. 127–135. Halsted Press, New York.
13. Ozanne, B., Fulton, J., and Kaplan, P. L. (1980): Kirsten murine sarcoma virus transformed cell lines and a spontaneously transformed rat cell-line produce transforming factors. *J. Cell. Physiol.*, 105:163–180.
14. Rinderknecht, E., and Humbel, R. E. (1976): Amino-terminal sequences of two polypeptides from human serum with nonsuppressive insulin-like and cell-growth-promoting activities: evidence for structural homology with insulin B chain. *Proc. Natl. Acad. Sci. U.S.A.*, 73:4379–4381.
15. Rinderknecht, E., and Humbel, R. E. (1978): The amino acid sequence of human insulin-like growth factor I and its structural homology with proinsulin. *J. Biol. Chem.*, 253:2769–2776.
16. Roberts, A. B., Lamb, L. C., Newton, D. L., Sporn, M. B., De Larco, J. E., and Todaro, G. J. (1980): Transforming growth factors: isolation of polypeptides from virally and chemically transformed cells by acid/ethanol extraction. *Proc. Natl. Acad. Sci. U.S.A.*, 77:3494–3498.
17. Shin, S., Freedman, V. H., Risser, R., and Pollack, R. (1975): Tumorigenicity of virus-transformed cells in nude mice is correlated specifically with anchorage-independent growth in vitro. *Proc. Natl. Acad. Sci. U.S.A.*, 72:4435–4439.
18. Spector, D. H., Smith, K., Padgett, T., McCombe, P., Roulland-Dussoix, D., Moscovici, C., Varmus, H. E., and Bishop, J. M. (1978): Uninfected avian cells contain RNA related to the transforming gene of avian sarcoma viruses. *Cell*, 13:371–379.

19. Sporn, M. B., Newton, D. L., Roberts, A. B., De Larco, J. E., and Todaro, G. J. (1981): Retinoids and the suppression of the effects of polypeptide transforming factors—A new molecular approach to chemoprevention of cancer. In: *Molecular Actions and Targets for Cancer Chemotherapeutic Agents*, edited by A. C. Sartorelli, J. R. Bertino, and J. S. Lazo. Academic Press, New York *(in press)*.

20. Stehelin, D., Varmus, H. E., Bishop, J. M., and Vogt, P. K. (1976): DNA related to the transforming gene(s) of avian sarcoma virus is present in normal avian DNA. *Nature*, 260:170–173.

21. Todaro, G. J., and De Larco, J. E. (1978): Growth factors produced by sarcoma virus-transformed cells. *Cancer Res.*, 38:4147–4154.

22. Todaro, G. J., and De Larco, J. E. (1980): Properties of sarcoma growth factors (SGFs) produced by mouse sarcoma virus-transformed cells in culture. In: *Control Mechanisms in Animal Cells: Specific Growth Factors*, edited by L. Jimenez de Asua, R. Levi-Montalcini, R. Shields, and S. Iacobelli, Vol. 1, pp. 223–243. Raven Press, New York.

23. Todaro, G. J., De Larco, J. E., and Cohen, S. (1976): Transformation by murine and feline sarcoma viruses specifically blocks binding of epidermal growth factor (EGF) to cells. *Nature*, 264:26–31.

24. Todaro, G. J., De Larco, J. E., Nissley, S. P., and Rechler, M. M. (1977): MSA and EGF receptors on sarcoma virus transformed cells and human fibrosarcoma cells in culture. *Nature*, 267:526–528.

25. Todaro, G. J., and Huebner, R. J. (1972): The viral oncogene hypothesis: new evidence. *Proc. Natl. Acad. Sci. U.S.A.*, 69:1009–1015.

Maturation Factors and Cancer,
edited by Malcolm A. S. Moore.
Raven Press, © New York 1982.

Role of the Thymosins as Immunomodulating Agents and Maturation Factors

Teresa L. K. Low and Allan L. Goldstein

Department of Biochemistry, The George Washington University School of Medicine and Health Sciences, Washington, D.C. 20037

The importance of the thymus to cell-mediated immunity (CMI) was first demonstrated in 1961 by Miller (96) and Good (58). Subsequent studies by many investigators (11,57,97,127,145) led to the understanding of the essential role of thymus in the development, growth, and function of lymphoid system and in the maintenance of immune balance. Investigations of the *in vivo* and *in vitro* effects of thymic extracts (31,66,67,72,73) and the effects of thymus grafts in cell impermeable millipore diffusion chambers (79,102,134) have established the endocrine function of the thymus.

Previous studies demonstrated that a partially purified thymic extract termed thymosin fraction 5 was effective in partially or fully reconstituting immune functions in thymic-deprived or immunodeprived animals (14,36,60,71,115,124,148), as well as in humans with immunodeficiency diseases and cancer (28,30,52,80, 112,113,138,139). Furthermore, ongoing studies (87) indicate that there are several chemically distinct biologically active peptides within fraction 5 that act on various pre-T and T-cell subpopulations to maintain normal immunological reactivity. A number of other laboratories have also succeeded in isolating and purifying factors with thymic hormone-like activity from thymus tissue (5,20,55,68,74,82,89,92,93,98), blood (8,14,25), and thymic epithelial cell cultures (70,76). Most thymic factors reported are of a protein nature.

Since patients with primary immunodeficiency diseases and neoplastic diseases frequently manifest abnormalities in both T-cell number and function, agents which restore normal T-cell physiology, such as thymic hormones, have been used in an attempt to restore immune competence. To date, a number of clinical trials, with thymosin and other thymic preparations, have been reported.

Although most clinical trials with thymic hormones cannot be critically evaluated at present, since either the number of treated patients was too small to permit proper statistical analysis of the finding, or subjects receiving placebo were not included. Nevertheless, the positive results with thymosin in immunodeficient children (49,138–140) and patients with oat cell carcinoma (28,30,80), as well as studies with other thymic preparations (4,5,34,59,68,81,135) offer a strong rationale for rapidly confirming the clinical studies and expanding the basic research program with thymic hormones.

In this chapter, we will discuss our recent progress in chemical and biological studies of thymosin. In addition, we will summarize the properties of other thymic preparations. Finally, we will review the therapeutic applications of thymosin.

PREPARATION AND BIOLOGICAL STUDIES OF FACTORS WITH THYMIC HORMONE-LIKE ACTIVITY

Beginning as early as 1896 with the report by Abelous and Billard (1), describing restoration of muscle tone in thymectomized frogs given crude thymic extracts, and continuing today, many investigators have attempted to isolate putative thymic hormones and have examined effects of a variety of thymic extracts in both normal and thymectomized animals (43,44,46,84,127,144). A chronological list of some thymic extracts and their reported biological effects has been given by Low and Goldstein (84). In the following sections, the chemistry and biology of thymosin, as well as some of the other better studied thymic factors, will be described in some detail.

From Thymus

Thymosin

A lymphocytopoietic factor in rat and mouse thymus extracts was first described in 1965 (72,73). A stable form containing the biologically active fraction was isolated from calf thymic tissue in 1966 and was termed thymosin (45). In 1972, after further fractionation of the crude extract, the preparation and characterization of a more purified fraction was achieved (47). In 1975, the isolation procedure was modified in order to prepare larger quantities of the partially purified preparation termed thymosin fraction 5 (61) for clinical trials.

Isolation and Chemical Characterization of Thymosin Partially Purified Preparations: Thymosin Fractions 5 and 5A

Thymosin fractions 5 and 5A are prepared from calf thymus, as outlined in Fig. 1 (88). The preparations are obtained by homogenization of thymus tissue, followed by an 80° C heat denaturation step, an acetone precipitation step, an ammonium sulfate precipitation step, and finally, an ultrafiltration step. An analytical isoelectric focusing gel of thymosin fraction 5 in the pH range of 3.5 to 9.5 has revealed the presence of a number of components. To facilitate the identification and comparison of all the thymic peptides, we have proposed (51) a nomenclature based on the isoelectric pattern of thymosin fraction 5. As shown in Fig. 2, the separated peptides are divided into three regions: the α region, which consists of peptides with pI below 5; the β region, 5.0 to 7.0; and the γ region, above 7.0. The subscripts

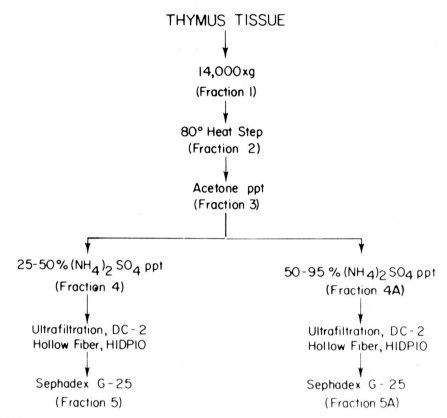

FIG. 1. Purification of bovine thymosin fractions 5 and 5A. One kg of thymus tissue homogenized in 3 liters of saline solution provides the sample to initiate the procedure. (From Low et al., ref. 88.)

($_{1,2,3,4}$, etc) are used to identify the peptides from that region as they are isolated. For comparative purposes, other well-defined thymic factors, such as thymic humoral factor (THF), facteur thymique serique (FTS), and thymopoietin are also included in the figure. They are directed on the thymosin fraction 5 gel pattern based on their reported isoelectric points. Thymosin fraction 5A appears to contain mostly the β region peptides and very few peptides from the α region (T. L. K. Low and A. L. Goldstein, unpublished data). So far, most of our biological studies and all of our clinical studies have been carried out using thymosin fraction 5, since this preparation appears to possess a wide spectrum of biological activities. From the limited biological data that we have, fraction 5A is not active in some bioassays, indicating that it is devoid of some biologically active components. Nevertheless, since fraction 5A is enriched in β region peptides, it appears that this fraction is a better source for isolation of β region peptides, such as $β_1$ (51) or $β_4$ (T. L. K. Low and A. L. Goldstein, unpublished data).

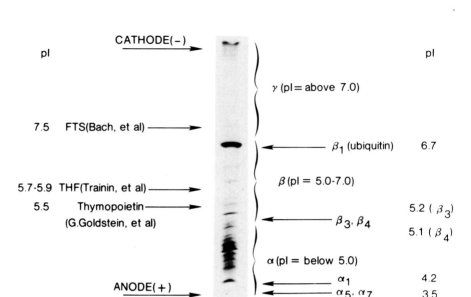

FIG. 2. Isoelectric focusing of thymosin fraction 5 in LKB PAG$_{plate}$ (pH 3.5–9.5). Purified thymosin peptides from the α, β, and γ regions are identified. The isoelectric points of several other well-characterized thymic factors are illustrated for comparison.

Purified Components of Thymosin Fraction 5

Thymosin α$_1$

The first thymosin polypeptide isolated from fraction 5 has been termed thymosin α$_1$ (51,85,88). This peptide is very active in several bioassay systems (88), including the human E-rosette assay (139), macrophage migration inhibitory factor (MIF) assay (125), murine Lyt 1,2,3 induction and helper cell assay (2,3), and *in vitro* TdT (terminal deoxynucleotidyl transferase) suppression assay (64). The amino acid sequence of thymosin α$_1$ has been elucidated (51,85) and is shown in Fig. 3. It is composed of 28 amino acid residues with an isoelectric point of 4.2 and a molecular weight of 3,108. The N-terminal end of the molecule is blocked by an acetyl group. The yield of thymosin α$_1$ from fraction 5 is about 0.6%.

Thymosin α$_1$ has been chemically synthesized by several laboratories, including that of Wang and co-workers (136,137), Bier and Stollenwerk (22), and Folkers (39), using both solution and solid-phase procedures. The synthetic material prepared by Wang et al. (136) has been tested by *in vitro* MIF, E-rosette, and TdT suppression assays, and *in vivo*, both experimentally and clinically, and appears to have an activity similar to the natural material. Recently, Wetzel et al. (143) have accomplished the synthesis of N^α-desacetyl thymosin α$_1$, utilizing recombinant DNA

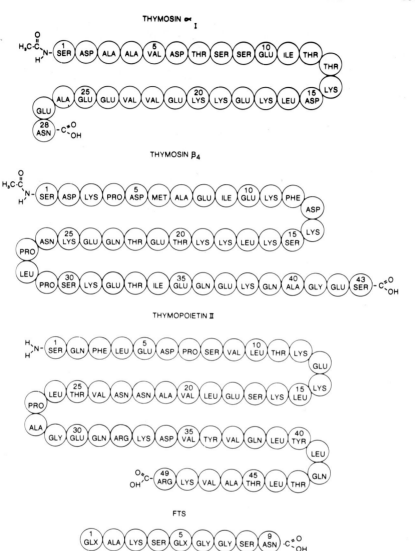

FIG. 3. Sequence analysis of well-characterized thymic hormones: thymosin α_1 (85), thymosin β_4 (86), thymopoietin II (116), and facteur thymique serique (FTS) (35).

techniques. The purified material was shown to exhibit activity similar to the natural α_1 in MIF and TdT suppression assays.

Thymosin α_1 from other species

To evaluate the species variation of thymosin polypeptides, we have prepared fraction 5 from thymus tissues of different species including human, pig, sheep, chinchilla, and mouse. The human thymus tissue was excised during open heart surgery and from selected autopsies. Thymosin α_1, from several animal species, was prepared from fraction 5, using a modification of the extraction and fractionation procedures developed for the isolation of bovine α_1. Human (84), porcine, and ovine (T. L. K. Low et al., unpublished data) thymosin α_1 have also been partially sequenced. From the results obtained, they appear to have an identical sequence to bovine α_1.

Thymosin α_7

This peptide was isolated from fraction 5 by ion-exchange chromatography on CM-cellulose and DEAE-cellulose and gel filtration on Sephadex G-75 (T. L. K. Low and A. L. Golstein, unpublished results). The peptides are highly acidic, with isoelectric points around 3.5, and a molecular weight of 2,200.

Polypeptide β_1

The predominant band on isoelectric focusing of thymosin fraction 5 is poly-peptide β_1 (Fig. 2). This peptide was isolated from fraction 5A by chromatography on DEAE-cellulose and gel filtration on Sephadex G-75 (88). The amino acid sequence of β_1 has been determined (85). It is composed of 74 amino acid residues with molecular weight 8,451 and isoelectric point 6.7. It is believed that this peptide is not involved in thymic hormone action, based on the observation that this peptide was not active in any of our assay systems. The sequence of β_1 was found to be identical to ubiquitin (117). It has been postulated that ubiquitin is a degradative product of protein A24, a nuclear chromosomal protein (65). Furthermore, a non-histone protein of trout testis chromatin was found to have a sequence identical to ubiquitin (141).

Most recently, Wilkinson et al. (147) provided evidence that ATP-dependent proteolysis factor 1 (APF-1) of rabbit reticulocytes is ubiquitin. Thus, although polypeptide β_1 (or ubiquitin) is not involved in thymic hormone action, it is likely that this peptide is an essential component of the ATP-dependent system in retic-ulocytes and possibly in degradation and proteolytic processing in other cells.

Thymosin β_3 and β_4

Both preparations were isolated from fraction 5 by chromatography on CM-cellulose and gel filtration on Sephadex G-50 (86, T. L. K. Low and A. L. Gold-stein, unpublished results). They were found to induce terminal deoxynucleotidyl transferase positive cells (63,105). Thymosin β_3 has an isoelectric point of 5.2 and a molecular weight of approximately 5,500. Thymosin β_4 has an isoelectric point of 5.1 and a molecular weight of 4,982. The amino acid sequence of thymosin β_4 has recently been elucidated (86) and is shown in Fig. 3.

Biological Activities of Thymosin

As summarized in Table 1, thymosin fraction 5 has been found to induce T-cell differentiation and enhance immunologic functions in genetically athymic mice (124), in adult thymectomized mice (14,124), in NZB mice with autoimmune reactions (36,124), in tumor-bearing mice (60,148), and in mice with casein-induced amyloidosis (115). Thymosin fraction 5 is also effective in inducing the differentiation of specific subclasses of T lymphocytes (helper and suppressor cells) (36,90,115,121,124), certain cell markers (TdT, Thy-1, and Lyt) (2,3,104), and functional expressions of lymphocyte maturation (29,87,125).

Also shown in Table 1 are the biological properties of purified thymosin components. Thymosin α_1 is active in a mouse mitogen assay (123), a MIF assay (125), a human E-rosette assay (139), the surface marker assay (2), and the TdT suppression assay (64). Thymosin α_7 is capable of expressing Lyt 1,2,3 positive cells (2). It also induces T cells with suppressive functions. Thymosin β_3 and β_4 can induce TdT expression in bone marrow cells (105) and thymocytes of immunosuppressed mice (64).

Thymic Humoral Factor

Using assays of lymphocytopoiesis induction and immune reconstitution in normal and thymectomized mice, Trainin and co-workers (128,129) have isolated from sheep, calf, and rabbit thymuses active factors which they named thymic humoral factor (THF). The molecule was determined to be a heat stable polypeptide with a pI of 5.7 to 5.9 and a molecular weight of around 3,000. It has been reported (132) that this molecule is composed of 31 amino acid residues. However, its primary structure has not been delineated.

THF was shown to increase the cytotoxic reactivity of lymphoid cells against syngeneic tumors *in vitro* and *in vivo* (26,133). It was also shown to restore cellular graft versus host (GvH) reactivity and the ability of spleen cells from neonatal thymectomized mice to produce a primary immune response to sheep red blood cells (83,131,132).

Thymopoietin

Thymopoietin was first isolated by G. Goldstein (54,56) and was initially named thymin. The preparation of this peptide was an outgrowth of experimental studies related to the human disease myasthenia gravis. This disease is characterized by a deficit in neuromuscular transmission and thymic malfunction (56). Based on the impairment of neuromuscular transmission with thymin, the neuromuscular blocking substance was isolated from thymus tissue and was renamed thymopoietin (55). It can also induce differentiation of bone marrow cells to T cells *in vitro* and, hence, has been claimed to be a putative thymic hormone. Thymopoietin has a molecular weight of 5,562 daltons and a pI of 5.5. The sequence of this molecule has been established (116) (Fig. 3). It is composed of 49 amino acid residues.

TABLE 1. *Some biological properties of thymosin fraction 5 and its component polypeptides*

Thymosin Fraction 5

In vitro enhancement of:
   Number of azathioprine-sensitive E-rosette forming spleen cells from adult, thymec-
      tomized mice
   Appearance of phenotypic T-cell markers on mouse spleen and bone marrow cells
   Responsivity to mitogens
   Mixed lymphocyte reaction
   Conversion of bone marrow cells into cells reactive in the graft vs host reaction *in vivo*
   Production of suppressor T cells
   Production of macrophage inhibitory factor
   Production of antibody to sheep erythrocytes by spleen cells of normal and thymec-
      tomized mice
   Intracellular cyclic GMP levels of mouse spleen cells
   Terminal deoxynucleotidyl transferase (TdT) activity
   Specific antibody production to tetanous, meningococcal, and gonococcal antigens

In vivo enhancement of:
   Lymphocytopoiesis in normal, germ-free, adrenalectomized, neonatally thymecto-
      mized, and athymic mice
   Rate of allograft rejection in normal and neonatally thymectomized mice
   Resistance to progressive growth of Moloney virus-induced sarcoma in normal mice
   Mixed lymphocyte reaction (*in vivo-in vitro*) by lymphoid cells from normal or neonatally
      thymectomized mice
   Lymphoid cell response to mitogens (*in vivo-in vitro*) by cells of normal and athymic
      mice
   Resistance to growth of allogeneic and xenogeneic tumors in athymic mice
   Delay of abnormal thymocyte differentiation (loss of suppressor function) in NZB mice
   Antibody production to sheep erythrocytes (*in vivo* + *in vitro*)
   Survival in tumor bearing mice (in conjunction with chemotherapy)
   Interferon production following viral challenge

Thymosin α_1

In vitro enhancement of:
   Numbers of E-rosette-forming cells in cancer patients
   Percentage of autologous rosette-forming cells in cancer patients
   Secondary T-cell dependent IgG, IgM, and IgA antibody responses
   Percentage of macrophage inhibitory factor (MIF)
   Expression of Thy 1.2 and Lyt 1,2,3 positive cells
   T-cell dependent specific antibody production
   Helper T cells activity
   TdT$^+$ cells in the bone marrow and spleen (at high concentrations of thymosin α_1)

In vitro suppression of:
   TdT activity in murine thymocytes at low concentrations
   Elevated Tγ/Tμ ratios in peripheral blood of cancer patients

In vivo enhancement of:
   Lymphoid cell responses to mitogens (*in vivo* + *in vitro*)
   Lymphotoxin production (*in vivo* + *in vitro*)
   Survival in tumor bearing mice

Thymosin α_7

In vitro enhancement of:
   Suppressor T cells
   Expression of Lyt 1,2,3 positive cells

Thymosin β_3 *and* β_4

In vitro and *in vivo* induction of TdT in separated bone marrow cells from normal or
   athymic mice
In vivo induction of TdT levels in thymocytes of immunosuppressed mice
In vivo reconstitution of immune responses in immunosuppressed mice

Chemical synthesis of a tridecapeptide of thymopoietin (residues 29–41) has been reported (118). This molecule was found to have 3% activity by comparison with thymopoietin in inducing the differentiation of T lymphocytes. The synthesis of the entire molecule of thymopoietin was reported by Fujino and co-workers (40) in Japan using the conventional liquid phase coupling method. The synthetic material was found to induce Thy-1 on prothymocytes. However, the biologic evaluation and activity confirmation for the synthetic preparation *in vivo* has not been studied. Most recently, Bliznakov et al. (23) also reported the total synthesis of thymopoietin by solid-phase methodology on a Beckman 990 peptide synthesizer. It was found that the suppression of the primary hemolysin immune response in old mice was partially reversed by the subcutaneous administration of the synthetic material. However, no natural thymopoietin was employed for comparison in these studies.

Other Thymic Extracts

The preparation of other thymic extracts, such as thymic factor X (TFX), thymostimulin (TS), bovine and porcine thymic preparations, homeostatic thymic hormone (HTH), lymphocytopoietic factors (LSH_h and LSH_r), hypocalcemic and lymphocytopoietic substance (TP_1 and TP_2), thymic polypeptide preparation (TP), and thymosterin have been reported by various laboratories. Table 2 summarizes their reported chemical and biological properties.

From Blood

Facteur Thymique Serique (FTS)

Following their studies with Goldstein and White showing thymosin induction of theta (Θ) antigen and increase in azathioprine sensitivity in rosette-forming T cells (RFC) from adult thymectomized mice (13), Bach and co-workers isolated a serum factor from normal mouse and human serum (14). They named this isolate circulating thymic factor (TF). Recently, this factor has been purified and the amino acid sequence determined (Fig. 3) (16,35), and it has been renamed the facteur thymique serique (FTS). This molecule was reported to be stable at 37° C for 8 hr and is relatively pH resistant. FTS has been shown to enhance mitogen response in cells of nude mice *in vitro* (111), to induce suppressor T cells in NZB mice (12), and to normalize the abnormally high level of autologous erythrocyte-binding cells in adult thymectomized mice (27).

FTS was chemically synthesized using solid-phase techniques (91). The synthetic peptide was reported (13) to be active in the rosette assay, resembling natural FTS. When given *in vivo* for 2 months, it is also active in normalizing the abnormally high level of autologous erythrocyte-binding cells in adult thymectomized mice, and in enhancing the *in vitro* generation of alloantigen-reactive T cells (13). Bliznakov et al. (23) also reported the synthesis of FTS and a dodecapeptide analogue of FTS (Val-Lys-Arg-Gln-Ala-Lys-Ser-Gln-Gly-Gly-Ser-Asn-Asn) on a Beckman

TABLE 2. *Thymic preparations and their biological effects*

Thymic peparations	Principal investigators	Chemical properties	Biological effects	References
		I. *From Thymus Tissue*		
Thymosin fraction 5	Hooper, A. Goldstein et al.	Family of heat stable, acidic polypeptides, MW 1,000–15,000	Induces T-cell differentiation and enhances immunological function in animal models and in humans	48,53,62,84, 87,90,141
Thymosin α₁	Low, A. Goldstein et al.	Polypeptide of 28 residues MW 3,108, pI 4.2, sequence determined	Increases mitogenic responsiveness of murine lymphocytes; induces enhancement of MIF production; increases Thy 1.2 and Lyt 1,2,3 positive cells and helper T cells; modulates TdT activity	2,64,88,125
Thymosin β₄	Low, A. Goldstein et al	Polypeptide of 43 residues, MW 4,982, pI 5.1, sequence determined	Induces TdT *in vivo* and *in vitro* in bone marrow cells from normal and athymic mice; *in vivo* induction of TdT in thymocytes of immuno-suppressed mice	63,105
Thymosin α₇	Low, A. Goldstein et al.	Acidic polypeptide, MW 2,500 pI ~ 3.5	*In vitro* enhancement of suppressor T cells; expression of Lyt 1,2,3 positive cells	2,3
Thymic humoral factor (THF)	Trainin et al.	Polypeptide of MW 3,200, pI 5.7, amino acid composition determined	Restoration of ability of spleen cells from neonatally thymectomized donors to induce an *in vivo* graft vs host reaction; enhancement of ability of normal spleen cells to respond to PHA and Con A	26,127,128, 129,130, 132,133
Thymopoietin	G. Goldstein et al.	Polypeptide of 49 residues, MW 5,562, pI 5.5, sequence determined	Causes delayed impairment of neuromuscular transmission *in vivo*; induces bone marrow cells to develop intrathymic lymphocytes	41,54–56,69, 114,122,142
Thymic polypeptide preparation (TP)	Milcu, Potop et al.	Mixture of polypeptides and amino acids	Elevation of serum calcium concentration and decrease in serum inorganic phosphate; stimulation of antibody synthesis in immunized, x-ray irradiated rabbits	92,93
Thymosterin	Potop et al.	Lipids or lipoproteins, one purified component termed IIB₃ is C₂₈ steroid with methyl groups at C-21 and C-28	Antiproliferative action on KB tumor cells in culture; repairs the specifically altered metabolism of normal or thymectomized tumor-bearing animals	94,95,106,107
		II. *From Blood*		
Facteur thymique serique (FTS)	Bach, Dardenne et al.	Nonapeptide. MW 857, pI 7.5, sequence determined	Enhancement of the generation of effector cytotoxic T cells both in *in vitro* and *in vivo*; inhibition of contact sensitivity in normal mice	17,18,24,3, 15,37

Name	Author	Characterization	Biological activity	Ref.
Protein fraction from human plasma	White et al.	Protein MW 57,700, properties analogous to prealbumin	Enhances ability of neonatally thymectomized mice to reject an allogeneic skin graft, enhances MLR of mouse spleen cells incubated with the blood fraction	25
Human serum factor (SF)	Astaldi et al	Adenosine (possibly other small molecular weight components)	Increases the intracellular cyclic AMP level of human and mouse thymocytes; increases the population of hydrocortisone-resistant cells	7,8,9,146

III. *From Thymic Epithelial Supernatants*

Name	Author	Characterization	Biological activity	Ref.
Thymic epithelial supernatant (TES)	Kruisbeek et al.	Crude extract, chemical nature not characterized	Augments the proliferative responses of rat thymocytes to PHA or Con A; stimulates mixed lymphocyte reactivity and antibody production to sheep erythrocytes by spleen cells from nude mice	75,76,77
Human thymic epithelial medium (HTEM)	Kater et al.	Crude extract, chemical nature not clear	Augments the mitogen responsiveness of thymocytes	70
Thymic factor X (TFX)	Aleksandrowicz, Skotnicki et al.	Polypeptide, MW 4,200, amino acid composition reported	*In vitro* restoration of the azathioprine sensitivity of spleen rosette-forming cells from adult thymectomized mice; *in vivo* increase in blood T-cell number and return of delayed hypersensitivity	5,120
Thymostimulin (TS)	Falchetti et al.	Mixture of polypeptides	Induced markers and specific functions of T lymphocytes both in immunosuppressed animals and in immunodeficient patients; stimulated interferon production in mice following challenge with Poly I : Poly C	4,21,38, 108,126
Porcine thymic preparation	Jin et al.	Mixture of polypeptides, MW 9,000–68,000, pI 5.0–7.5	Increased rosette formation in fetal thymocytes	68
Bovine thymic preparation	Liu et al.	Mixture of polypeptides	Increased rosette formation in umbilical cord blood lymphocytes	81,82
Homeostatic thymic hormone (HTH)	Comsa et al.	Glycopeptide, MW 1,800–2,500	Suppression of deleterious consequences of thymectomy in young guinea pigs; restoration of delayed hypersensitivity of thymectomized rats	20,32,33
Lymphocytopoietic factors (LSH_h and LSH_r)	Luckéy et al.	Polypeptides, MW 80,000 (LSH_r) and 15,000 (LSH_h); amino acid composition of LSH_r is available	Enhances antibody production to sheep erythrocytes and induces a lymphocytosis	89
Hypocalcemic and lymphocytopoietic substances (TP_1 and TP_2)	Mizutani et al.	Polypeptides	Enhances production of antibody to sheep erythrocytes in neonatal mice; hypocalcemic activity in normal rabbits	98,99,100, 101

990 peptide synthesizer. Both synthetic peptides were found to reverse the marked suppression of the primary humoral hemolysin immune response in old mice.

Protein Fraction from Human Plasma

Using the azathioprine-rosette assay, White and his colleagues isolated an active protein component from human plasma (25). The mobility of this fraction, its amino acid composition, amino terminal end group analysis, as well as its subunit structure, were all identical with prealbumin. No chemical relationship of prealbumin to FTS is apparent.

Thymus-dependent Human Serum Factor (SF)

Astaldi and his colleagues (8) demonstrated the presence in human serum of a thymus-dependent factor which they designated as SF. This factor was characterized by its ability to increase the intracellular cyclic AMP level of human and mouse thymocytes when the cells were incubated with human serum. SF activity appears to be due to a molecule with molecular weight 500. Most recently, it has been reported that the molecule responsible for stimulating cAMP in this fraction is adenosine (A. Astaldi, personal communication).

From Thymic Epithelial Supernatants

Kater and colleagues (70) reported the preparation of thymic hormonelike activity from cell-free supernatant of thymic epithelial cell cultures, which they termed HTEM (human thymus epithelium media). Kruisbeck et al. (76) also reported the preparation of active thymic epithelial culture supernatants, which were termed TES. Both HTEM and TES augment the mitogen responsiveness of thymocytes. TES also shows a stimulatory effect on mixed lymphocyte reactivity and on antibody production to sheep erythrocytes by nu/nu mouse spleen cells. Most recently, it was found that TES can induce alloreactive and H-2 restricted cytotoxic T lymphocyte responses in PNA^+ thymocytes (77).

THERAPEUTIC APPLICATIONS OF THYMOSINS

Thymosin fraction 5 has been utilized in the largest number of clinical trials to date. The patients who have been treated with thymosin include those with a variety of disorders such as immunodeficiency and autoimmune diseases, as well as cancer. We will review results of the initial clinical trials with thymosin in the following sections.

Immunodeficiency Patients

Over 100 children have received thymosin fraction 5 for primary immunodeficiency diseases (19,42,49,50,109,119,138–140). Most of the patients have received 60 mg/m^2 thymosin by subcutaneous injection. There was a close correlation between the number of patients who responded *in vitro* in the E-rosette assay and those patients who have also responded *in vivo* with increased absolute T-cell numbers and clinical improvements. In recent studies, Barrett et al. (19) and Wara et al. (140) have found that good correlation between changes in MLC with thymosin can be used as an indicator of the *in vivo* efficacy of thymosin to enhance T-cell function.

Autoimmune Disorders

Six patients with autoimmune diseases have been treated with thymosin fraction 5 (78). Five of the patients had systemic lupus erythematosus (SLE), and the sixth rheumatoid arthritis. Significant changes in peripheral blood T-cell and null cell percentages and a major decrease in a cytotoxic serum factor that is present in many patients with autoimmune diseases were seen.

Phase I and Phase II Cancer Trials

More than 200 cancer patients have been treated according to Phase I or Phase II protocols. No major side effects have been seen in the majority of patients treated with thymosin fraction 5.

Phase I trials of thymosin in cancer patients were first initiated in 1974 at the University of Texas Medical Branch in Galveston. Greater than 75% of the Phase I cancer patients who responded to thymosin *in vitro* have shown increased numbers of T cells following thymosin treatment (52,111–113). Furthermore, the first efficacy trial of thymosin has now been completed in patients with nonresectable small cell carcinoma of the lungs by P. B. Chretien and M. Cohen and their associates at the National Cancer Institute and the V.A. Hospital in Washington, D.C. (28,30,80). In this trial, thymosin fraction 5 was found to significantly prolong the survival of cancer patients when given in conjunction with intensive chemotherapy. Thymosin effects in cancer patients might be due to an increase in mature T cells, which would then enhance endogenous antitumor activity. In addition, thymosin may function in immunosuppressed cancer patients to increase T-cell reactivity and thus help in reducing the high incidence of infection that often accompanies treatment with radiotherapy and chemotherapy. Table 3 summarizes the clinical trials of thymosin.

PERSPECTIVES

Our ongoing basic research on the chemical characterization of thymosin has demonstrated that thymosin fraction 5 is a mixture of many components. Since fraction 5 is prepared from a homogenate of the whole thymus tissue, we postulate that there are three classes of peptides existing in the fraction 5 preparation: One class of peptides is the product of thymic epithelial cells, which should be termed thymic hormones; the second class of peptides is produced by thymocytes, which are more likely to be lymphokines; the third class of peptides are tissue products and are not thymic specific.

TABLE 3. Current status of therapeutic applications of thymosin

Type of disorder (agent used)	No. of patients	Treatment duration	Immunological/clinical results	References
Immunodeficiency diseases (Thymosin fraction 5)				
Immunodeficient children	82	1 week–5 years	Increase in T-cell numbers, mitogenic and MLC responsiveness, decreased infections	139,49,109,42, 138,10,19,140, 119,50
Chronic mucocutaneous candidiasis	4	6 months	Increase in PBL responses in MLC; one patient had marked clearing of cutaneous candidiasis	138
Ataxia-telangiectasia	3	6–12 months	One patient had increase in PBL responses to PHA and in MLC; two patients remained stable	138
Wiskott-Aldrich syndrome	3	6–30 months	All had increased total T-cell numbers; one increased in PBL response to PHA and two increased in MLC response; all had clinical improvements	138
Severe combined immunodeficiency disease	1	5 months	No immunological or clinical improvement	138
DiGeorge syndrome	2	20 days–3 months	One had no immunological or clinical improvement; the other had increased T cells and PBL responses to PHA and in MLC	138
Thymic hypoplasia	2	6–33 months	One had increased T-cell numbers and PBL responses to PHA and in MLC; however, therapy discontinued due to complication; the other had increased T-cell numbers and general clinical improvement	138
Acquired hypogammaglobulinemia	1	18 months	Total T-cell number increased; clinically stable	138
Cartilage hair hypoplasia	1		No significant alteration in T-cell function	138
DiGeorge syndrome	5		Three patients who responded in vitro (MLC) also responded in vivo	19

Disease	No.	Dose	Duration	Results	Ref.
DiGeorge syndrome Thymic hypoplasia and nucleoside phosphorylase	1 1		9 months	Improvement of cellular immunity; Increased % E-RFC and total T cells; increased PHA and MLC responses; therapy discontinued due to systemic type 1 reactions	119 6
Adenosine deaminase deficiency and combined immunodeficiency	1			Improved clinical course when given with red-cell transfusions; improvement immunologically	110

Autoimmune diseases (Thymosin fraction 5)

Disease	No.	Dose	Duration	Results	Ref.
Systemic lupus erythematosus and rheumatoid arthritis	5 1		4–16 months	Significant changes in peripheral blood T-cell and null cell percentages; major decrease in a cytotoxic serum factor	78

Cancer Trials

Disease	No.	Dose	Duration	Results	Ref.
Oat cell carcinoma of the lung (Phase II) (Thymosin fraction 5)	55		2 years	Patients receiving 60 mg/m^2 (21 patients) had prolonged survival rate over placebo (19) or low dose (20 mg/m^2) (15 patients) thymosin treatment	28,30,80
Brain tumors, anaplastic gliomas (synthetic thymosin α_1 vs thymosin fraction 5, phase I)	3 (60 mg/m^2 fraction 5) 4 (900 μg/m^2 α_1) 5 (600 μg/m^2 α_1) 2 (300 μg/m^2 α_1)			No clinical or hematological toxic effects noted with α_1 therapy; increase in T cells and α_2 HS glycoprotein	Dr. A Ommaya, Natl. Institute of Neurological Diseases, and Dr. P. Chretien, Natl. Cancer Inst.
Stage III B melanoma (thymosin fraction 5)	28 (4 or 40 mg/m^2)			High dose thymosin treatment improved disease-free survival of the immunoincompetent group; immunocompetent patients relapsed earlier with high dose thymosin plus BCG than those treated with low dose thymosin and BCG	103

The isolation and purification of several components in fraction 5 provide the opportunity for the study of the biological activity of individual components. Thymosin α_1 has shown great activity in many of our assay systems and should be termed a thymic hormone. However, this peptide is not active in some other assays in which fraction 5 is active, indicating that there is more than one active component in fraction 5. Indeed, the isolation and biological studies of other peptides, such as thymosin α_7, β_3, and β_4 indicate that these peptides also possess thymic hormone activity. Figure 4 shows the postulated role of thymosin polypeptide components in T-cell maturation. It appears that individual active polypeptides in fraction 5 are acting on different subpopulations of T cells in the maturation sequence. Thymosin α_1 appears to act at both early and late stages of thymocyte maturation. Thymosin α_7 converts immature T cells to cells with suppressor function. Thymosin β_3 and β_4 appear to act at very early stages of the maturation sequence on TdT-negative bone marrow stem cells to form TdT-positive prothymocytes. So far, of all the polypeptides we have purified from fraction 5, only polypeptide β_1, which is equivalent structurally to ubiquitin, does not show any activity in our assay systems, indicating that this polypeptide is not involved in thymic hormone action. In fact, the recent report (147) that ubiquitin is the ATP-dependent proteolysis factor 1 of rabbit reticulocytes has specified a unique function of polypeptide β_1 (or ubiquitin) which is not related to thymic hormone action.

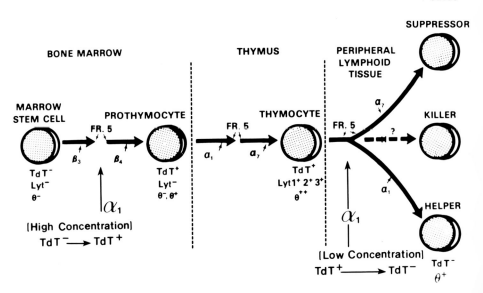

FIG. 4. Proposed role of thymosin peptides in T-cell maturation. Thymosin β_3 and β_4 promote early stem cell differentiation to the prothymocyte stage. Thymosin α_1 induces both early and late stages of T-cell differentiation. Thymosin α_7 is associated with the generation of functionally mature suppressor T cells and α_1 with the generation of helper T cells.

The most important contribution of thymic hormone research resides in its application to the clinical management of thymus-dependent diseases. Our ongoing clinical trials of thymosin have suggested that thymosin has a major role in restoring immune responsiveness and augmenting specific lymphocyte activities in children with hypothymic function, and in patients with secondary T-cell deficiencies resulting from a variety of disorders, including cancer and autoimmune disease.

Most of the clinical trials with thymosin have been carried out using thymosin fraction 5. The complete elucidation of the structure of thymosin α_1, thymosin β_4, and other thymic factors, and successful chemical synthesis of these molecules renders the clinical trials of purified thymic polypeptide hormones feasible. The ability of thymosin to trigger maturation events at several stages of T-cell development and to augment the reactive capacity of mature T cells renders thymosin superior to many other forms of immunomodulation. The eventual isolation of all biologically active thymosin polypeptides and acquisition of a full understanding of their biological activities will make possible the treatment of different diseases with different components or a combination of them. This approach should prove to be extremely useful in the area of immunotherapy. In anergic cancer patients, thymosin or other thymic hormones may be of importance as an adjunct to conventional treatments by increasing T-cell function in response not only to tumor cells, but also to pathogens, thus reducing the high incidence of infection that often accompanies cancer treatment.

ACKNOWLEDGMENTS

This study was supported in part by grants from the National Cancer Institute (CA 25017 and CA 24974), the Battelle Memorial Foundation, and Hoffman–La Roche, Inc.

REFERENCES

1. Abelous, J. E., and Billard, A. (1896): Recherches sur les fonctions de thymus. *Arch. Physiol. Norm. Pathol.*, 28:898–902.
2. Ahmed, A., Smith, A. H., Wong, D. M., Thurman, G. B., Goldstein, A. L., and Sell, K. W. (1978): *In vitro* induction of Lyt surface markers on precursor cells incubated with thymosin polypeptides. *Cancer Treat. Rep.*, 62:1739–1747.
3. Ahmed, A., Wong, D. M., Thurman, G. B., Low, T. L. K., Goldstein, A. L., Sharkis, S. J., and Goldschneider, I. (1979): T-lymphocyte maturation: cell surface markers and immune function induced by T-lymphocyte cell-free products and thymosin polypeptides. *Ann. N.Y. Acad. Sci.*, 332:81–94.
4. Aiuti, F., Ammirati, P., Fiorilli, M., D'Amelio, R., Franchi, F., Calvani, M., and Businco, L. (1979): Immunologic and clinical investigation on a bovine thymic extract. Therapeutic application in primary immunodeficiency. *Pediatr. Res.*, 13:797–802.
5. Aleksandrowicz, J., and Skotnicki, A. B. (1976): The role of the thymus and thymic humoral factors in immunotherapy of aplastic and proliferative diseases of the hemopoietic system. *Acta Med. Pol.*, 17:1–12.
6. Ammam, A. J., Wara, D. W., and Allen, T. (1978): Immunotherapy and immunopathologic studies in a patient with nucleoside phosphorylase deficiency. *Clin. Immunol. Immunopathol.*, 10:262–269.

7. Astaldi, A., Astaldi G. C. B., Wijermans, P., Groenewoud, M., Van Bemael, T., Schillekens, P. T. A., and Eijsvoogel, V. P. (1975): Thymus-dependent serum factor activity on the precursors of mature T cells. In: *Cell Biology and Immunology of Leukocyte Function*, edited by M. R. Quastel, pp. 221–228. Academic Press, New York.

8. Astaldi, A., Astaldi, G. C. B., Schellekens, P. T. A., and Eijsvoogel, V. P. (1976): Thymic factor in human sera demonstrable by a cyclic AMP assay. *Nature*, 260:713–715.

9. Astaldi, G. C. B., Astaldi, A., Groenwoud, M., Wijermans, P., Schellekens, P. T. A., and Eijsvoogel, V. P. (1977): Effect of a human serum thymic factor on hydrocortisone-treated thymocytes. *Eur. J. Immunol.*, 7:836–840.

10. Astaldi, A., Astaldi, G. C. B., Wijermans, P., Groenwoud, M., Schellikens, P. T. A., and Eijsvoogel, V. P. (1978): Thymosin-induced human serum factor increasing cyclic AMP. *J. Immunol.*, 119:1106–1108.

11. Bach, J. F. (1977): Thymic hormones: biochemistry, biological and clinical activities. *Ann. Rev. Pharmacol. Toxicol.*, 17:281–291.

12. Bach, M. A., and Niaudet, P. (1976): Thymic function in NZB mice. II. Regulatory influence of a circulating thymic factor on antibody production against polyvinylpyrrolidone in NZB mice. *J. Immunol.*, 117:760–764.

13. Bach, J. F., Dardenne, M., Goldstein, A., Guha, A., White, A. (1971): Appearance of T cell markers in bone marrow after incubation with purified thymosin, a thymic hormone. *Proc. Natl. Acad. Sci. U.S.A.*, 68:2734–2738.

14. Bach, J. F., Dardenne, M., Pleau, J. M., and Bach, M. A. (1975): Isolation, biochemical characteristics and biological activity of a circulating thymic hormone in the mouse and in the human. *Ann. N.Y. Acad. Sci.*, 249:186–210.

15. Bach, M. A., Fournier, C., and Bach J. F. (1975): Regulation of Θ-antigen expression by agents altering cyclic AMP level and by thymic factor. *Ann. N.Y. Acad. Sci.*, 249:316–327.

16. Bach, J. F., Dardenne, M., and Pleau, J. M. (1977): Biochemical characterization of a serum thymic factor. *Nature*, 266:55–57.

17. Bach, J. F., Bach, M. A., Blanot, D., Bricus, E., Charreire, J., Dardenne, M., Fournier, C., and Pleau, J. M. (1978): Thymic serum factor. *Bull. Inst. Past.*, 76:325–398.

18. Bach, M. A. (1977): Lymphocyte-mediated cytotoxicity: effects of aging, adult thymectomy and thymic factor. *J. Immunol.*, 119:641–647.

19. Barrett, D. J., Wara, D. W., Ammann, A. J., and Cowan, M. J. (1980): Thymosin therapy in the DiGeorge Syndrome. *J. Pediatr.*, 97:66–71.

20. Bernardi, G., and Comsa, J. (1965): Purification de l' hormone thymique par chromatographie sur colonne. *Experentia*, 21:416–417.

21. Bernengo, M. G., Capella, G., De Matteis, A., Tovo, P. A., and Zina, G. (1979): In vitro effect of a calf thymus extract on the peripheral blood lymphocytes of 66 melanoma patients. *Clin. Exp. Immunol.*, 36:279–284.

22. Birr, C., and Stollenwerk, U. (1979): Synthesis of thymosin α_1, a polypeptide of the thymus. *Angew. Chem. (Engl.)*, 18.394–395.

23. Bliznakov, E. G., Wan, Y., Chang, D., and Folkers K. (1978): Partial reactivation of impaired immune competence in aged mice by synthetic thymus factors. *Biochem. Biophys. Res. Commun.*, 80:631–636.

24. Briscas, E., Martinez, T., Blanot, D., Auger, G., Dardenne, M., Pleau, J. M., and Bach, J. F. (1977): The serum thymic factor and its synthesis. In: *Proceedings 5th International Peptide Symposium*, edited by M. Goodman and J. Meienhofer, pp. 564–574. John Wiley & Sons, New York.

25. Burton, P., Iden, S., Mitchell, K., and White, A. (1978): Thymic hormone-like restoration by human prealbumin of azathioprine sensitivity of spleen cells from thymectomized mice. *Proc. Natl. Acad. Sci. U.S.A.*, 75:823–827.

26. Carnaud, C., Ilfeld, D., Brook, I., and Trainin, N. (1973): Increased reactivity of mouse spleen cells sensitized *in vitro* against syngeneic tumor cells in the presence of a thymic humoral factor. *J. Exp. Med.*, 138:1521–1532.

27. Charriere, J., and Bach, J. F. (1975): Binding of autologous erythrocytes to immature T-cells. *Proc. Natl. Acad. Sci. U.S.A.*, 72:3201–3205.

28. Chretien, P. B., Lipson, S. D., Makuch, R., Kenady, D. E., Cohen, M. H., and Minna, J. D. (1978): Thymosin in cancer patients: *in vitro* effects and correlations with clinical response to thymosin immunotherapy. *Cancer Treat. Rep.*, 62:1787–1790.

29. Cohen, G. H., Hooper, J. A., and Goldstein, A. L. (1975): Thymosin-induced differentiation of murine thymocytes in allogeneic mixed lymphocyte cultures. *Ann. N.Y. Acad. Sci.*, 249:145–153.
30. Cohen, M. H., Chretien, P. B., Ihle, D. C., Fossicek, B. E., Makuch, R., Bunn, P. A., Johnston, A. V., Shackney, S. E., Matthews, M. J., Lipson, S. O., Kenady, D. E., and Minna, J. D. (1979): Thymosin fraction 5 and intensive combination chemotherapy prolonging the survival of patients with small cell lung cancer. *J.A.M.A.*, 241:1813–1815.
31. Comsa, J. (1955): Action of the purified thymic hormone in thymectomized guinea pigs. *Am. J. Med. Sci.*, 250:79–85.
32. Comsa, J. (1957): Consequences of thymectomy upon the leukopoiesis in guinea pigs. *Acta Endocrinol.*, 26:361–364.
33. Comsa, J. (1973): Thymus substitution and HTH, the homeostatic thymus hormone. In: *Thymic Hormones*, edited by T. D. Luckey, pp. 39–58. University Park Press, Baltimore.
34. Dardenne, M., and Bach, J. F. (1976): Thymic hormone in immunological diseases. In: *C.R. 5eme Journees Montpellieraines de Pneumologie*, edited by B. Michael, pp. 1–12. Masson, Paris.
35. Dardenne, M., Pleau, J. M., Man, N. K., and Bach, J. F. (1977): Structural study of circulating thymic factor, a peptide isolated from pig serum. I. Isolation and purification. *J. Biol. Chem.*, 252:8040–8044.
36. Dauphinee, M. J., Talal, N., Goldstein, A. L., and White, A. (1974): Thymosin corrects the abnormal DNA synthetic response of NZB mouse thymocytes. *Proc. Natl. Acad. Sci. U.S.A.*, 71:2637–2641.
37. Erard, D., Charreire, J., Auffredou, M. T., Galanaud, P., and Bach, J. F. (1979): Regulation of contact sensitivity to DNFB in the mouse. Effects of adult thymectomy and thymic factor. *J. Immunol.*, 123:1573–1576.
38. Falchetti, R., Bergesi, G., Eishkof, A., Cafiero, G., Adorini, L., and Caprino, L. (1977): Pharmacological and biological properties of a calf thymus extract (TP-1). *Drugs Exp. Clin. Res.*, 3:39–43.
39. Folkers, K. A., Leban, J., Sakura, N., Rampold, G., Lundanes, E., Dahmen, J., Lebek, M., Ohta, M., and Bowers, C. Y. (1980): Current advances on biologically active synthetic peptides. In: *Polypeptide Hormones*, edited by R. F. Beers, Jr., and E. G. Bassett, pp. 149–159. Raven Press, New York.
40. Fujino, M., Shinagawa, W., Fukuda, T., Takaoki, M., Kawaii, H., and Sugino, Y. (1977): Synthesis of the nonatetracontapeptide corresponding to the sequence proposed for thymopoietin II. *Chem. Pharm. Bull. (Tokyo)*, 25:1486–1489.
41. Gupta, S., and Good, R. A. (1977): Subpopulations of human T lymphocytes. II. Effect of thymopoietin, corticosteroids and irradiation. *Cell. Immunol.*, 34:10–18.
42. Goldstein, A. L., and Rossio, J. L. (1978): Thymosin for immunodeficiency diseases and cancer. *Comp. Therap.*, 4:49–57.
43. Goldstein, A. L., and White, A. (1970): The thymus as an endocrine gland. In: *Biochemical Actions of Hormones*, edited by G. Litwak, pp. 456–502. Academic Press, New York.
44. Goldstein, A. L., and White, A. (1971): Role of thymosin and other thymic factors in the development, maturation and functions of lymphoid tissue. In: *Current Topics in Experimental Endocrinology*, edited by V. H. T. James and L. Martini. pp. 121–149. Academic Press, New York.
45. Goldstein, A. L., Slater, F. D., and White, A. (1966): Preparation, assay and partial purification of a thymic lymphocytopoietic factor (thymosin). *Proc. Natl. Acad. Sci. U.S.A.*, 56:1010–1017.
46. Goldstein, A. L., Asanuma, Y., and White, A. (1970): The thymus as an endocrine gland: Properties of thymosin, a new thymus hormone. In: *Recent Progress in Hormone Research*, Vol. 26, edited by E. B. Astwood, pp. 505–538. Academic Press, New York.
47. Goldstein, A. L., Guha, A., Zatz, M. M., Hardy, A., and White, A. (1972): Purification and biological activity of thymosin, a hormone of the thymus gland. *Proc. Natl. Acad. Sci. U.S.A.*, 69:1800–1803.
48. Goldstein, A. L., Thurman, G. B., Cohen, G. H., and Hooper, J. A. (1975): Thymosin: chemistry, biology and clinical applications. In: *The Biological Activity of Thymic Hormones*, edited by D. W. Van Bekkum, pp. 173–197. Kooyker Scientific Publications, Rotterdam.
49. Goldstein, A. L., Wara, D. W., Ammann, A. J., Sakai, H., Harris, N. S., Thurman, G. B., Hooper, J. A., Cohen, G. H., Goldman, A. S., Costanzi, A. S., and McDaniel, M. C. (1975): First clinical trial with thymosin: Reconstitution of T cells in patients with cellular immunodeficiency diseases. *Transplant. Proc.*, 7:681–686.

50. Goldstein, A. L., Cohen, G. H., Rossio, J. L., Thurman, G. B., Brown, C. N., and Ulrich, J. T. (1976): Use of thymosin in the treatment of primary immunodeficiency diseases and cancer. *Med. Clin. North Am.*, 60:591–606.

51. Goldstein, A. L., Low, T. L. K., McAdoo, M., McClure, J., Thurman, G. B., Rossio, J. L., Lai, C-Y., Chang, D., Wang, S-S., Harvey, C., Ramel, A. H., and Meienhofer, J. (1977): Thymosin α_1: isolation and sequence analysis of an immunologically active thymic polypeptide. *Proc. Nat. Acad. Sci. U.S.A.*, 74:725–729.

52. Goldstein, A. L., Thurman, G. B., Rossio, J. L., and Costanzi, J. J. (1977): Immunological reconstitution of patients with primary immunodeficiency diseases and cancer after treatment with thymosin. *Transplant. Proc.*, 9:1141–1144.

53. Goldstein, A. L., Thurman, G. B., Low, T. L. K., Rossio, J. L., and Trivers, G. E. (1978): Hormonal influences on the reticuloendothelial system: current status of the role of thymosin in the regulation and modulation of immunity. *J. Reticuloendothel. Soc.*, 23(4):253–266.

54. Goldstein, G. (1974): Isolation of bovine thymin: a polypeptide hormone of the thymus. *Nature*, 247:11.

55. Goldstein, G. (1978): The isolation of thymopoietin (thymin). *Ann. N.Y. Acad. Sci.*, 249:177–185.

56. Goldstein, G., and Mananaro, A. (1971): Thymin: a thymic polypeptide causing the neuromuscular block of myasthenia gravis. *Ann. N.Y. Acad. Sci.*, 183:230.

57. Good, R. A., and Gabrielson, A. E., Editors (1964): *The Thymus in Immunobiology: Structure, Function and Role in Disease*, Hoeber-Harper, New York.

58. Good, R. A., Dalmasso, A. P., Martinez, G., Archer, O. K., Pierce, J. C., and Papermaster, B. W. (1962): The role of the thymus in development of immunologic capacity in rabbits and mice. *J. Exp. Med.*, 116:773–796.

59. Handzel, Z. T., Dolfin, Z., Levin, S., Altman, T., Hahn, T., Trainin, N., and Godot, N. (1979): Effect of thymic humoral factor on cellular immune functions of normal children and of pediatric patients with ataxia telangiectasia and Down's syndrome. *Pediatr. Res.*, 13:803–812.

60. Hardy, M. A., Zisblatt, M., Levine, N., Goldstein, A. L., Lilly, F., and White, A. (1971): Reversal by thymosin of increased susceptibility of immunosuppressed mice to Moloney sarcoma virus. *Transplant. Proc.*, 3:926–928.

61. Hooper, J. A., McDaniel, M. C., Thurman, G. B., Cohen, G. H., Schulof, R. S., and Goldstein, A. L. (1975): The purification and properties of bovine thymosin. *Ann. N.Y. Acad. Sci.*, 249:125–144.

62. Horowitz, S., Borcherding, C. O., Moorthy, A. V., Chesney, R., Schulte-Wisserman, H., Hong, R., and Goldstein, A. L. (1977): Induction of suppressor T cells in systemic lupus erythematosus by thymosin and cultured thymic epithelium. *Science*, 197:999–1001.

63. Hu, S. K., Low, T. L. K., and Goldstein, A. L. (1979): *In vivo* induction of terminal deoxynucleotidyl transferase (TdT) by thymosin of hydrocortisone acetate (HCA) treated mice. *Fed. Proc.*, 38:1079A.

64. Hu, S. K., Low, T. L. K, and Goldstein, A. L. (1980): Modulation of terminal deoxynucleotidyl transferase (TdT) *in vitro* by thymosin fraction 5 and purified thymosin α_1 in normal thymocytes. *Fed. Proc.*, 39:1133 (1980).

65. Hunt, L. T., and Dayhoff, M. O. (1977): Amino-terminal sequence identity of ubiquitin and the nonhistone component of nuclear protein A-24. *Biochem. Biophys. Res. Commun.*, 74:650–655.

66. Jankovic, B. D., Waksman, B. H., and Arnason, B. G. (1962): Role of the thymus in immune reactions in rats. I. The immunologic response to bovine serum albumin (antibody formation, Arthus reactivity, and delayed hypersensitivity) in rats thymectomized or splenectomized at various times after birth. *J. Exp. Med.*, 116:159–175.

67. Jankovic, B. D., Isakovic, K., and Horvat, J. (1965): Effect of a lipid fraction from rat thymus on delayed hypersensitivity reactions of neonatally thymectomized rats. *Nature*, 208:356–357.

68. Jin, Y., Xu, X., Zhu, J., Wang, Y., Zhu, A., and Zhang, H. (1979): A preliminary study on the isolation, property and function of porcine thymic hormone. *J. Nanking Univ.*, 1:115–124.

69. Kagan, W. A., Siegal, F. P., Gupta, S., Goldstein, G., and Good, R. A. (1979): Early stages of human marrow lymphocyte differentiation: Induction *in vitro* by thymopoietin and ubiquitin. *J. Immunol.*, 122:686–691.

70. Kater, L., Oosterom, R., McClure, J. E., and Goldstein, A. L. (1979): Presence of thymosin-like factors in human thymic epithelium conditioned medium. *Int. J. Immunopharmacol.*, 1:273–284.

71. Khaw, B. A., and Rule, A. H. (1973): Immunotherapy of the Dunning leukaemia with thymic extracts. *Br. J. Cancer*, 28:288–292.

72. Klein, J. J., Goldstein, A. L., and White, A. (1965): Enhancement of *in vivo* incorporation of labeled precursors into DNA and total protein of mouse lymph nodes after administration of thymic extracts. *Proc. Natl. Acad. Sci. U.S.A.*, 53:812–817.

73. Klein, J. J., Goldstein, A. L., and White, A. (1966): Effects of the thymus lymphocytopoietic factor. *Ann. N.Y. Acad. Sci.*, 135:485–495.

74. Kook, A. I., Yakir, Y., and Trainin, N.: Isolation and partial chemical characterization of THF, a thymus hormone involved in immune maturation of lymphoid cells. *Cell. Immunol.*, 19:151–157.

75. Kruisbeek, A. M., Kohose, T. C. J. M., and Ziglstra, J. J. (1977): Increase in T cell mitogen responsiveness in rat thymocytes by thymic epithelial culture supernatants. *Eur. J. Immunol.*, 7:375–381.

76. Kruisbeek, A. M., Astaldi, G. C. B., Blankwater, M. J., Ziglstra, J. J., Leverb, L. A., and Astaldi, A. (1978): The *in vitro* effect of a thymic epithelial culture supernatant on mixed lymphocyte reactivity and intracellular cAMP levels of thymocytes on antibody production of Nu/Nu spleen cells. *Cell. Immunol.*, 35:134–147.

77. Kruisbeek, A. M., Ziglstra, J. J., and Krose, T. J. M. (1980): Distinct effects of T cell growth factors and thymic epithelial factors on the generation of cytotoxic T lymphocytes by thymocyte subpopulations. *J. Immunol.*, 125:995–1002.

78. Lavastida, M. T., and Daniels, J. C. (1978): The use of thymosin (fraction 5) in autoimmune disorders: a preliminary report. *Fed. Proc.*, 37:1669.

79. Levey, R. H., Trainin, N., and Law, L. W. (1963): Evidence for function of thymic tissue in diffusion chambers implanted in neonatally thymectomized mice. Preliminary report. *J. Natl. Cancer Inst.*, 31:199–217.

80. Lipson, D. S., Chretien, P. B., Makuch, R., Kenady, D. E., and Cohen, M. H. (1979): Thymosin immunotherapy in patients with small cell carcinoma of the lung. *Cancer*, 43:863–870.

81. Liu, S.-L. (1979): Use of calf thymosin fraction 5 in the treatment of 7 cases with acquired immunodeficiency diseases. *Peking Med.*, 1:219–222.

82. Liu, S.-L., Hsu, C.-S., Tsuel, L.-H., Yang, K.-C., and Chang, S.-C. (1978): Modification of the purification method and *in vitro* bioassay of thymosin fraction 5. *Acta Biochem. Biophys. Sinica*, 10:413–416.

83. Lonai, P., Mogilner, B., Rotter V., and Trainin, N. (1973): Studies on the effect of a thymic humoral factor on differentiation of thymus-derived lymphocytes. *Eur. J. Immunol.*, 3:21–26.

84. Low, T. L. K., Goldstein, A. L. (1978): Structure and function of thymosin and other thymic factors. In: *The Year in Hematology*, edited by R. Silber, J. LoBue, and A. S. Gordon, pp. 281–319. Plenum Press, New York.

85. Low, T. L. K., and Goldstein, A. L. (1979): The chemistry and biology of thymosin. II. Amino acid sequence analysis of thymosin α_1 and polypeptide β_1. *J. Biol. Chem.*, 254:987–995.

86. Low, T. L. K., Hu, S. K., and Goldstein, A. L.: Complete amino acid sequence of bovine thymosin β_4: A thymic hormone that induces terminal deoxynucleotidyl transferase activity in thymocyte populations. *Proc. Natl. Acad. Sci. U.S.A.*, 78:1162–1166.

87. Low, T. L. K., Thurman, G. B., Chincarini, C., McClure, J. E., Marshall, G. D., Hu, S. K., and Goldstein, A. L. (1979): Current status of thymosin research: Evidence for the existence of a family of thymic factors that control T cell maturation. *Ann. N.Y. Acad. Sci.*, 332:33–48.

88. Low, T. L. K., Thurman, G. B., McAdoo, M., McClure, J., Rossio, J. L., Naylor, P. H., and Goldstein, A. L. (1979): The chemistry and biology of thymosin. I. Isolation, characterization and biological activities of thymosin α_1 and polypeptide β_1 from calf thymus. *J. Biol. Chem.*, 254:981–986.

89. Luckey, T. D., Robey, W. G., and Campbell, B. J. (1973): LSH, a lymphocyte-stimulating hormone. In: *Thymic Hormones*, edited by T. D. Luckey, pp. 167–183. University Park Press, Baltimore.

90. Marshall, G. D., Thurman, G. B., and Goldstein, A. L. (1980): Regulation of *in vitro* generation of cell-mediated cytotoxicity. *In vitro* induction of suppressor T lymphocytes by thymosin. *J. Reticuloendothel. Soc.*, 28:141–149.

91. Merrifield, R. B. (1963): Solid phase peptide synthesis. I. The synthesis of a tetrapeptide. *J. Am. Chem. Soc.*, 85:2149–2154.

92. Milcu, S. M., and Potop, I. (1973): Biologic activity of thymic protein extracts. In: *Thymic Hormones*, edited by T. D. Luckey, pp. 97–134. University Park Press, Baltimore.

93. Milcu, S. M., and Simionescu, N. (1953): Rolul sistemului nerves central in desfasurarea hipertrofiei de compensatie a glandei suprarenale le animalele tratate cu extract de timus. *Stud. Cercet. Endocr.*, 6:535–538.

94. Milcu, S. M., Potop, I., Peterscu, R., and Ghinea, E. (1976): Effect of thymosterin on lymphocytes *in vitro*. *Endocrinologie*, 14:283–286.
95. Milcu, S. M., Potop, I., Petrescu, R., and Ghinea, E. (1977): Effect of thymosterin on desocyribonucleic acid in KB tumor cell cultures *in vitro*. *Endocrinologie*, 15:105.
96. Miller, J. F. A. P. (1961): Immunological function of the thymus. *Lancet*, 2:748–749.
97. Miller, J. F. A. P. (1965): Effect of thymectomy in adult mice on immunological responsiveness. *Nature*, 208:1337–1338.
98. Mizutani, A. (1973): A thymic hypocalcemic component. In: *Thymic Hormones*, edited by T. D. Luckey, pp. 193–204. University Park Press, Baltimore.
99. Mizutani, A., and Tanaka, M. (1978): Sequence determination of amino and carboxyl-terminal residues of hypocalcemic protein TP extracted from bovine thymus glands. *Chem. Pharm. Bull.*, 26:2630.
100. Mizutani, A., Suzuki, I., Matsushita, Y., and Hayakawa, K. (1977): Effect of bovine thymic hypocalcemic factor on increasing antibody-producing cells in mice. *Chem. Pharm. Bull.*, 25:2156–2162.
101. Ogato, A., and Ito, Y. (1944): Studies on salivary gland hormones. V. Bioassay method based on the hypocalcemic activity in rabbits. *J. Pharm. Soc. Japn.*, 64:332–337.
102. Osoba, D., and Miller, J. F. A. P. (1964): The lymphoid tissues and immune responses of neonatally thymectomized mice bearing thymus tissue in Millipore diffusion chambers. *J. Exp. Med.*, 119:177–194.
103. Patt, Y. Z., Hersh, E. M., Schafer, L. A., Smith, T. L., Burgess, M. A., Gutterman, J. U., Goldstein, A. L., and Mavligit, G. M. (1979): The need for immune evaluations prior to thymosin-containing chemoimmunotherapy for melanoma. *Cancer Immunol. Immunother.*, 7:131–136.
104. Pazmino, N. H., Ihle, J. N., and Goldstein, A. L. (1978): Induction *in vivo* and *in vitro* of terminal deoxynucleotidyl transferase by thymosin in bone marrow cells from athymic mice. *J. Exp. Med.*, 147:708–718.
105. Pazmino, N. H., Ihle, J. N., McEwan, R. N., and Goldstein, A. L. (1978): Control of differentiation of thymocyte precursors in the bone marrow by thymic hormones. *Cancer Treat. Rep.*, 62:1749–1755.
106. Potop, I. (1979): Structure and properties of thymosterin. *Endocrinologie*, 17:2–8.
107. Potop, I., and Milcu, S. M. (1973): Isolation, biologic activity and structure of thymic lipids and thymosterin. In: *Thymic Hormones*, edited by T. D. Luckey, pp. 205–273. University Park Press, Baltimore.
108. Pugliese, A., and Tovo, P. A. (1980): Potentiation of Poly I:C induced interferon production in mice using a cell thymus extract TP-1. *Thymus*, 1:305–309.
109. Rossio, J. L., and Goldstein, A. L. (1977): Immunotherapy of cancer with thymosin. *World Surg.*, 1:605–616.
110. Rubenstein, A., Hirschorn, R., Sicklick, M., and Murphy, R. A. (1979): *In vivo* and *in vitro* effects of thymosin and adenosine deaminase on adenosine-deaminase deficient lymphocytes. *N. Engl. J. Med.*, 300:387–392.
111. Schafer, L. A., Goldstein, A. L., Gutterman, J. U., and Hersh, E. M. (1976): *In vitro* and *in vivo* studies with thymosin in cancer patients. *Ann. N.Y. Acad. Sci.*, 277:609–620.
112. Schafer, L. A., Gutterman, J. U., Hersh, E. M., Mavligit, G. M., Dandridge, K., Cohen, G. H., and Goldstein, A. L. (1976): Partial restoration by *in vivo* thymosin of E-rosettes and delayed-type-hypersensitivity reactions in immunodeficient cancer patients. *Cancer Immunol. Immunother.*, 1:259–264.
113. Schafer, L. A., Gutterman, J. U., Hersh, E. M., Mavligit, G. M., and Goldstein, A. L. (1977): *In vitro* and *in vivo* studies of thymosin activity in cancer patients. In: *Progress in Cancer Research and Therapy*, Vol. 2, edited by M. A. Chirigos, pp. 329–346. Raven Press, New York.
114. Scheid, M. P., Goldstein, G., and Boyse, E. A. (1975): Differentiation of T cells in nude mice. *Science*, 190:1211–1213.
115. Scheinberg, M. A., Goldstein, A. L., and Cathcart, E. S. (1976): Thymosin restores T cell function and reduces the incidence of amyloid disease in casein-treated mice. *J. Immunol.*, 116:156–158.
116. Schlesinger, D. H., and Goldstein, G. (1975): The amino acid sequence of thymopoietin II. *Cell*, 5:361–365.
117. Schlesinger, D. H., Goldstein, G., and Niall, H. D. (1975): The complete amino acid sequence of ubiquitin, an adenylate cyclase stimulating polypeptide probably universal in living cells. *Biochemistry*, 14:2214–2218.

118. Schlesinger, D. H., Goldstein, G., Scheid, M. P., and Boyse, E. A. (1975): Chemical synthesis of a peptide fragment of thymopoietin II that induces selective T cell differentiation. *Cell*, 5:367.

119. Sharp, M. R., and Peterson, D. A. (1978): Improvement of cellular immunodeficiency with thymosin. *Clin. Res.*, 26:818A.

120. Skotnicki, A. B. (1978): Biologiczna okthwnosc i wlasciwosci fizykochemiczne wyciagu grasiczego TFX. *Pol. Tyg. Lek.*, 28:1119–1124.

121. Strausser, H. R., Bober, L. A., Busci, R. A., Schillcock, J. A., and Goldstein, A. L. (1971): Stimulation of the hemagglutinin response of aged mice by cell-free lymphoid tissue fractions and bacterial endotoxin. *Exp. Gerontol.*, 6:373–378.

122. Sunshine, G. H., Basch, R. S., Coffey, R. G., Cohen K. W., Coldstein, G., and Hadden, J. W. (1978): Thymopoietin enhances the allogeneic response and cyclic GMP levels of mouse peripheral, thymus-derived lymphocytes. *J. Immunol.*, 120:1594–1599.

123. Thurman, G. B., and Goldstein, A. L. (1975): Mitogen bioassay for thymosin: increased mitogenic responsiveness of murine lymphocytes *in vitro* following *in vivo* treatment with thymosin. In: *The Biological Activity of Thymic Hormones*, edited by D. W. van Bekkum, pp. 261–264. Kooyker Scientific Publications, Rotterdam.

124. Thurman, G. B., Ahmed, A., Strong, D. M., Gershwin, M. E., Steinberg, A. D., and Goldstein, A. L. (1975): Thymosin-induced increase in mitogenic responsiveness of lymphocytes of C57B16J, NZB/W and nude mice. *Transplant. Proc.*, 7:299–303.

125. Thurman, G. B., Rossio, J. L., and Goldstein, A. L. (1977): Thymosin-induced enhancement of MIF production by peripheral blood lymphocytes of thymectomized guinea pigs. In: *Regulatory Mechanisms in Lymphocyte Activation*, edited by O. Lucas, pp. 629–631. Academic Press, New York.

126. Tovo, P. A., Bernengo, M. G., di Montezemolo, L. Cordero, Del Piano, A., Saitta, M., and Nicola, P. (1980): Thymus extract therapy in immunodepressed patients with malignancies and herpes virus infections. *Thymus*, 2:41–49.

127. Trainin, N. (1974): Thymic hormones and the immune response. *Physiol. Rev.*, 54:272–315.

128. Trainin, N., Begerano, A., Strahilevitch, M., Goldring, D., and Small, M. (1966): A thymic factor preventing wasting and influencing lymphopoiesis in mice. *Israel J. Med. Sci.*, 2:549–559.

129. Trainin, N., Burger, M., and Kaye, A. (1967): Some characteristics of a thymic humoral factor determined by assay *in vivo* of DNA synthesis in lymph nodes of thymectomized mice. *Biochem. Pharmacol.*, 16:711–720.

130. Trainin, N., Burger, M., and Linker-Israeli, M. (1967): Restoration of homograft response in neonatally thymectomized mice by a thymic humoral factor (THF). In: *Proceedings of the International Congress, Transplantation Society, First Advance in Transplantation*, edited by J. Dausset, J. Hamburger, and G. Mathe, pp. 91–105. Munksgaard, Copenhagen.

131. Trainin, N., Small, M., and Globerson, A. (1969): Immunocompetence of spleen cells from neonatally thymectomized mice conferred *in vitro* by a syngeneic thymus extract. *J. Exp. Med.*, 130:765–776.

132. Trainin, N., Small, M., Zipori, D., Umiel, T., Kook, A. I., and Rotter, V. (1975): Characteristics of THF, a thymic hormone. In: *Biological Activity of Thymic Hormones*, edited by D. K. van Bekkum, pp. 117–144. Kooyker Scientific Publications, Rotterdam.

133. Trainin, N., Rotter, V., Yakir, Y., Leve, R., Handzel, Z., Shohat, B., and Zaizov, R. (1979): Biochemical and biological properties of THF in animal and human models. *Ann. N.Y. Acad. Sci.*, 332:9–22.

134. Trench, C. A. H., Watson, J. W., Walker, F. C., Gardner, P. S., and Green, C. A. (1966): Evidence for a humoral thymic factor in rabbits. *Immunology*, 10:187–191.

135. Varsano, I., Danon, Y., Jaber, L., Livni, E., Shohat, B., Yakir, Y., Schneyoun, A., and Trainin, N. (1976): Reconstitution of T-cell function in patients with subacute sclerosing periencephalitis treated with thymus humoral factor. *Isr. J. Med. Sci.*, 12:1168–1175.

136. Wang, S. S., Kulesha, I. D., and Winter, D. P. (1978): Synthesis of thymosin α_1. *J. Am. Chem. Soc.*, 101:253–254.

137. Wang, S. S., Makofske, R., Bach, A. E., and Merrifield, R. B. (1980): Solid phase synthesis of thymosin α_1. *Int. J. Pept. Protein Res.*, 15:1–4.

138. Wara, D., and Ammann, A. J. (1978): Thymosin treatment of children with primary immunodeficiency diseases. *Transplant. Proc.*, 10:203–209.

139. Wara, D. W., Goldstein, A. L., Doyle, W., and Ammann, A. J. (1975): Thymosin activity in patients with cellular immunodeficiency. *N. Engl. J. Med.*, 292:70–74.

140. Wara, D. W., Barrett, D. J., Ammann, A. J., and Cowan, M. J. (1980): *In vitro* and *in vivo* enhancement of mixed lymphocyte culture reactivity by thymosin in patients with primary immunodeficiency disease. *Ann. N.Y. Acad. Sci.*, 332:128–134.

141. Watson, D. C., Levy, W. B., and Dixon, G. H. (1978): Free ubiquitin is a nonhistone protein of trout testis chromatin. *Nature*, 276:196–198.

142. Weksler, M. C., Innes, J. D., and Goldstein, G. (1978): Immunological studies of aging. IV. The contribution of thymic involution to the immune deficiencies of aging mice and reversal with thymopoietin. *J. Exp. Med.*, 148:996–1006.

143. Wetzel, R., Heyneker, H. L., Goeddel, D. V., Jhurani, P., Shapiro, J., Crea, R., Low, T. L. K., McClure, J. E., and Goldstein, A. L. (1980): Production of biologically active N$^{\alpha}$-desacetyl thymosin α_1 through expression of a chemically synthesized gene. *Biochemistry*, 19:6096–6104.

144. White, A., and Goldstein, A. L. (1968): Is the thymus an endocrine gland? Old problem, new data. *Perspect. Biol. Med.*, 11:475–489.

145. White, A., and Goldstein, A. L. (1975): The endocrine role of the thymus and its hormone, thymosin, in the regulation of the growth and maturation of host immunological competence. *Adv. Metab. Disorders*, 8:359–374.

146. Wijermans, P., Astaldi, G. C. B., Facehini, A., Schellekens, P. T. A., and Astaldi, A. (1979): Early events in thymocyte activation. I. Stimulation of protein synthesis by a thymus-dependent human serum factor. *Biochem. Biophys. Res. Commun.*, 86:88–96.

147. Wilkinson, K. D., Urban, M. K., and Haas, A. L. (1980): Ubiquitin is the ATP-dependent proteolysis factor I of rabbit reticulocytes. *J. Biol. Chem.*, 255:7529–7532.

148. Zisblatt, M., Goldstein, A. L., Lilly, F., and White, A. (1970): Acceleration by thymosin of the development of resistance to murine sarcoma virus-induced tumor in mice. *Proc. Natl. Acad. Sci. U.S.A.*, 66:1170–1174.

Maturation Factors and Cancer,
edited by Malcolm A. S. Moore.
Raven Press, © New York 1982.

T-Cell Growth Factor and the Establishment of Cell Lines from Human T-Cell Neoplasias

F. W. Ruscetti, B. J. Poiesz, C. Tarella, and R. C. Gallo

Laboratory of Tumor Cell Biology, National Cancer Institute, National Institutes of Health, Bethesda, Maryland 20205

Normal human B-lymphocytes can be established in long-term culture relatively easily (21,26). These lymphoblastoid cell lines are diploid, polyclonal B-lymphocytes transformed *in vitro* by Epstein-Barr virus present in the blood or tissues of sero-positive donors (24,31). Malignant lymphoid cells, with the exception of Burkitt's lymphoma, are difficult to grow in long-term culture (25,26). Few of these cell lines have been established from T-cell malignancies, and most have been from young patients with acute lymphoblastic leukemia (21,25). These cell lines contain high levels of terminal deoxynucleotidyl transferase (TdT), a marker for either immature T-cells or early lymphoid precursors (1), and they possess varying amounts of receptors which bind sheep red blood cells (E-rosette), a marker for more mature T-cells (15). Also, these cell lines retain little immune reactivity.

In previous studies, normal human T-cells activated by either antigen or lectin have been maintained in continuous culture for over 1 year, provided that they were supplemented every 3 to 5 days with conditioned media from lectin-stimulated mononuclear cells (22,23). Subsequent studies have shown that a protein designated T-cell growth factor (TCGF) is responsible for this growth promotion (34,40). These cells were over 90% E-rosette positive, negative for TdT, and retained all immune reactivity associated with T-cells. Thus for the first time, continuously proliferating clones of lymphocytes, which retained functional specificity and responsiveness to normal humoral regulation, were developed.

One objective of our laboratory is to compare the properties of specific kinds of normal human hematopoietic cells with their transformed counterparts, especially in regard to their growth control. We were, therefore, interested in studying the growth of neoplastic T-lymphocytes and in determining their response to TCGF.

Although there are various clinical presentations of T-lymphocytic neoplasias in man, including approximately 25% of both childhood and adult acute lymphocytic leukemia, rare cases of chronic lymphocytic leukemia, hairy cell leukemia, diffuse non-Hodgkin's lymphoma, and all patients with cutaneous T-cell lymphomas (mycosis fungoides, Sezary syndrome, and nodular papulosis), only in rare cases have investigators reported successful cell growth. As noted above, these were cell lines which were TdT-positive and often did not form rosettes. In general, mature T-cell lines were not established. In view of the ability of TCGF to propagate normal activated T-cells, our initial attempts to develop cell lines from patients with T-cell neoplasias, in fact, concentrated on those cells which represent a more mature form of the disease, namely, the cutaneous T-cell lymphomas (CTCL) and E-rosette-positive T-cell acute lymphoblastic leukemia (ALL). The use of mitogenic and crude TCGF (5) and especially purified TCGF (29) resulted in the long-term growth of these cells for the first time. The growth, morphological and histochemical characteristics, and the immunoregulatory capability of these cells are summarized in this chapter.

MATERIALS AND METHODS

Tumor Source

Malignant lymphoblasts were obtained from peripheral blood or bone marrow of patients with ALL. CTCL cells were obtained from biopsies of involved lymph nodes or skin lesions of patients with MF and from circulating cells from patients with Sezary syndrome. Lymph node cells were disaggregated by passing through a sieve (pore size 80 μm). Mononuclear blood cells were prepared by Ficoll-hypaque density gradient centrifugation.

T-cell Growth Factor

The detailed purification scheme and properties of the purified TCGF are de-scribed elsewhere (20). Here we summarize the basic steps to achieve the partially purified human TCGF used in this work. Crude TCGF was prepared from human lymphocytes combined from multiple healthy donors as described elsewhere (30,35). $(NH_4)_2SO_4$ fractionation of this material yielded over 90% of the TCGF between 50 and 75% saturated solution. The precipitate was dissolved in and dialyzed against 10 mM Tris-HCl, pH 8.0. Subsequently, this material was fractionated on a DEAE-Scpharose column by elution at approximately 0.07 M with a linear NaCl gradient. Each different preparation of pp-TCGF used was first tested for its inability to grow fresh peripheral blood leukocytes (PBL) from normal donors (29). The biochemical characteristics of TCGF are summarized in Table 1.

Cell Culture Methods

The mononuclear cells were placed in tissue culture flasks at 10^6 cells/ml under the following conditions: (a) RPMI 1640 with 20% FCS, (b) RPMI 1640 with 20% FCS and 50% crude TCGF, and (c) RPMI 1640 with 20% FCS and 20% pp-TCGF. The media in the flasks was changed twice weekly and the number and viability of the cells were monitored periodically. If a sample achieved a saturation density of 1 to 2 × 10^6 cells/ml, it was diluted with an equal amount of its particular media and continued in culture. Once continuous culture was achieved with added growth factor, routine attempts were made to grow the cells without the factor and in RPMI-

TABLE 1. *Some characteristics of purified human TCGF*

1. Nature of molecule	Protein
2. Size	About 13,000 daltons
3. pI	6.8
4. Glycosyl moiety	None detected
5. Target cell	Activated T-lymphocyte
6. Mode of action	Unknown
7. Cell or origin	Probably a subset of activated T-lymphocytes, distinct from the target T-cell
8. Stability	Very labile unless stored in albumin or PEG

FCS alone. PHA-stimulated normal peripheral blood lymphocytes (PBL) were also grown as cell lines with pp-TCGF, as above, and used as controls in the studies below.

Lymphocyte Characterization

Erythrocyte rosette tests were performed by slight modifications of established techniques, as detailed elsewhere (7,16). AET-treated sheep erythrocytes were used in the E-rosette assays. Fc and complement receptors were estimated using the EA and EAC-rosette tests, performed with sheep erythrocytes. Tests for surface immunoglobulins IgG, IgM, and IgA (SIg) were performed using an immunofluorescent method, as detailed elsewhere (16). The Epstein-Barr virus nuclear antigen (EBNA) test was performed by a modification of the Reedman-Klein technique (31). Histochemical properties of the cells were determined using napthol ASD chloracetate and α-naphthyl acetate esterases (nonspecific esterase) (43); Sudan black B and alkaline phosphatase (11); myeloperoxidase (11); acid phosphatases, with or without tartrate treatment (14); and the periodic acid Schiff (PAS) reaction (11) assayed according to published procedures. In addition, karyotype analyses were carried out initially on all fresh samples and periodically thereafter on the established cell lines according to previously published methods (29). Cell samples were also periodically removed from the cultures and centrifuged, and the cell pellets were prepared for thin section electron microscopy, as detailed below.

TCGF Assay

TCGF-dependent long-term (>20 days) cultured human T-cells served as target cells in all TCGF assays. These T-cells, washed free of growth media, were resuspended at 2×10^4 cells/ml in 96-well plates followed by serial dilutions of the sample to be assayed. After 48 hr of incubation, 0.5 μCi of ^{3}H-TdR (specific activity 3 Ci/mmole) was added to each well and cultured for an additional 4 hr. Cultures were harvested onto glass fiber filters and ^{3}H-TdR incorporation was determined. Units of TCGF activity were determined using probit analysis as previously described (8).

Hemapoietic Factor Production and Assay

Cultured T-cells, washed free of TCGF, were tested for their ability to release colony stimulatory activity (CSA), erythroid burst promoting activity (BPA), and TCGF by suspending the cells at 10^6 cells/ml in the following conditions: RPMI-1640-5% FCS; RPMI-1640-5% FCS + 10% pp-TCGF; RPMI-5% FCS + PHA; RPMI-1640-5% FCS + PHA + mitomycin-treated Daudi cells. Cell-free conditioned media (CM) were harvested daily for 72 hr. CSA (4) and BPA (12,13) were assayed according to standard procedures using methylcellulose as the semisolid media.

RESULTS

Cell Lines Derived From Patients With T-cell Neoplasias

As previously described, purified TCGF does not stimulate the growth of freshly isolated normal T-cells (20,29). If malignant T-cells were activated during the process of transformation, these cells could be selectively grown by treatment with the purified TCGF. In fact, this was observed. Long-term growth of T-cells from tissue samples from 12 of 14 patients with cutaneous T-cell lymphoma (CTCL) and 8 of 11 patients selected as having ALL of a T-cell origin was achieved by using mitogen-free pp-TCGF (29). All these fresh samples began to proliferate after 24 to 48 hr and were in continuous culture for at least 4 months. Some have been maintained in culture for over a year. These cell lines remained E-rosette positive, TdT negative, and negative for B-cell markers, typing them as mature T-cells. There are some significant differences in the cultured CTCL and ALL cells.

Growth

The cell lines derived from CTCL and ALL cells differ in their growth characteristics. The CTCL cells grow rapidly to a high saturation density ($> 2 \times 10^6$ cells/ml), tend to grow in large clumps, and can be maintained in culture for a longer period. The ALL cells grow more slowly, have a lower saturation density ($1-1.2 \times 10^6$ cells/ml), grow in single cell suspension, and seem to have a culture life of only 3 to 4 months.

Morphology

The ALL cells have a fairly homogeneous morphology, while the cultured CTCL cells contain many giant multinucleated cells in addition to mono- and binucleated smaller cells (Fig. 1). Ultrastructural analysis of these cultures revealed the presence of highly convoluted nuclei in three CTCL cultures (Fig. 2). These cells are very

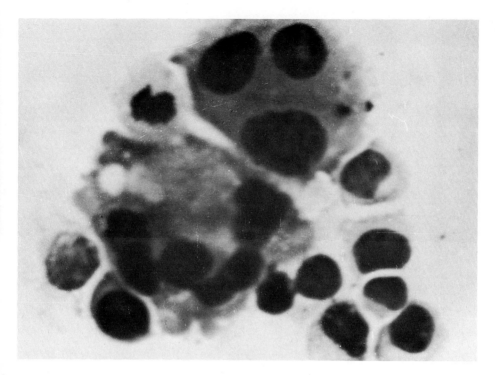

FIG. 1. Light microscopic appearance of cultured cutaneous T-cell lymphoma cells. Cytocentrifuge preparations of cultured CTCL-2 cells, illustrating the varying size and nuclear number of CTCL cells (Wright-Giemsa stain, × 1,800).

similar in morphology to the cells of primary tumors of these patients, and such cells are considered diagnostic for CTCL (18,19).

Cytochemical Characteristics

The CTCL, ALL, and normal cultured T-cells can be distinguished from one another by cytochemical procedures. All the CTCL cell lines (and only those T-cell lines) were strongly positive for nonspecific esterase, utilizing assay conditions which only stain monocytes (43). The presence of markers for both T-cell and monocytoid characteristics on these CTCL cultured cells is puzzling, but it probably means they are neoplastic T-cells with aberrant properties. The large multinucleated cells are able to form E-rosettes, suggesting their T-cell origin. Normal cultured T-cells exhibited a mild granular cytoplasmic staining for acid phosphatase which is typical of freshly isolated T-cells. The majority of the cultured ALL cells showed a strong concentration of the staining pattern in the Golgi region of the cells (Fig. 3), which together with E-rosette receptors has been reported to be a strong indication of malignant T-cells in fresh ALL samples (3,37). The CTCL lines have a strong diffuse cytoplasmic granular staining pattern (Fig. 3).

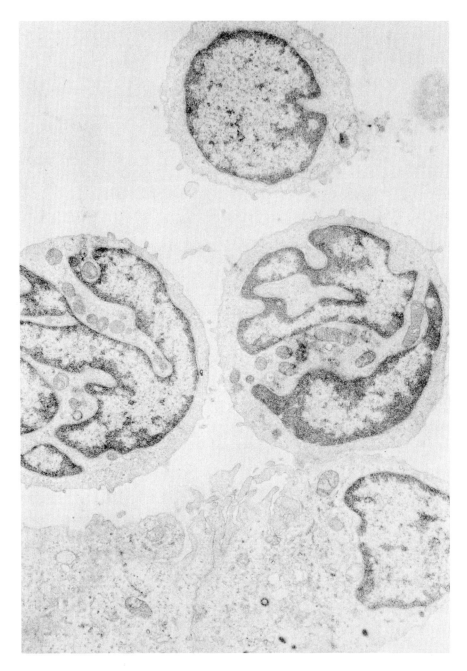

FIG. 2. Electron micrograph of cultured CTCL-8 cells (passage 5) showed cells with highly convoluted nuclei. Cells were fixed for 1 hr in 28% gluteraldehyde, washed 5 times in 0.2 M Na cacodylate buffer and postfixed in Dalton's chrome osmium. Following dehydration, the cell pellets were embedded, and sections were cut on an LKB Ultramicrotome.

Karyotypic Abnormalities

The cultured cells of CTCL-3 have chromosomal alterations which are the same as found in the fresh tumor cells. The characteristics of these cell lines are summarized in Table 2.

Production of TCGF by Malignant T-cells

Two cell lines (HUT102 and CTCL-2), originally dependent on addition of TCGF for *in vitro* growth, sequentially become independent of TCGF for growth (5,29). If a subset of T-cells do, in fact, have the capacity to elaborate TCGF, and malignant T-cells retain their ability to respond to it, then self-replicating malignant T-cells could have a selective growth advantage. In fact, cell lines are constitutive producers of low levels of TCGF (Table 3), whereas normal T-cells require another cell and antigen/lectin to produce TCGF (35). Conditioned media (CM) from HUT102 concentrated $20 \times$ by ammonium sulfate precipitation can maintain the growth of normal T-cells. No CM from B-cell lines (10 samples), factor independent ALL cell lines (15 samples), or two other CTCL cell lines that we tested are able to support growth of T-cells (Table 3).

Hematopoietic Factor Production by Cultured T-cells

There is evidence that T-lymphocytes are involved in the regulation of myeloid (28,30,32) and erythroid (23,38) colony formation. A continuous T-cell line from a patient with hairy cell leukemia (10) releases these factors, but it can be argued that this is a unique malignant T-cell line and its products have no relationship to normal control mechanisms. The ability to grow normal and malignant T-cells still responsive to normal growth regulation provides an opportunity to study pure populations of T-cells of several origins for factor production. The ability of these cultured T-cells to release hematopoietic factors is summarized in Table 4. Some, but not all the cell lines derived from patients with ALL, mycosis fungoides, and Sezary syndrome constitutively released CSA. Cell lines from normal individuals released CSA only after mitogen stimulation. Factor independent cell lines from CTCL also released CSA, but 15-factor independent cell lines derived from ALL (e.g., Molt-4, 8402) did not. The removal of adherent cells from the bone marrow used to assay the CM had no effect on the results. Four cell lines from patients with T-cell malignancies released BPA, which increased erythyroid burst formation two- to threefold.

DISCUSSION

A main observation concerning the control of T-cell proliferation was the demonstration that the proliferative stimulus is provided by TCGF rather than the lectin or antigen (for reviews, see refs. 34 and 40). The lectin or antigen is mitogenic only in situations where they stimulate the release of TCGF (41). The T-cell proliferative response and acquisition of effector cell function depends upon interactions

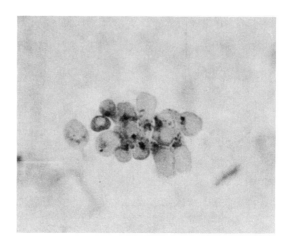

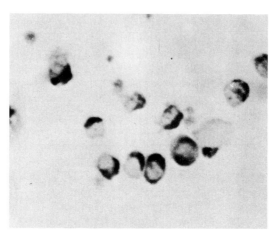

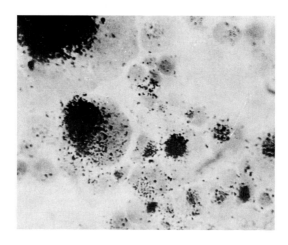

FIG. 3.

among at least three cell types. An adherent cell, most likely the macrophage, processes the antigen/lectin and releases a soluble product termed lymphocyte activating factor (LAF) (27). This activity is not in itself a proliferative stimulus, but it appears to stimulate the production and/or release of TCGF (17,41). However, once the T-cells are activated and TCGF is present, the T-cells will proliferate in the absence of antigen, adherent cells, or adherent cell products. This responsiveness appears to be a direct result of the development of TCGF-specific membrane receptors (2,39).

Several observations suggest that the TCGF-producing cell is a mature T-cell that is activated by antigen and stimulated by LAF to release TCGF: (a) highly purified T-cells produce TCGF when provided with these signals (36,41), (b) TCGF production required the maturational influence of the thymus (9), and (c) cloned T-helper cells can produce TCGF *in vitro* (6,36). It is not clear whether under normal circumstances the TCGF producer T-cell can respond to TCGF. All the mature T-cell lines reported to date have required the addition of exogenous TCGF for continuous proliferation in the absence of other cells, and no normal T-cell lines capable of making enough TCGF to be independent of it have been found.

The discovery that T-cells had to be activated before acquiring responsiveness to TCGF suggested that malignant T-cells activated by the transforming process could selectively proliferate in direct response to TCGF. Long-term growth dependent on the addition of TCGF was observed in 12 out of 14 cases of CTCL and in 8 out of 11 cases of T-cell ALL. We believe the evidence is strong that the cultured cells discussed in this report represent the neoplastic cells of the primary tumor. This interpretation is based upon (a) their abnormal cell morphology, (b) histochemical distinctions from cultured normal T-cells, and (c) karyotypic abnormalities in the cultured cells of CTCL-3, which is the same as the primary tumor. Other samples were karyotypically normal, but so were the primary tumor cells. Finally, in two cases, the cultured cell produced TCGF, becoming independent of its addition for growth. All T-cell lines from normal donors continually require TCGF for growth. Since these lines, which are producing TCGF, are not cloned cell lines, it is not known whether the same cell line that is producing TCGF is also responding to it. It is possible that these malignant cells are self-replicating in response to their own TCGF. Neoplastic T-cells may have TCGF receptor(s) on their cell surface at all times, thereby explaining their ability to grow when TCGF is produced by the same or different T-cells. This could be due to either chronic stimulation by some ill-defined antigen or cellular membrane changes which lead to exposure of a receptor or its synthesis *de novo*.

T-lymphocytes have been implicated in the regulation of hematopoiesis through the release of CSA and BPA activities (23,28,30,38). The establishment of a human

FIG. 3. Acid phosphatase cytochemical appearance of cultured T-lymphocytes. Acid phosphatase staining was performed as described in Materials and Methods. Cells were grown in growth media supplemented with 10% pp-TCGF. *Top,* cultured T-cells from a normal donor after 35 days of culture; *middle,* cultured T-cells from a patient with T-cell-ALL after 23 days in culture; *bottom,* cultured T-cells from a patient with CTCL after 75 days in culture.

TABLE 2. *Comparative properties of continuously cultured human T-cells*

Source	Requirements for growth			Morphology	TdT	EBV, IgG	E-rosette	Acid phosphatase	Nonspecific esterase	Karyology
	No additions	TCGF alone	TCGF + PHA initiation							
Normal	–	–	+	Normal lymphoblasts	–	–	+	+ Mild granular cytoplasmic	–	Normal diploid
ALL[a]	– (rarely +)	+	+	Homogeneous lymphoblasts, sometimes with multiple nucleoli in nucleus	–	–	+	++ Concentrated in Golgi region	–	Variable and like primary cells
CTCL[b]	– (rarely +)	+	+	Heterogeneous giant multinucleated cells and other smaller lympho-blasts, mono- or binucleated; some with convoluted nuclei	–	–	+	+++ Diffuse intense reaction	Diffuse intense reaction in a few cells; majority small para-nuclear cyto-plasmic granule	Variable and like primary cells

[a]ALL refers to acute lymphoblastic leukemia. The cells were from peripheral blood of patients with T-cell disease.
[b]CTCL refers to cutaneous T-cell lymphomas. Cells were from either peripheral blood or lymph nodes.

TABLE 3. *Production of TCGF by human cell lines*

Cell line	Origin[a]	TCGF activity[b]	
		CM (cpm)	Stimulated CM[c] (cpm)
HUT102	MF	3,200 ± 650	3,800 ± 700
CTCL-2	SS	1,200 ± 220	2,100 ± 450
HUT78	MF	150 ± 40	380 ± 100
YT4E	SS	90 ± 70	190 ± 100
HSB, Molt-4	ALL	55 ± 40	170 ± 120
CCRF, 8402	ALL	80 ± 30	120 ± 70
Daudi, Raji	BL	65 ± 50	75 ± 40
NPB-32	Normal	320 ± 90	3,200 ± 580
		75 ± 20	180 ± 50

[a]MF refers to mycosis fungoides, SS to Sezary syndrome, ALL to acute lymphocytic leukemia, and BL to Burkitt's lymphoma.

[b]TCGF activity was measured as ^{3}H-TdR incorporation into cultured T-cells using a microassay as described in Materials and Methods.

[c]Conditioned media was collected 72 hr after culturing the cell lines at 5×10^5 cells/ml in fresh growth media. In order to prepare stimulated CM, PHA-p at 0.05 λ/ml and Daudi cells at 2×10^5 cells/ml were added to the growth media.

TABLE 4. *Production of hematopoietic factors by malignant T-cells*

Cell type[a]	Time in culture[b] (days)	Growth requirement[c]	CSA[d] (# pos.)	BPA[d] (# pos.)
8 T-cell-ALL	15–85	TCGF	6	3
15 T-cell-ALL	NA		0	0
4 MF	15–150	TCGF	3	1
8 Sezary	15–200	TCGF	4	0
4 CTCL	NA		3	0
10 Normal T-cells	15–50	TCGF	5	0

[a]T-cell ALL refers to T-cell variant of acute lymphocytic leukemia, MF to mycosis fungoides, SS to Sezary syndrome, and CTCL to cutaneous T-cell lymphoma.

[b]Time in culture refers to the earliest and longest length of time in culture that the cells were tested for producing CSA and BPA.

[c]TCGF was partially purified as described in Materials and Methods. It was used at 10% (v/v) with RPMI-1640-15% FCS. The cell lines that do not require TCGF were grown in RPMI-1640-10% FCS.

[c]The CM from cells growing in RPMI-1640-5% FCS and 10% pp-TCGF were harvested 72 hr after subculturing the cells. These CM were assayed for CSA (4) and BPA (12,13) using standard procedures. pp-TCGF did not have any CSA or BPA activity.

T-cell line from hairy cell leukemia (1) suggested that certain malignant T-cells retain this stimulatory capacity. We have been able to demonstrate that malignant cells (from a variety of T-cell diseases) grown in the presence of the normal regulator-TCGF release both CSA and BPA (42). Cell lines from normal donors release CSA only after mitogen stimulation. The removal of adherent cells from the bone marrow used to assay these CM do not affect the results, suggesting that these CM did not stimulate macrophage to release these mediators. The constitutive release of these factors by T-cells proliferating in the presence of the putative physiological regulator lends further credence to the role of the T-cell in regulating hematopoiesis.

Finally, we think these cell systems will be useful for (a) comparative studies between normal and neoplastic T-cells, (b) possible predictive value in patients in remission by utilizing the direct response of transformed T-cells to TCGF as an indication of the presence of residual neoplastic cells, and (c) providing malignant T-cells for biochemical and virological studies relating to etiology.

REFERENCES

1. Bollum, F. J. (1979): Terminal deoxynucleotidyl transferase as a hematopoietic cell marker. *Blood*, 54:1203–1218.
2. Bonnard, G. D., Yasaka, K., and Jacobson, D. (1979): Ligand-activated T-cell growth factor-induced proliferation: Absorption of T-cell growth factor by activated T-cells. *J. Immunol.*, 123:2704–2712.
3. Catousky, D., Cheshi, M., and Greaves, M. F. (1978): Acid-phosphatase reaction in acute lymphoblastic leukemia. *Lancet*, 1:749–751.
4. Chervenick, P. A., and Boggs, D. R. (1971): *In vitro* growth of granulocytic and mononuclear cell colonies from blood of normal individuals. *Blood*, 37:131–135.
5. Gazdar, A. F., Carney, D. N., Bunn, P. A., Russell, E. F., Jaffe, E. S., Schecter, G. P., and Guccion, J. G. (1980): Mitogen requirements for *in vitro* propagation of cutaneous T-cell lymphomas. *Blood*, 55:409–417.
6. Glasebrook, A. L., and Fitch, F. W. (1980): I. Interactions between cloned amplifier and cytolytic T-cell lines. *J. Exp. Med.*, 151:876–895.
7. Blick, J. E. (1980): *Human Lymphocyte Cell Culture: The Fundamentals*. Marcel Dekker, New York.
8. Gillis, S., Ferm, M. M., Ou, W., and Smith, K. A. (1978): T-cell growth factor: parameters for production and a quantitative microassay for activity. *J. Immunol.*, 120:2027–2035.
9. Gillis, S., Baker, P. E., Union, N. A., and Smith, K. A. (1979): The *in vitro* generation and sustained culture of nude mouse cytolytic T-lymphocytes. *J. Exp. Med.*, 149:1460–1473.
10. Golde, D. W., Quan, S. G., and Cline, M. J. (1978): Human T-lymphocyte cell line producing colony-stimulating activity. *Blood*, 52:1068–1071.
11. Hayhoe, F. G. J., Quaglino, D., and Doll, R. (1964): *Cytology and Cytochemistry of Acute Leukemias*. Her Majesty's Stationery Office, London.
12. Iscove, N. N., Silber, F., and Winterhalter, K. H. (1974): Erythroid colony formation in culture of mouse and human bone marrow: analysis of the requirements for erythropoietin by gel filtration and affinity chromatography on agarose-concanavalin A. *J. Cell Physiol.*, 83:309–322.
13. Iscove, N. N. (1978): Erythropoietin-independent stimulation of early erythropoiesis in adult marrow culture by conditioned media from stimulated spleen cells. In: *Hematopoietic Cell Differentiation*, edited by D. W. Golde, M. J. Cline, D. Metcalf, and C. F. Fox, pp. 37–56. Academic Press, New York.
14. Janckila, A. J., Li, C. Y., Lam, K. W., and Yam, L. T. (1978): The cytochemistry of tartrate-resistant acid phosphatase. *Am. J. Clin. Pathol.*, 70:45–55.
15. Jondal, J., Wigzell, H., and Aiuti, F. (1973): Human lymphocyte subpopulations: classification according to surface markers and/or functional characteristics. *Transplant. Rev.*, 16:63–98.

16. Kaplan, M. E., and Clark, C. (1974): An improved rosetting assay for detection of human T-lymphocytes. *J. Immunol. Methods*, 5:131–135.

17. Larsson, E. L., Iscove, N. N., and Coutinho, A. (1980): Two distinct factors are required for induction of T-cell growth. *Nature*, 283:664–666.

18. Lutzner, M. A., Hobbs, J. W., and Horvath, P. (1971): Ultrastructure abnormal cells in Sezary syndrome, mycosis fungoides, and parapsoriasis. *Arch. Dermatol.*, 103:375–386.

19. Lutzner, M. A., and Jordan, H. (1968): The ultrastructure of an abnormal cell in Sezary syndrome. *Blood*, 31:719–726.

20. Mier, J. W., and Gallo, R. C. (1980): Purification and some characteristics of human T-cell growth factor (TCGF) from PHA-stimulated lymphocyte conditioned media. *Proc. Natl. Acad. Sci., U.S.A.*, 77:6134–6138.

21. Minowada, J., Ohnuma, T., and Moore, G. E. (1972): Rosette-forming human lymphoid cell lines. I. Establishment and evidence for origin of thymus derived lymphocytes. *J. Natl. Cancer Inst.*, 49:891–895.

22. Morgan, D. A., Ruscetti, F. W., and Gallo, R. C. (1976): Selective *in vitro* growth of T-lymphocytes from normal human bone marrows. *Science*, 193:1007–1008.

23. Nathan, D. G., Chess, L., Hillman, D. G., Clarke, B., Beard, J., Merler, E., and Housman, D. E. (1978): Human erythroid burst-forming unit: T-cell requirement for proliferation *in vitro*. *J. Exp. Med.*, 147:324–339.

24. Nilsson, K., Klein, G., Henle, W., and Henle, G. (1971): The establishment of lymphoblastoid lines from adult and fetal human lymphoid tissue and its dependency on EBV. *Int. J. Cancer*, 8:443–450.

25. Nilsson, K., and Ponten, J. (1975): Classification and biological nature of established human hematopoietic cell lines. *Cancer*, 15:321–341.

26. Nilsson, K. (1976): Establishment of permanent human lymphoblastoid cell lines *in vitro*. In: *In Vitro Methods in Cell Mediated and Tumor Immunity*, edited by B. R. Bloom and J. R. David, pp. 713–721. Academic Press, New York.

27. Oppenheim, J. J., Mizel, S. B., and Meltzer, M. S. (1979): Biological effects of lymphocyte and macrophage-derived "amplification" factors. In: *Biology of the Lymphokines*, edited by S. Cohen, E. Pick, and J. J. Oppenheim, pp. 291–328. Academic Press, New York.

28. Parker, J. W., and Metcalf, D. (1974): Production of colony-stimulating factors in mitogen stimulated lymphocyte cultures. *J. Immunol.*, 112:502–510.

29. Poiesz, B. J., Ruscetti, F. W., Mier, J. W., Woods, A. M., and Gallo, R. C. (1980): T-cell lines established from human T-lymphocytic neoplasias by direct response to T-cell growth factor. *Proc. Natl. Acad. Sci., U.S.A.*, 77:6815–6819.

30. Prival, J. T., Paran, M., Gallo, R. C., and Wu, A. M. (1974): Colony stimulating factors in cultures of human peripheral blood cells. *J. Natl. Cancer Inst.*, 53:1583–1591.

31. Reedman, B. M., and Klein, G. (1973): Cellular localization of an Epstein-Barr virus (EBV)-associated complement-fixing antigen in producer and non-producer lymphoblastoid cell lines. *Int. J. Cancer*, 11:499–520.

32. Ruscetti, F. W., and Chervenick, P. A. (1975): Release of colony stimulating activity from thymus-derived lymphocytes. J. Clin. Invest., 55:520–529.

33. Ruscetti, F. W., Morgan, D. A., and Gallo, R. C. (1977): Functional and morphological characterization of human T-cells continuously grown *in vitro*. *J. Immunol.*, 119:131–138.

34. Ruscetti, F. W., and Gallo, R. C. (1980): Human T-lymphocyte growth factor: regulation of growth and function of T-lymphocytes. *Blood*, 57:379–394.

35. Ruscetti, F. W., Mier, J. W., and Gallo, R. C. (1980): Human T-cell growth factor: parameter for production. *J. Supramol. Struct.*, 13:229–241.

36. Schrier, M. H., Iscover, N. N., Tees, R., Aardon, L., and von Boehmer, H. (1980): Clones of killer and helper T-cells: Growth requirements, specificity and retention of function in long-term culture. *Immunol. Rev.*, 51:315–336.

37. Schwarce, W. W. (1975): T-cell origin of acid-phosphatase positive lymphoblasts. *Lancet*, 2:1264–1266.

38. Sharkis, S. J., Spivak, J. L., Ahmed, A., Misiti, J., Stuart, R. K., Wiktor-Jedrzejczak, W., Sell, K. W., and Sensenbrenner, L. L. (1980): Regulation of hematopoiesis: helper and suppressor influence of the thymus. *Blood*, 55:524–527.

39. Smith, K. A., Gillis, S., Baker, P. E., McKenzie, D., and Ruscetti, F. W. (1979): T-cell growth factor mediated T-cell proliferation. *Ann. N.Y. Acad. Sci.*, 332:423–432.

40. Smith, K. A. (1980): T-cell growth factor. *Immunol. Rev.*, 51:337–357.
41. Smith, K. A., Lachman, L. B., Oppenheim, J. J., and Favata, M. F. (1980): The functional relationship of the interleukins. *J. Exp. Med.*, 151:1551–1556.
42. Tarella, C., Ruscetti, F. W., Poiesz, B. J., Gazdar, A. F., and Gallo, R. C. (1982): Factors regulating human hematopoiesis are produced by normal and neoplastic T-cells grown in long-term culture by t-cell growth factor. *Blood*, 59.
43. Yam, L. T., Li, C. Y., and Crosby, W. W. (1971): Cytochemical identification of monocytes and granulocytes. *Am. J Pathol.*, 55:283–288.

Maturation Factors and Cancer,
edited by Malcolm A. S. Moore.
Raven Press, © New York 1982.

Interleukin 2 Produced by Murine and Human T Cell Tumors: A Perspective on Leukemogenesis

*Steven Gillis, **Steven B. Mizel, and †James Watson

*Basic Immunology Program, Fred Hutchinson Cancer Research Center, 1124 Columbia Street, Seattle, Washington 98104; **Department of Microbiology, Cell Biology, Biochemistry, and Biophysics, The Pennsylvania State University, University Park, Pennsylvania, 16802; †Department of Microbiology, California College of Medicine, University of California at Irvine, Irvine, California 92717

Recent studies conducted in several laboratories have confirmed that a soluble protein, interleukin 2 (IL-2, formerly referred to as T cell growth factor) is present in tissue culture medium conditioned by mouse, rat, or human mononuclear leukocytes (1–4).[1] Purified IL-2 has been found to greatly influence several *in vitro* and *in vivo* immune responses. Most reproducibly, purified IL-2 has been found (a) to markedly enhance thymocyte mitogenesis, (b) to induce cytotoxic T cell (CTL) generation in either alloantigen-stimulated thymocyte or nude mouse spleen cell cultures, and (c) to promote antierythrocyte plaque forming cell (PFC) responses in nude mouse spleen cell cultures (1,2). Furthermore, Wagner and colleagues recently observed that *in vivo* administration of IL-2 in concert with antigen allowed for elaboration of alloantigen-specific directly cytolytic nude mouse splenic T cells (5).

In each of these assay systems, IL-2 presumably acts by fostering the exponential proliferation of any ligand activated pre-T or mature T cell. Such a hypothesis is consistent with the observation that IL-2 has been found to be the only biological mediator capable of promoting the sustained *in vitro* proliferation of antigen-specific helper or killer T cell lines (1,2,6).

Unfortunately, given current methods for IL-2 preparative purification (1,2), hundreds of liters of conventionally prepared conditioned medium would be required to isolate milligram quantities of pure IL-2 for further molecular characterization or for experiments aimed at determining the physiologic role of this potent regulatory molecule. Based primarily on the observations of Ralph et al. (7) (who showed

---

[1]Abbreviations used: Con-A, concanavalin A; CTL, cytotoxic T lymphocyte; CTLL, cytotoxic T lymphocyte line; IL-1, interleukin 1; IL-2, interleukin 2; LAF, lymphocyte activating factor; NaGO, neuraminidase galactose oxidase; PBL, peripheral blood leukocyte; PFC, plaque forming cell; PHA, phytohemagglutinin; PMA, phorbol myristate acetate; TCGF, T cell growth factor.

that mitogen stimulation of murine tumor cell lines led to elaboration of the biological mediator of myelopoiesis, colony stimulating factor), we undertook the long screening of human and murine T cell leukemias for both constitutive and lectin-induced IL-2 production.

We report in this chapter identification of two potent IL-2 producer tumor cell lines. One, designated LBRM-33 (a splenic lymphoma from the B10.BR mouse) generates (upon stimulation with T cell mitogens) between 1,000 and 5,000 times the amount of IL-2 present in conventionally prepared rat or murine spleen cell conditioned medium (8). The second IL-2 producer (designated Jurkat-FHCRC) is a human T cell leukemia which generates similar high titer IL-2 containing conditioned medium when stimulated with phytohemagglutin (PHA) (9). In addition to serving as an excellent source for biochemically defined IL-2, we have used these cell lines, along with nonproducer variants cloned from them, to dissect the mechanism of monokine (interleukin 1) mediated control of T cell activation and to formulate new hypotheses regarding the involvement of aberrant IL-2 proliferation control in the etiology of T cell leukemia.

MATERIALS AND METHODS

Screening of T Cell Lines for IL-2 Production

In vitro and *in vivo* passaged murine T cell leukemia and lymphoma cell lines were collected from tissue culture sources at the Memorial Sloan-Kettering Cancer Center, New York, and the University of California at Irvine. Human leukemic T cell lines designated SKI were obtained either from Dr. Roland Mertelsmann, Laboratory of Developmental Hematopoiesis, or Dr. Peter Ralph, both from the Memorial Sloan-Kettering Cancer Center, New York. Cell lines designed FHCRC were obtained from Dr. John Hansen, Histocompatibility Laboratory, Puget Sound Blood Center, Fred Hutchinson Cancer Research Center, Seattle, Wash. (10). After harvest from exponential proliferative culture, cell line samples (2×10^6 cells/ml) were resuspended in Click's medium (supplemented with 10% FCS, 25 mM HEPES Buffer, 16 mM $NaHCO_3$, 50 units/ml penicillin, 50 μg/ml streptomycin, and 300 μg/ml fresh L-glutamine) and seeded in 100 μl aliquots in replicate flat-bottom microplate wells (#3596 Costar Inc., Cambridge, Mass.). Triplicate microwell cultures were then stimulated by 100 μl addition of either (a) tissue culture medium; (b) Con A (20 μg/ml, Miles Biochemicals Inc., Elkhart, Ind.); or (c) PHA-M (2% by volume, Grand Island Biologicals, Grand Island, N.Y.). After the time periods indicated (see Results), supernate samples from triplicate cultures were pooled and assayed for IL-2 activity in a standard microassay as detailed below. Optimal mitogen dose, harvest time, and cell concentration for Jurkat-FHCRC and LBRM-33 mediated IL-2 production was determined in separate experiments conducted either in 200 μl microwell cultures as detailed above or in 5 ml volumes in tissue culture flasks (#3013, Falcon Plastics, Oxnard, Calif.). All IL-2 production cultures were conducted at 37°C in a humidified atmosphere of 5% CO_2 and air.

IL-2 Microassay

IL-2 activity was determined using a standard T cell growth factor microassay (11) monitoring the IL-2 dependent cellular proliferation of a mouse T cell line (CTLL 2) (12). Briefly, 3,000 CTLL cells were seeded in replicate 200 μl volumes (in 96 well flat-bottom microtiter plates) in the presence of a $\log_2$ dilution series of a given IL-2 containing sample. Following 24 hr of culture (at 37°C in a humidified atmosphere of 5% and air), microwell cultures were pulsed for 4 hr with 0.5 μCi of tritiated thymidine (^{3}H-Tdr, specific activity 20 mCi/mmole, New England Nuclear, Boston, Mass.), after which time, the cultures were harvested onto glass fiber filter strips with the aid of a multiple automated sample harvester. ^{3}H-Tdr incorporation was determined by liquid scintillation counting. Using these methods, only CTLL cells cultured in the presence of IL-2 incorporated ^{3}H-Tdr in a dose-dependent manner. CTLL cells cultured in the absence of IL-2 incorporated only scintillant control levels of ^{3}H-Tdr and were greater than 95% trypan blue positive following 24 hr of IL-2 deprivation. Units of IL-2 activity were determined by probit analysis of ^{3}H-Tdr incorporation data (11). A 1 unit/ml standard was defined as the amount of IL-2 activity present in 48 hr tissue culture medium conditioned by the Con A (5 μg/ml) stimulation of normal rat spleen cells (10^6 cells/ml). Assay of 1 unit/ml standard routinely stimulated 10,000 cpm of CTLL ^{3}H-Tdr incorporation at a dilution of 1:2.

To confirm that the IL-2 activity produced by PHA-stimulated Jurkat-FHCRC cells would support the sustained *in vitro* proliferation of human activated T cells, identical T cell growth factor (TCGF) microassays were conducted using an IL-2 dependent human T cell line as the indicator cell (10^5 cells/ml). This cell line, designated MLR-FHCRC-1, was developed from effector cells harvested from a 10 day mixed lymphocyte reaction and had been in IL-2 dependent culture for 4 to 6 weeks prior to use in IL-2 microassays.

The amount of IL-2 activity generated by Jurkat-FHCRC cells was compared to that present in several other sources of conditioned medium. Conditioned media were prepared by the T cell mitogen stimulation of normal murine or rat spleen cells. IL-2 containing supernates were also generated from single donor human peripheral blood leukocytes (PBL) stimulated with (a) PHA; (b) PHA and allogeneic cells from an *in vitro* cultured B lymphoblastoid cell line (AR-77, obtained from Dr. R. Mertelsmann); or (c) neuraminidase and galactose-oxidase (NaGO). Additional IL-2 containing supernates were produced by the 1% PHA stimulation of either normal human spleen cells (obtained from Dr. Michael Bean, Virginia Mason Research Center, Seattle, Wash.) or the mouse lymphoma LBRM-33. Methods for production of all of the above IL-2 containing tissue culture media have been detailed elsewhere (1,2,11,13–15).

IL-2 Producer Cell Cloning

LBRM-33 cells were subcloned by limiting dilution in flat-bottom microplate wells. Cells were seeded in 200 μl volumes of FCS supplemented RPMI 1640 at a concentration of 0.1 cell/ml. After 10 days of culture, microplate wells were screened for viable cell growth. Positive wells were harvested and subcultured in 25 cm² tissue culture flasks (#3013, Falcon Plastics, Oxnard, Calif.) in FCS supplemented RPMI 1640. 50 to 70% plating efficiency was observed in cloning trials of LBRM-33. Once the subcultures reached sufficient densities (10^6 cells/ml), the clonal cultures were harvested and retested for both constitutive and mitogen-induced IL-2 production as detailed above. In some experiments, LBRM-33 parent and cloned cell lines (10^6 cells/ml) were stimulated with either phorbol myristate acetate (PMA, 10 ng/ml, Sigma Chemical Co., St. Louis, Mo.) or interleukin 1 (IL-1, 10 units/ml) either alone or in concert with 1% PHA. Twenty-four hr supernates from such dual stimulation cultures were harvested and assayed for IL-2 activity as detailed above. IL-1 was purified (as previously described) from tissue culture medium conditioned by PMA stimulated $P388D_1$ mouse macrophage tumor cells (16,17).

IL-1 Absorption

To test the capacity of LBRM-33 cell line derivatives to IL-1, cloned LBRM-33 cell lines (10^8 cells) were washed and resuspended in RPMI 1640, 2% FCS containing either 100 or 0.5 units/ml of IL-1. Following a 4 hr incubation at 4° or 37°C, the cells were pelleted by a 10 min centrifugation at $300 \times g$, and the supernatants were tested for residual IL-1 activity by their capacity to enhance thymocyte mitogenesis (16). In some experiments, cloned LBRM-33 cell lines were fixed with 2% glutaraldehyde (15 min, 4°C) and washed extensively prior to use in absorption tests. IL-1 assays (enhancement of PHA-initiated thymocyte mitogenesis) were conducted as detailed elsewhere (16). Briefly, C3H/HeJ (4–6 weeks old, Jackson Laboratories, Bar Harbor, Maine) thymocytes were cultured in 200 µl volumes in flat-bottom microplate wells (1.5×10^6 cells/well) in the presence of a $\log_2$ dilution series of a putative IL-1 containing sample. Under these conditions, a standard preparation of IL-1 (100 units/ml) induced approximately 10,000 to 15,000 cpm of thymocyte ³H-Tdr incorporation at a dilution of 1:4 (medium control stimulation = 300 cpm of ³H-Tdr incorporation). Fifty percent of maximum thymocyte proliferation was routinely observed with 5 to 10 units/ml IL-1.

RESULTS

Comparison of Conventional IL-2 Production Protocols

Table 1 displays mitogen-induced IL-2 production data from several lymphocyte sources. Mitogen doses selected were those which generated peak proliferation as measured by 4 hr, ³H-Tdr incorporation by full-term cultures (generally 2–3 days following mitogen sensitization). All cultures were conducted in RPMI 1640 medium supplement with 10% fetal calf serum, 2-mercaptoethanol, and antibiotics unless otherwise specified. It should be stressed that murine T-cell clones (such as

TABLE 1. *Relative capacity of conditioned media to support proliferation of long-term cultured murine effector T cells*

Lymphocyte source	Mitogen	Cell concentration[a]	Units/ml interleukin-2 (TCGF) activity in filtered medium	
			24 hr supernate	48 hr supernate
Mouse spleen	Con-A (1.25 µg/ml)	10^6/ml	0.10	0.35
Mouse spleen	Con-A (2.5 µg/ml)	10^7/ml	1–4	0.5–1.5
Rat spleen	Con-A (5 µg/ml)	10^6/ml	0.68	1.0 (standard)
Rat spleen	Con-A (5 µg/ml)	10^7/ml	10–35	6–15
Human PBL	PHA (1%)	10^6/ml	2–4	4–7
Human PBL	B-LCL[b] (Daudi or AR-77 cells, 2–5 × 10^5/ml live or irradiated)	10^6/ml	0.63	1.2
Human PBL	B-LCL + 1.0% PHA	10^6/ml	10–22	15–31
Human PBL	Na-GO[c]	10^6/ml	4.1	0.73
Human spleen	1% PHA	10^7/ml	25.0	12.6

[a]Fifty ml volumes in 250 ml flasks, lying flat in a humidified atmosphere of 5% CO_2 and air.
[b]B-lymphoblastoid cell line.
[c]Neuraminidase-galactose oxidase treatment (see ref. 14).

those described earlier; ref. 6) have been maintained for over 3 years in tissue culture medium containing 0.5-IU/ml IL-2 activity.

In comparative production protocols, IL-2 activity was measured in a standard microassay based on its ability to trigger ^{3}H-Tdr incorporation (exponential proliferation) by cloned helper and/or cytotoxic murine T cells as detailed above (11). Because mouse T cell lines grow using condioned medium from either mouse, rat, or human sources (1,2,11), use of a murine T cell clone as an indicator in IL-2 microassays allows for measurement of IL-2 activity from any species source. Use of a human T cell line as an indicator would allow measurement of only human IL-2 production, in that human T cells will not proliferate in culture in the presence of IL-2 derived from mouse or rat lymphocytes (11).

As is clear from examination of the data displayed in Table 1, harvest of conditioned medium with peak IL-2 activity was cell concentration and culture duration dependent. This was most likely due to the well-documented observation that IL-2 supernate titer depended upon two competing reactions, the first being IL-2 production by a subpopulation of T cells, the second being the binding of IL-2 by a proliferating mitogen-activated T cell subset in the same culture (15). To obtain maximal IL-2 concentration in the supernate, it was imperative that conditioned medium be harvested after a majority of the IL-2 had been produced, but prior to the time when activated T cells had proliferated to the extent where they had begun to exhaust the IL-2 supply.

Optimal murine IL-2 titer was obtained in culture supernates harvested after 24 hr Con-A stimulation of spleen cells (10^7 cells/ml). A greater than 10-fold increase in supernate IL-2 titer was routinely witnessed when rat spleen cells (10^7 cells/ml) were substituted for mouse T cells. It was of interest that if after 24 hr Con-A stimulation, rat spleen cells were resuspended in additional, mitogen-containing, tissue culture medium and recultured in their original stimulation flasks, it was possible to obtain a second pool of conditioned medium with identical titer IL-2 activity. However, further repetitive cycling of mitogen activated cells was unsuccessful in increasing IL-2 production yield. One further advantage to using rat conditioned medium (10^7 cells/ml) as an IL-2 source was that identical titer IL-2 activity was obtained in supernates harvested from cultures supplemented with only 2% fetal calf or 2% adult bovine serum.

Optimal production of human IL-2 activity was achieved either by PHA stimulation of human spleen cells or by PHA and allogeneic B lymphoblastoid cell line stimulation of peripheral blood mononuclear cells (as originally reported by Bonnard and his colleagues; ref. 18). Use of human spleen was of considerable advantage given the ability to recycle human spleen cells in an identical fashion to that described above for obtaining repetitive rounds of IL-2 production from rat spleen cell cultures. It should be stressed that an excellent source of mitogen-free IL-2 could be obtained via neuraminidase/galactose oxidase (NaGL) treatment of human peripheral blood cells. Originally described by Novogrodsky and his coworkers (14) as a procedure for triggering human T cell proliferation, we have recently found that NaGO treatment of human PBL produces supernates with considerable IL-2 activity.

Tumor Cell Line IL-2 Production

Unfortunately, given current methods for IL-2 preparative purification and any of the lymphocyte stimulation protocols detailed in Table 1, literally hundreds of liters of conditioned medium would be required for isolation of pure IL-2 for either further molecular characterization or for use in *in vivo* experimentation. Because of the limitation that poor yields of IL-2 placed on further research, clearly more efficient means of factor production and recovery had to be developed. In hopes of establishing a system in which to produce initial conditioned medium with a significantly higher IL-2 titer, we screened some 40 murine and human T cell leukemia and lymphoma cell lines for both constitutive and mitogen-induced IL-2 production. Of the cell lines tested, only two parent tumor lines (one each in both human and mouse systems) were found to produce high titer IL-2 upon mitogen stimulation. As summarized in Table 2 (only a portion of the cell lines tested is displayed), of the murine T cell lines tested, 1% PHA stimulation of LBRM-33 cells resulted in the generation of culture supernates which contained between 1,000 and 5,000 times the amount of biologically active IL-2 that was routinely generated by identical numbers (10^6 cells/ml) of optimally stimulated rat or mouse splenocytes (8). Similarly, only PHA stimulation of the human leukemia T cell line Jurkat-FHCRC produced between 100 and 300 times the amount of human IL-2/ml normally generated by lectin-stimulated human PBL or spleen cells (Table 1) (9).

Because the experiments detailed in Tables 1 and 2 monitored IL-2 activity on the basis of its capacity to sustain the *in vitro* proliferation of murine activated T cells, it was not necessarily clear that PHA stimulated Jurkat-FHCRC cells produced significant amounts of human IL-2 activity. To approach this problem, both Jurkat-FHCRC and LBRM-33 cell, PHA conditioned media were tested for relative capacities to induce proliferation of both murine CTLL and human antigen-specific T cells harvested from long-term IL-2 dependent cultures. IL-2 microassays using human CTLL (10^5 cells/ml) were conducted as previously described (11). Results of these experiments are displayed in Fig. 1 in terms of ^{3}H-Tdr incorporation observed in cultures containing various concentrations of conditioned medium. Jurkat-FHCRC derived IL-2 activity was capable of sustaining the *in vitro* proliferation of both murine and human CTLL. LBRM-33 generated conditioned medium proved effective only when tested on murine CTLL. Tissue culture medium containing 1% PHA was incapable of inducing proliferation of either mouse or human activated T cells. These data were consistent with our previous studies detailing the species specificity of IL-2 (11) and confirmed that Jurkat-FHCRC conditioned medium was an excellent source of human IL-2 activity.

LBRM-33 and Jurkat-FHCRC IL-2 Production Parameters

To determine the production kinetics of tumor cell line elicited IL-2, both Jurkat-FHCRC and LBRM-33 cells were harvested from *in vitro* cultures and seeded in replicate microplate wells at 10^6 cells/ml in the presence of 1% PHA. After 2, 4, 6, 12, 18, 24, and 48 hr of culture, supernates were harvested and assayed for IL-

TABLE 2. *Screening of leukemia and lymphoma cells for IL-2 production*

Cell line	IL-2 activity[a] present in 48 hr supernate following activation with		
	Medium[b]	Con-A[c]	PHA[d]
Murine T cell tumors			
RBL-5	0.0	0.0	0.0
EL-4	0.0	0.0	0.0
L51784	0.0	0.0	0.0
S49	0.0	0.0	NT[e]
BW5147	0.0	0.0	NT
RDM 4	0.0	0.0	0.0
ASL-1	0.0	0.0	0.0
RLo-1	0.0	0.0	0.0
HRST 34	0.0	0.0	0.0
LBRM-33	0.0	26.0	517.0
LBRM-33 1A5	0.0	0.0	0.0
LBRM-33 4CI	0.0	0.1	4.3
LBRM-33 5A4	0.0	35.0	866.0
LBRM-33 4A2	0.0	42.0	1,163.0
LBRM-33 6BI	0.0	32.0	927.0
Human T cell leukemias			
CEM-SKI	0.0	0.0	0.0
CEM-FHCRC	0.0	0.0	0.0
8402-FHCRC	0.0	0.0	0.0
HSB2-SKI	0.0	0.0	0.0
HSB2-FHCRC	0.0	0.0	0.0
MOLT-4-SKI	0.0	0.0	0.0
MOLT-4-FHCRC	0.0	0.0	0.0
Ke37-FHCRC	0.0	0.0	0.0
T-45-SKI	0.0	0.0	0.0
R-2-SKI	0.0	0.0	0.0
PEER-SKI	0.0	0.0	0.0
HPB-ALL-SKI	0.0	0.0	0.0
JURKAT-FHCRC	0.0	93.7	225.0

[a]Units/ml.
[b]RPMI 1640,10% FCS.
[c]Ten μg/ml.
[d]1.0% PHA by volume.
[e]Not tested.

2 activity. Tumor cell line IL-2 production kinetics were similar to those previously detailed for cultures of lectin-stimulated rat, mouse, and human mononuclear leukocytes (11). Measurable IL-2 activity was detected within 6 hr after mitogen stimulation and reached peak concentrations 16 to 24 hr after induction. However, in addition to the magnitude of factor produced, LBRM-33 and Jurkat-FHCRC IL-2 production kinetics were somewhat different from normal production profiles in that the amount of IL-2 present in postpeak cultures did not significantly decline over time. In a sense, it was not surprising that postpeak culture duration had little

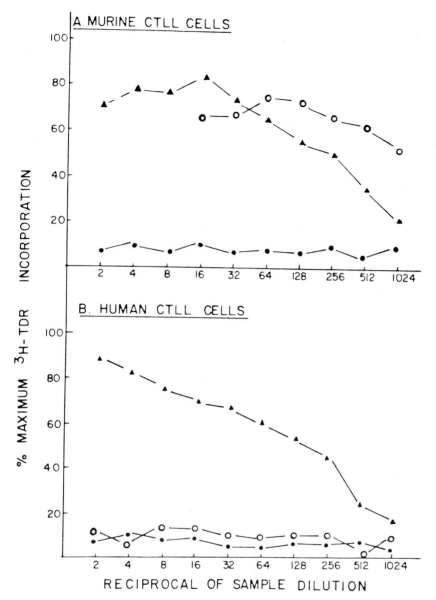

FIG. 1. ^{3}H-Tdr incorporation (4 hr pulse) by murine (**A**) and human (**B**) CTLL cells following 24 hr culture in a $\log_2$ dilution series of medium conditioned by 1% PHA stimulated Jurkat-FHCRC (▲) or LBRM-33 cells (○). Response is also indicated after culture in 1% PHA (●). Maximal ^{3}H-Tdr incorporation witnessed by murine and human CTLL cells was 10,984 and 6,530 cpm, respectively. LBRM-33 derived supernate contained 936 units/ml IL-2, whereas Jurkat-FHCRC generated conditioned medium contained 225 units/ml IL-2 activity.

effect on IL-2 concentration, as neither tumor cell line was dependent on IL-2 for its own proliferation.

Similar experiments were also conducted to determine optimal cell and mitogen concentration for LBRM-33 and Jurkat-FHCRC induced IL-2 production. In studies conducted with both cell lines (see Table 3), peak IL-2 containing supernates were harvested from 24 hr cultures (10^6 cells/ml) stimulated with either 1% PHA or 20 μg/ml Con-A. LBRM-33 cells stimulated in such a manner routinely generated conditioned medium containing greater than 1,000 units/ml IL-2 activity. Similarly prepared Jurkat-FHCRC supernates contained greater than 300 units/ml IL-2. It should be stressed that identical high titer IL-2 containing supernates could be produced by Jurkat-FHCRC or LBRM-33 cells under these conditions (10^6 cells/ml, 1% PHA stimulation) regardless of the presence of serum.

As further detailed in Table 3, one of the most interesting facets of Jurkat-FHCRC or LBRM-33 cell IL-2 production was the consistent observation that peak production by 24 hr lectin-stimulated cultures was consistently accompanied by poor cell viability. In fact, both LBRM-33 and Jurkat-FHCRC cells were greater than 95% trypan blue positive following 24 hr of 1% PHA stimulation. At present, it is difficult to distinguish whether Jurkat-FHCRC and LBRM-33 cells die as a result of IL-2 production or whether IL-2 is released as a result of mitogen toxicity. Attempts to isolate active IL-2 from supernates of nonstimulated cells (via sonication or heat treatment) have been unsuccessful. Therefore, it is questionable whether IL-2 is preformed in the cytoplasm of Jurkat-FHCRC and LBRM-33 cells and is released into the medium following mitogen sensitization. The observation that increasing concentrations of IL-2 were found over a 16 hr time period in supernates of stimulated tumor cells also argues against the hypothesis that mitogen activation simply stimulates cell death and concomitant release of preformed IL-2. Regardless of the mechanism behind mitogen-stimulated LBRM-33 and Jurkat-FHCRC cell

TABLE 3. *Tumor cell line IL-2 production: mitogen dose responses*

Culture stimulant	Concentration	Units/ml IL-2 activity present in 24 hr supernatant (% viable cells remaining after stimulation)	
		LBRM-33 culture	JURKAT-FHCRC
PHA	10.0%	163 (67)	101 (46)
PHA	5.0%	415 (25)	135 (25)
PHA	1.0%	1,216 (0)	252 (0)
PHA	0.5%	970 (10)	234 (0)
PHA	0.1%	486 (32)	39 (65)
Con-A	100 μg/ml	612 (22)	124 (39)
Con-A	50 μg/ml	785 (12)	171 (16)
Con-A	25 μg/ml	1,116 (0)	207 (0)
Con-A	10 μg/ml	372 (31)	121 (42)
Con-A	2 μg/ml	26 (85)	11 (79)

death, tumor cell line-derived, serum-free, IL-2 rich supernates should prove to be of significant value for biochemical characterization and bulk purification of this lymphocyte regulatory molecule.

In fact, we have recently found that LBRM-33 derived IL-2 is biochemically indistinguishable from conventionally prepared mouse spleen generated factor (19). Mouse tumor cell line derived IL-2 appears to be localized in a 30,000 MW protein, isolatable by net charge into two electrophoretically distinct species with isoelectric points of 4.3 and 4.9, respectively. Each molecular species has the capacity to (a) enhance thymocyte mitogenesis, (b) sustain IL-2 dependent T cell line proliferation, and (c) induce CTL and PFC responses in thymocyte and nude spleen cell populations, respectively. Enzymatic analysis of conventionally generated murine spleen and LBRM-33 derived IL-2 activity further confirms the identity of the two molecules. Regardless of the source, murine IL-2 was found to be extremely sensitive to proteolytic enzyme treatment. Exposure to trypsin, subtilisin, and chymotrypsin completely destroyed both IL-2 activities. IL-2 activity purified from either LBRM-33 or murine spleen cells was remarkably stable to chemical modification. Only treatment with 8 M urea or prolonged exposure to high temperature (70°C for 30 to 60 min) resulted in a significant diminution of IL-2 activity. Of the two preparations tested, it appeared that LBRM-33 generated IL-2 activity was consistently more resistant to pH, urea, and heat treatment than splenic derived material.

Use of Cloned T Cell Lymphomas for Dissection of Lymphokine Mediated Immune Reactivity

As indicated above in Table 2, limiting dilution (0.1 cell/microculture well) subcloning of the murine IL-2 producer lymphoma LBRM-33 resulted in the isolation of several viable sublines. Of the clones harvested, several (5A4, 4A2, and 6B1, for example) produced even greater quantities of IL-2 upon lectin stimulation than did the parent line LBRM-33. Interestingly, only one isolate (LBRM-33 1A5) was identified as incapable of producing IL-2 in response to PHA stimulation. Quite surprisingly, further study of LBRM-33 5A4 and 1A5 sublines has revealed a remarkable relationship between IL-2 production and the effects of another interleukin (IL-1, previously referred to as lymphocyte activating factor or LAF; ref. 20).

Due to the well-documented macrophage requirement for mitogen stimulated IL-2 production (15,21,22) and the observation that IL-1 is a macrophage product (16,17), it has been hypothesized that IL-1 may be an essential signal required by IL-2 producer T cells. Such a hypothesis was first suggested by the observations of Smith and his co-workers, who found that IL-1 producer tumor cell line supernates could restore adherent cell depleted, mitogen stimulated murine spleen cell cultures to normal levels of IL-2 production (21). IL-1 involvement in IL-2 production was also suggested by the studies of Farrar and Fuller-Bonar (22), who showed that the saturated fatty acid tumor promoter, phorbol myristate acetate (PMA, previously shown to act as a replacement for IL-1 in several immune response assays; refs.

23 and 24) could substitute for the macrophage requirement of IL-2 production by murine T cells. Finally, addition of IL-1 to mitogen activated, adherent cell depleted spleen cell cultures has been shown to reconstitute IL-2 production to normal levels (25,26). Although the involvement of IL-1 in the production of IL-2 by ligand stimulated T cells cannot be questioned, the precise mechanism by which IL-1 functions in this capacity remains unknown. It occurred to us that IL-2 producer and nonproducer LBRM-33 clones might prove to be useful reagents in dissecting the mechanism behind the IL-1 requirement for IL-2 production.

As shown in Table 4, addition of purified IL-1 to cultures of PHA-stimulated, LBRM-33 5A4 and 1A5 cell lines had profound effects on IL-2 production. As was the case with PMA (10 ng/ml), addition of 10 units/ml IL-1 to suboptimally mitogen stimulated 5A4 cells resulted in restoration of peak levels of IL-2 production. Furthermore, 10 units/ml IL-1 supplementation of PHA-stimulated 1A5 cultures allowed for the production of IL-2 in concentrations equal to that produced by optimally stimulated 5A4 cells. Addition of IL-1 to cultures of nonstimulated 1A5 cells was not sufficient for conversion of the 1A5 cell line to IL-2 production.

One interpretation of the experiments detailed above was that exposure of 1A5 cells to IL-1 resulted in an alteration of the 1A5 cells themselves, which led to their capacity to later produce IL-2 in response to mitogen stimulation. In an attempt to dissociate requirements for IL-1 and mitogen sensitization, multiple cultures were conducted in which 1A5 cells were either treated in concert with PHA and IL-1 (10 units/ml) or in which 1A5 cells were first exposed to IL-1 for 4 hr at 37°C, and following exhaustive washing, were cultured either in the absence or presence of additional IL-1 and PHA. We found that brief exposure of 1A5 cells to IL-1 resulted in their capacity to produce IL-2 upon subsequent exposure to PHA. In

TABLE 4. *Effects of IL-1 and PMA on LBRM-33 5A4 and IA5 cell line IL-2 production*

	Culture stimulant				Units/ml IL-2
Cell line	IL-1 (10 units/ml)	PMA (10 ng/ml)	1.0% PHA	0.1% PHA	present in 24 hr supernate
LBRM-33 5A4	−	−	+	−	565.0
"	−	−	−	+	35.0
"	+	−	−	−	0.0
"	+	−	+	−	604.0
"	+	−	−	+	525.0
"	−	+	−	−	0.0
"	−	+	+	−	576.0
"	−	+	−	+	612.0
LBRM-33 1A5	−	−	+	−	0.0
"	−	−	−	+	0.0
"	+	−	−	−	0.0
"	+	−	+	−	476.0
"	+	−	−	+	513.0
"	−	+	−	−	0.0
"	−	+	+	−	36.0
"	−	+	−	+	18.0

fact, pretreatment of 1A5 cells with IL-1 allowed for IL-2 production identical in magnitude to that generated by 1A5 cells cultured for 24 hr in the presence of IL-1 and PHA. These results suggested that perhaps 1A5 cells possessed a particular responsiveness to IL-1, which was saturated in a short period of time, leading to conversion to IL-2 production upon subsequent mitogen stimulation.

Based on our previous studies, which have demonstrated the capacity of activated T cells to absorb IL-2 from cultures where it was present (15), we questioned whether 1A5 and/or 5A4 cells possessed a similar cell surface responsiveness (presumably mediated by receptors) for IL-1. To test this hypothesis, 10^8 1A5 and 5A4 cells were harvested from *in vitro* cultures, washed extensively, and resuspended in a known amount of IL-1. Following a 4 hr incubation at 4°C, the cells were pelleted and the supernate tested for remnant IL-1 activity (assayed by enhancement of thymocyte mitogenesis).

As detailed in Fig. 2, both 1A5 and 5A4 cell lines (either live or fixed with 2% glutaraldehyde for 15 min prior to testing) could absorb IL-1 from cultures where it was present. 1A5 possessed a greater cell surface responsiveness to IL-1 than did the 5A4 cell line in that 10^8 1A5 cells absorbed away 90% of the biologic activity present in a 280 units/ml solution of IL-1. Identical absorption trials using

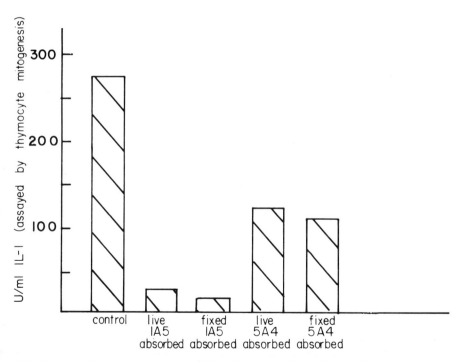

FIG. 2. Absorption of IL-1 activity by LBRM-33 1A5 and 5A4 cells. IL-1 (282 units/ml) was incubated for 4 hr at 4°C either alone (control) or in the presence of 10^8 live or fixed (2% glutaraldehyde, 15 min, 9°C) 1A5 or 5A4 cells. After 4 hr, the cells were removed and the supernatants tested for residual IL-1 activity by their ability to enhance thymocyte mitogenesis.

5A4 cells resulted in removal of only 55% of the biologic activity (20). We feel confident that such absorption studies were detailing reactivity of cell surface receptors for IL-1 and not the cell surface degradation of the monokine. First, absorption experiments were conducted at 4°C (a temperature which does not normally allow for high levels of cellular degradation metabolism), and second, fixed 1A5 cells absorbed IL-1 activity to the same extent as did live 1A5 cells (Fig. 2).

DISCUSSION

The experiments detailed in this chapter demonstrate the capacity of both murine LBRM-33 and human Jurkat-FHCRC malignant T cells to produce IL-2. Jurkat-FHCRC derived IL-2 induced T cell proliferation as tested on both murine and human cultured T cell lines. Both tumor cell lines were observed to produce IL-2 upon stimulation with appropriate concentrations of T cell mitogens; however, the quantities of factor generated far exceeded those routinely obtained from more conventional modes of IL-2 production. Peak titers of IL-2 (150–1,000 units/ml) were present in 16 to 24 hr cultured supernates of either 1% PHA or 20 μg/ml Con A stimulated Jurkat-FHCRC or LBRM-33 cells (10^6 cells/ml). This compares with titers of approximately 10 to 15 units/ml of IL-2 activity produced either by (a) mitogen stimulated spleen or (b) PHA and allogeneic B lymphoblastoid cell line stimulation of normal human PBL.

In addition to providing a new source for the isolation and characterization of human IL-2, the capacity of a continuously cultured T cell leukemia line to produce IL-2 may provide additional insight into normal IL-2 production and the role that aberrant IL-2 regulation might play in the etiology of human leukemia. For example, the observation that Jurkat-FHCRC and LBRM-33 lymphoma cells died following release of IL-2 may have some relationship to the normal condition. No evidence has been presented to date either in the mouse or human system to suggest that following ligand activation, the IL-2 producer T cell responds to IL-2 or even survives. If IL-2 producer cells were capable of responding to IL-2, one would expect that following mitogen/antigen sensitization, these cells would continue to proliferate by their own accord; if not indefinitely, at least to the point where they would represent a substantial proportion of the cells surviving ligand stimulation. Clearly, this is not the case. Activated T cells have been grown in culture only by the continual addition of IL-2. In all cases, such cell lines have been shown to mediate effector T cell function and have not been found to demonstrate capacity for IL-2 production (6,7,12).

The hypothesis that T cell leukemia may represent a population of IL-2 producer cells which respond to their own factor is an intriguing one. One might, therefore, envision a leukemic T cell as a cell with both IL-2 production and response (surface receptor) capacities. Such autostimulatory roles for factor production and use have recently been invoked in the relationship of sarcoma growth factor to the sustained *in vitro* proliferation of sarcoma virus transformed cells (27). Similar autostimulatory viral antigen presentation has been suggested as a possible explanation for the proliferation observed in virus induced murine thymomas (28). Given the knowledge that IL-2 is responsible for antigen-initiated T cell replication (1,2), the potential involvement of IL-2 in the uncontrolled replication of leukemic T cells may be considerable. For example, in screening 49 samples of adult human leukemic blasts, we observed that greater than 95% of those patients whose malignant cells tested positive for cytosol terminal deoxynucleotidyl transferase (TDT) produced significant amounts of IL-2 (greater than 20 units/ml) upon mitogen stimulation (29). Furthermore, IL-2 production by TDT (+) leukemic blasts was accompanied by extremely poor mitogen induced T cell proliferation (29). One possible (among several) hypotheses for such a finding might be that leukemic T cell IL-2 receptors were previously saturated by cellular factor production. Therefore, upon increased synthesis of IL-2, one would expect little, if any, effect on already active replicatory processes. Alternatively, poor T cell proliferation in the face of high IL-2 production might suggest a lack of IL-2 receptors on the surface of leukemic blasts or perhaps an IL-2 induced dedifferentiation effect (cessation of proliferation) on human leukemia cell replication. This possibility was further suggested by the observation that addition of exogenous purified human IL-2 to TDT (+) leukemic cells resulted in a significant diminution of leukemic cell proliferation as monitored by ^{3}H-Tdr incorporation in 24 to 72 hr cultures. Finally, it is possible to interpret the above findings simply by cell death upon IL-2 release as we have noted for both Jurkat-FHCRC and LBRM T cell malignancies (Table 2).

In addition to serving as a useful model system for studying the involvement of IL-2 production and use in leukemogenesis, cloned IL-2 producer cells were extremely useful in delineating the mechanism of action of the monokine, IL-1. We found that IL-1 has the capacity to modify the PHA-unresponsive LBRM-33 1A5 clone in some manner, which rendered it capable of producing IL-2 upon subsequent ligand activation. Such modification occurred after brief exposure to IL-1 at approximately a 10-fold lower concentration than has been shown to be active in conventional IL-1 assays (enhancement of thymocyte mitogenesis). Such an observation, however, was not totally surprising if one reconsiders what is truly being measured in a conventional IL-1 assay. It has been well documented that IL-1 in and of itself is incapable of triggering the sustained proliferation of activated T lymphocytes (30). This is a property uniquely applicable to IL-2. Therefore, the enhanced mitogenesis observed when an entire thymocyte preparation is stimulated with PHA and IL-1 must be promulgated somehow upon production of IL-2. Because only the relatively small, cortisol resistant population of the thymus (i.e., the mature T cell compartment) has been shown to produce IL-2 (21), when an entire thymocyte preparation is stimulated with mitogen (in the absence of exogenous IL-1), very little IL-2 is produced and concomitant T cell proliferation is poor. However, in the presence of IL-1, presumably more T cells (perhaps immature thymocytes) are converted to a state where they can produce IL-2 and, in doing so, result in a marked augmentation of thymocyte mitogenesis.

To this end, the observation that 1A5 cells, and to a lesser extent, 5A4 cells possessed a cell surface responsiveness to IL-1 is extremely important. 1A5 cells were shown to be converted to a state of lectin-inducible IL-2 production following only brief exposure to IL-1. Identical cell populations were also shown to be capable of actively removing IL-1 from cultures where it was present. In fact, both live and fixed 1A5 cells mediated identical absorption of IL-1 activity in 4 hr cultures conducted at 4°C. These results argue in favor of the existence of a 1A5 cell surface responsiveness to IL-1 (presumably mediated via the existence of cell surface receptors). Taken in total, it appears that the monokine IL-1 mediates its effects on immune responses via induction of the differentiation of a putative IL-2 producer cell (more than likely an immature T cell) to the point where subsequent ligand activation triggers the production and release of IL-2. Such a pathway truly separates the effects of the maturation inducing monokine IL-1 from the proliferation inducing lymphokine IL-2.

ACKNOWLEDGMENTS

Steven Gillis is a Special Fellow of The Leukemia Society of America and is supported by NCI grant #CA-28419, grant I-724 from The National Foundation, and a grant from The National Leukemia Association, Inc. James Watson is the recipient of a Research Career Development Award (AI-00182) and is supported by NIAID grant AI-13383 and a grant (I-469) from The National Foundation.

REFERENCES

1. Watson, J., Gillis, S., Marbrook, J., Mochizuki, D., and Smith, K. A. (1979): Biochemical and biological characterization of lymphocyte regulatory molecules. I. Purification of a class of murine lymphokines. *J. Exp. Med.*, 150:849.
2. Gillis, S., Smith, K. A., and Watson, J. (1980): Biochemical and biological characterization of lymphocyte regulatory molecules. II. Purification of a class of rat and human lymphokines. *J. Immunol.*, 124:1954.
3. Farrar, J. J., Simon, P. L., Koopman, W. J., and Fuller-Bonar, J. (1978): Biochemical relationship of thymocyte mitogenic factor and factors enhancing humoral and cell-mediated response. *J. Immunol.*, 121:1353.
4. Shaw, J., Monticone, V., Miller, G., and Paetkau, V. (1978): Effects of costimulator on immune responses *in vitro*. *J. Immunol.*, 120:1974.
5. Wagner, H., Hardt, C., Heeg, K., Rollinghoff, M., and Pfizenmaier, K. (1980): T cell derived helper factor allows *in vivo* induction of cytotoxic T cells in nu/nu mice. *Nature*, 284:278.
6. Watson, J. (1979): Continuous proliferation of murine antigen-specific helper T lymphocytes in culture. *J. Exp. Med.*, 150:1510.
7. Ralph, P., Broxmeyer, H., Nakoinz, I., and Moore, M. A. S. (1978): Induction of myeloid colony-stimulating activity (CSA) in murine monocyte tumor cell lines by macrophage activators, and in a T cell line by Con A. *Cancer Res.*, 38:1414.
8. Gillis, S., Scheid, M., and Watson, J. (1980): The biochemical and biological characterization of lymphocyte regulatory molecules. III. The isolation and phenotypic characterization of interleukin 2 producing T cell lymphomas. *J. Immunol.*, 125:2570.
9. Gillis, S., and Watson, J. (1980): Biochemical and biological characterization of lymphocyte regulatory molecules. V. Identification of an interleukin 2 producer human leukemia T cell line. *J. Exp. Med.*, 152:1709.
10. Hansen, J. A., Martin, P. J., and Nowinski, R. C. (1980): Monoclonal antibodies identifying a novel T cell antigen and Ia antigens of human lymphocytes. *Immunogenetics*, 10:247.
11. Gillis, S., Ferm, M. M., Ou, W., and Smith, K. A. (1978): T cell growth factor: parameters of production and a quantitative microassay for activity. *J. Immunol.*, 120:2027.
12. Gillis, S., and Smith, K. A. (1977): Long-term culture of tumor-specific cytotoxic T cells. *Nature*, 268:154.

13. Gillis, S., Baker, P. E., Ruscetti, F. W., and Smith, K. A. (1978): Long-term culture of human antigen-specific cytotoxic T cell lines. *J. Exp. Med.*, 148:1093.

14. Novogrodsky, A., Suthanthiran, M., Saltz, B., Newman, D., Rubin, A. L., and Stenzel, K. H. (1980): Generation of a lymphocyte growth factor by treatment of human cells with neuraminidase and galactose-oxidase. *J. Exp. Med.*, 151:755.

15. Smith, K. A., Gillis, S., Ruscetti, F. W., Baker, P. E., and McKenzie, D. (1979): T cell growth factor: the second signal in the T cell immune response. *Proc. N. Y. Acad. Sci.*, 332:423.

16. Mizel, S. B., Oppenheim, J. J., and Rosenstreich, D. L. (1978): Characterization of lymphocyte-activating factor (LAF) produced by the macrophage cell line, P388D. *J. Immunol.*, 120:1497.

17. Mizel, S. B. (1979): Biochemical and biological characterization of lymphocyte activating factor (LAF) produced by the murine macrophage line P388D. *Proc. N. Y. Acad. Sci.*, 332:539.

18. Alvarez, J. M., de Landazuri, M. O., Bonnard, G. D., and Herberman, R. B. (1978): Cytotoxic activities of normal cultured human T cells. *J. Immunol.*, 121:1270.

19. Mochizuki, D., Watson, J., and Gillis, S. (1980): The biochemical and biological characterization of lymphocyte regulatory molecules. IV. Purification of interleukin 2 from a murine T cell lymphoma. *J. Immunol.*, 125:2579.

20. Gillis, S., and Mizel, S. B. (1980): T cell lymphoma model for the analysis of interleukin-1 mediated T cell activation, *Proc. Natl. Acad. Sci.*, 78:1133.

21. Smith, K. A., Gillis, S., and Baker, P. E. (1979): The role of soluble factors in the regulation of T cell immune reactivity. In: *The Molecular Basis of Immune Cell Function*, edited by J. G. Kaplan, pp. 223. Elsevier/North-Holland Biomedical Press, New York.

22. Farrar, J. J., and Fuller-Bonar, J. (1980): Regulation of the production of interleukin 2 (T cell growth factor). *Fed. Proc.*, 39:3.

23. Mastro, A. M., and Mueller, G. C. (1974): Synergistic action of phorbol esters in mitogen-activated bovine lymphocytes. *Exp. Cell. Res.*, 88:40.

24. Rosenstreich, D. L., and Mizel, S. B. (1979): Signal requirements for T lymphocyte activation. I. Replacement of macrophage function with phorbol myristic acetate. *J. Immunol.*, 123:1749.

25. Larsson, E. L., Iscove, N. N., and Coutinho, A. (1980): Two distinct factors are required for induction of T cell growth. *Nature*, 283:664.

26. Smith, K. A., Lachman, L. B., Oppenheim, J. J., and Favata, M. F. (1980): The functional relationship of the interleukins. *J. Exp. Med.*, 151:1551.

27. Todaro, G. J., de Larco, J. E., Marquardt, H., Bryant, M. L., Sherwin, S. A., and Sliski, A. H. (1979): Polypeptide growth factors produced by tumor cells and virus-transformed cells: a possible growth advantage for the producer cells. In: *Hormones and Cell Culture*, edited by G. H. Sato and R. Ross. Cold Spring Harbor Symposium, Academic Press, New York.

28. Weissman, I. L. (1980): Normal and neoplastic maturation of lymphocytes. *J. Supramol. Struct.*, 4:114.

29. Gillis, S., Mertelsmann, R., Clarkson, B., and Moore, M. A. S. (1980): Correlation of elevated terminal transferase (TdT) with production of T cell growth factor in human leukemia cells. *Proc. Am. Assoc. Cancer Res.*, 21:238.

30. Aarden, L. A., *et al.* (1979): Revised nomenclature for antigen-nonspecific T cell proliferation and helper factors. *J. Immunol.*, 123:2928.

Maturation Factors and Cancer,
edited by Malcolm A. S. Moore.
Raven Press, © New York 1982.

Abnormal T-Cell Growth Factor (Interleukin 2) Response Pattern in Human Leukemias Exhibiting High Terminal Transferase Activity

Roland Mertelsmann, *Steven Gillis, Benjamin Koziner, and
Malcolm A. S. Moore

Memorial Sloan-Kettering Cancer Center, New York, New York 10021

T-cell growth factor (TCGF, interleukin 2; refs. 1,2) is the agent responsible for both mitogen and antigen stimulated T-lymphocyte proliferation (3–9). Recent studies have shown that the presence of a particular subset of T-cells is required for TCGF production, while distinct subsets of antigen or mitogen activated T-lymphocytes bind TCGF and proliferate as a direct result of this interaction (10,11). Further analysis has shown that TCGF is an important regulator of primary immune reactivity, in that it can restore nude mouse T-cell function both *in vitro* (12) and *in vivo* (13) and can support the *in vitro* generation and long-term (greater than 3 years to date) culture of cytolytic and helper T cells (3–5,14–16). Recent studies have suggested that the mechanism behind glucocorticoid hormone induced immune suppression may be explained by the capacity of glucocorticoids to inhibit TCGF production (17,18).

While TCGF appears to be one of the more important proliferation-regulating molecules of the immune response, less is known about a possible differentiative effect of TCGF on T-cell precursors. Because both T-cell mediated immune response as well as T-cell differentiation appear to be of direct relevance to leukemogenesis and to the pathophysiology of T-cell related leukemias, we examined mononuclear blood cells from patients with various leukemias in assays testing mitogen-induced proliferation, TCGF production, and TCGF response. Since TCGF production and response appear to be properties restricted to lymphocytes of the T-cell lineage, we also evaluated TCGF production and response pattern with respect to the leukemic cell phenotype, as determined by other cell markers, including terminal deoxynucleotidyl transferase (TdT).

TdT is a unique DNA polymerase apparently restricted to normal and neoplastic cells of early T-cell lineage (19–23) and a subclass of pre-B cells (24). Since

*Current address: Basic Immunology Program, Fred Hutchinson Cancer Research Center, 1124 Columbia Street, Seattle, Washington 98104.

leukemic phenotypes appear to be "frozen" at discrete developmental stages of a given cell differentiation pathway (25,26), such multifunctional analysis should help to identify the physiological roles of both TCGF and TdT during normal T-cell ontogeny and to elucidate possible aberrant mechanisms in T-cell related neoplasias.

MATERIALS AND METHODS

Patients

Peripheral blood samples from 49 adult patients with various types of leukemia, 3 patients with nonhematological malignant tumors (2 melanomas, 1 breast carcinoma), and 7 healthy volunteers were studied. Mononuclear cells were isolated from 10 ml of anticoagulated venous blood (EDTA or heparin) using a standard flotation technique (23). Only leukemia patients with at least 85% leukemic cells by morphological criteria were included in this study, with the exception of four patients in complete remission on chemotherapy. All patients were studied at diagnosis prior to initiation of chemotherapy (Table 1). Morphological diagnoses were made based on standard clinical, morphological, and cytochemical criteria (27,28). All cases of CML exhibited the Philadelphia chromosome. The comparatively high number of cases with acute nonlymphocytic leukemia (ANLL) exhibiting high levels of TdT activity (Tables 1 and 2) reflects the case selection process. Although samples from cases with ALL and CML in blast crisis were routinely obtained for TdT determinations, ANLL samples were screened predominantly in cases with equivocal morphological and cytochemical findings, often carrying a clinical diagnosis of acute undifferentiated leukemia (AUL; refs. 28,29).

Mitogen and TCGF Stimulation Assays

Separated mononuclear blood cells (23) were resuspended (1×10^6 cells/ml) in Click's medium [supplemented with 10% heat-inactivated fetal calf serum (FCS), 25 μM/ml HEPES buffer, 16 μM/ml $NaHCO_3$, 50 units/ml penicillin, 50 μg/ml streptomycin, and 300 μg/ml fresh L-glutamine] and stimulated in triplicate 200 μl microwell cultures (#3596 culture plate, Costar, Inc., Cambridge, Mass.) with either (a) tissue culture medium, (b) Concanavalin-A (Con-A, 10 μg/ml), (c) phytohemagglutin (PHA-M, 1% by volume, Grand Island Biologicals Co.) or (d) purified human TCGF to which a mitogenic dose of PHA had been added. Human TCGF was purified from 48 hr culture medium from peripheral blood mononuclear leukocytes conditioned by 1% PHA and lymphoblastoid cell line stimulation (5). Purified human TCGF used in these studies was prepared by sequential 85% ammonium sulfate precipitation, Sephadex G-100 gel filtration chromatography, and DEAE ion-exchange chromatography using methods previously described (10,11). After varying time periods (see Results), 100 μl of supernate from stimulated cultures was removed and tested for TCGF activity. To assess cellular proliferation,

TABLE 1. *Clinical diagnoses, TdT activities, and TCGF parameters in response to concanavalin A[a]*

Clinical diagnosis	Cases (n)	TdT activity (units/10⁸ cell)	Stimulation index (S. I.)[b]	TCGF production (units/ml)	TCGF response index (F. I.)[c]
Acute leukemias					
ALL, TdT(+)	9	4.5 ± 6.6	4.7 ± 6.3	3.9–5.5	2.1 ± 2.1
ALL, TdT(−)	1	0.03	1.0	0.0	
ALL, CR, TdT(−)[d]	3	0.05	265	4.0	67.6
		(0.04–0.05)	(121–362)	(1.8–6.1)	(59.4–75.9)
ANLL, TdT(+)	7	6.4 ± 8.3	17.7 ± 32.6	8.5 ± 5.1	7.6 ± 15.5
ANLL, TdT(−)	9	0.05 ± 0.02	73.2 ± 65.3	1.8 ± 1.6	30.1 ± 16.8
ANLL, CR, TdT(−)	1	0.05	97.4	1.1	88.2
Chronic leukemias					
CML, TdT(−)	2	0.07	0.8	0.0	
		(0.05–0.09)	(0.5–1.1)		
CML, blastic, TdT(−)	3	0.04	0.9	0.0	
		(0.02–0.07)	(0.8–1.1)		
CML, blastic, TdT(+)	4	7.9 ± 5.4	2.0 ± 1.3	2.6 ± 0.9	0.7 ± 0.3
CLL, TdT(−)	3	0.04	69.7	1.2	66.1
		(0.02–0.05)	(8.9–186)	(0.1–3.1)	(49.0–89.0)
LSA-leukemia[e] TdT(−)	5	0.04 ± 0.02	206 ± 164	3.4 ± 2.6	60.8 ± 19.4
HCL, TdT(−)	2	0.02	38.5	0.5	36.8
		(0.01–0.03)	(35–42)	(0.1–0.9)	(33–40.6)
Controls, TdT(−)					
Solid tumors	3	0.04	312	13.7	33.1
		(0.02–0.05)	(60–469)	(1.5–24.0)	(29–40.1)
Normal blood	7	0.05 ± 0.02	146 ± 61	3.4 ± 1.4	42.7 ± 3.6

[a]All assays were performed under standard conditions as described in Materials and Methods. All values are expressed as mean values ± standard deviation (range). For three and less cases means (range) are given.
[b]Cpm stimulated cultures/cpm medium control.
[c]TCGF response index = stimulation index/TCGF produced (units/ml)
[d]TdT(+) ALL, tested in a TdT(−) complete remission sample.
[e]Leukemic phase of three cases of DPDL and two cases of NPDL.

identical cultures were pulsed for 4 hr with tritiated thymidine (³H-Tdr, 0.5 μCi/microplate well, specific activity 20 mCi/mmole, New England Nuclear, Boston, Mass.) and harvested onto glass fiber filter strips with the aid of a multiple sample harvester. Incorporated thymidine was counted by liquid scintillation and cellular proliferation, quantified in terms of stimulation indices (S.I.; cpm of ³H-Tdr incorporated by stimulated cultures divided by cpm incorporated in medium control cultures). In experiments designed to test the effects of malignant blasts on normal T-cell mitogen-induced TCGF production and proliferation, density separated normal mononuclear leukocytes were mixed prior to culture in various ratios (total final concentration 1 × 10⁶ cells/ml) with malignant T-lymphoma cells harvested from long term *in vitro* cultures (CEM or MOLT-4).

TCGF Microassay

Supernatants harvested from cultures of resting and stimulated leukemic blasts were tested for TCGF activity by their ability to maintain the proliferation of murine cytotoxic T cells (CTLL) harvested from long term TCGF-dependent cultures (4). Using a method previously described (1), 3,000 CTLL cells were cultured in 200 μl of supplemented Click's medium for 24 hr in the presence of a log2 dilution series of a putative TCGF-containing sample. Following a subsequent 4 hr pulse with ^{3}H-Tdr, only CTLL cells cultured in the presence of TCGF incorporated ^{3}H-Tdr in a dose-dependent manner (1). CTLL cells cultured in the absence of TCGF were >95% trypan blue positive and incorporated only scintillant control levels of ^{3}H-Tdr. TCGF activity was quantified by means of probit analysis of ^{3}H-Tdr incorporation data, which used a 1 unit/ml preparation of TCGF supernate from 48 hr Con A stimulated rat splenocytes (10^6 cells/ml) as a standard. Factor response index values (F.I.) were determined by dividing the S.I. observed in a particular stimulation culture by the amount of TCGF (units/ml) present in the supernate harvested from the same culture. F.I. was considered as an indicator of the proliferative response of the incubated cells in response to factor produced by these cells ("endogenous TCGF response"). The difference between S.I. observed in the presence of added TCGF + PHA and the S.I. determined in the presence of PHA alone (ΔS.I.; "exogenous TCGF response") was used as an indicator of the response of the test cells to the exogenous TCGF, purified from normal T-lymphocyte conditioned medium (cf. above).

Terminal Deoxynucleotidyl Transferase Assay

Terminal transferase activities were determined as recently described (30). Briefly, mononuclear cells were isolated after 1 : 1 dilution with normal saline using the standard Ficoll-Hypaque flotation technique. After separation, cells were washed once with normal saline and then suspended (10^7 cells/ml) in TGED (50 mM Tris HCL, pH 7.8, 0.5 mM K-EDTA, 1 mM DTT, 10% glycerol) with 0.5% Triton X-100 and 0.3 M KCl, sonicated, and cell debris removed by a 5 min 10,000 × g centrifugation (Beckman Minifuge). One hundred μl (equivalent to 1.0 × 10^6 cells) of the supernatant were mixed with 50 μl of a 30% phosphocellulose (PC) slurry, previously equilibrated in TGED. TdT binds to PC at the resulting salt concentration of 0.2 M KCl. The PC pellet was washed once in TGED and TdT was subsequently eluted with 50 μl 0.5 M KCl in TGED. TdT activity was determined in quadruplicate, using 5 μl PC eluate (equivalent to 100,000 cells) in a 50 μl reaction volume in the absence and presence of 50 μM ATP as a specific inhibitor for TdT (30). TdT activity was expressed in units [nmoles of (^{3}H) dGTP incorporated in 1 hr at 37°C] per 10^8 cells. Normal values for bone marrow mononuclear cells are <0.15 unit/10^8 cells. Approximately 95% of cases of lymphoblastic leukemia, lymphoblastic lymphoma, or lymphoblastic crisis of chronic myeloid leukemia exhibit activities over 1.0 unit/10^8 cells in this assay system (30).

Cell Surface Markers

Cell surface marker analysis was performed on separated peripheral blood mono-nuclear cells employing previously published techniques for demonstration of sur-face immunoglobulins, and of receptors for complement, Fc, and for mouse and sheep red blood cells (23).

RESULTS

Typical TCGF production and cellular proliferation kinetics of mitogen stimulated human blood lymphocytes are detailed in Fig. 1. Both Con-A and PHA stimulated cells produced significant quantities of TCGF (3–8 units/ml). Peak concentrations of TCGF were detected in 48 hr supernates, whereas maximal lectin-induced pro-liferation was observed 24 hr later (72 hr cultures). The previous observations that any population of ligand-stimulated T lymphocytes actively absorbs TCGF from tissue culture medium where it is present, and that upon absorption of TCGF, responsive T cells proliferate, are supported by these data, which show peak TCGF production preceding the TCGF-dependent T cell proliferation. Based on these data, we chose to assay 48 hr mitogen-induced supernates for TCGF activity and identical 72 hr cultures for lectin induced proliferation, when studying peripheral leukemic blasts for TCGF production and response.

The patients studied carried clinical diagnoses of acute lymphoblastic leukemia (ALL, $n = 13$), acute nonlymphoblastic leukemia (ANLL, $n = 17$), chronic myeloid leukemia, chronic phase (CML, $n = 2$), CML-blast crisis ($n = 7$), chronic

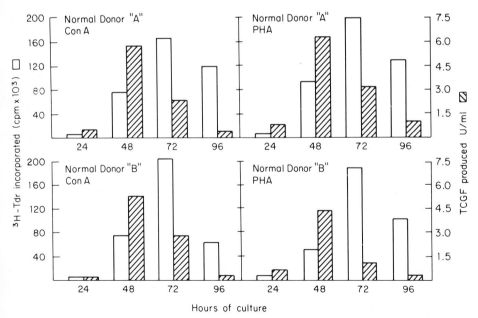

FIG. 1. Proliferation kinetics and TCGF production by normal human blood lymphocytes.

lymphocytic leukemia (CLL, $n = 3$), lymphosarcoma (LSA) leukemia ($n = 5$), and hairy cell leukemia (HCL, $n = 2$). The same peripheral blood samples which were received for TdT determination were further analyzed for TCGF production and response. In addition, cell surface marker analysis was performed in 10 patients, revealing 1 thymic and 2 "non-B, non-T" phenotypes in the ALL group, and 7 "non-B, non-T" phenotypes in the ANLL group. Data generated from all normal controls and patient samples tested are detailed in Tables 1 and 2 and are grouped by clinical diagnosis. Table 1 lists mean TdT expression by the leukemic blasts as well as mean Con-A induced cellular proliferation and TCGF production. TCGF response is also shown in Table 1 by calculation of the mean factor response index (S.I. observed in 72 hr cultures per unit/ml TCGF in 48 hr culture supernates). Table 2 details the data in response to stimulation with PHA observed in the same blood samples. In addition to listing the mean TCGF production and factor response index values (as a measure of endogenous TCGF response), Table 2 also details exogenous TCGF response in terms of ΔS.I. (the difference between the S.I. observed when leukemic or normal blood lymphocytes were cultured in the presence of PHA and additional TCGF, and the S.I. determined after 72 hr culture with PHA alone). These same data (mitogen-induced proliferation and TCGF production, TCGF response indices and ΔS.I.) are displayed graphically in Fig. 2 according to diagnosis and TdT phenotype. Factor response index values and ΔS.I. (exogenous factor response) for individual patients are shown in Figs. 3 and 4.

Mononuclear cell fractions containing predominantly T lymphocytes from healthy control persons revealed a reproducible and characteristic pattern of TCGF production and response. Spontaneous proliferation of normal lymphocytes was characteristically low (104–306 cpm incorporated in unstimulated medium control cultures). Unstimulated cultures did not produce detectable amounts of TCGF. In PHA or Con-A stimulated cultures, more than 0.5 unit/ml of TCGF was consistently produced. There was at least a 30-fold increase in proliferation in stimulated cultures compared to medium controls. A very pronounced response was observed following stimulation with endogenous as well as additional TCGF. Endogenous TCGF response indices (F.I.) were typically over 25. The exogenous TCGF response index (ΔS.I.) was always over 20 (Table 2), indicating that normal mitogen-activated human T cells used exogenously supplied TCGF to support their exponential proliferation. Neither unstimulated nor stimulated cultures revealed any detectable TdT activity, as previously reported (21).

Analysis of leukemic blast cell responses revealed three different TCGF production and response patterns, irrespective of their clinical diagnoses. Nineteen of 20 patients (9 ALL, 7 ANLL, 4 CML-blast crisis) exhibiting high levels of TdT activity in their leukemic blood cells [TdT(+)] showed a small proliferation increase in response to PHA or Con-A stimulation but produced exceptionally high levels of TCGF, resulting in very low TCGF indices (Tables 1 and 2; Figs. 2 and 4). The response to added purified human TCGF and PHA was also atypical, in that incorporation of ^{3}H-Tdr was found to actually decrease in the majority of TdT(+) leukemias, when compared to PHA-stimulated proliferation (Figs. 2 and 4). This

TABLE 2. Clinical diagnosis, TdT, and TCGF parameters in response to PHA and PHA + TCGF[a]

Clinical diagnosis, TdT	Cases (n)	PHA Stimulation index (S.I.)	PHA TCGF produced (units/ml)	TCGF response index (F.I.)	PHA + TCGF, stimulation index (S.I.)	S.I. (PHA + TCGF) −S.I. (PHA) Δ S.I.
Acute leukemias						
ALL, TdT(+)	8	5.3 ± 9.2	6.9 ± 5.6	0.8 ± 0.9	4.0 ± 5.2	−0.7 ± 1.4
ALL, TdT(−)	1	0.9	0.0		0.5	0.4
ALL, CR, TdT(−)	3	321 (132–436)	5.7 (2.0–8.3)	59 (48–66)	428 (255–562)	106 (70–126)
ANLL, TdT(+)	7	13.5 ± 22.9	9.9 ± 8.9	6.0 ± 13.8	19.7 ± 44.2	6.2 ± 20.6
ANLL, TdT(−)	9	100.3 ± 105.5	2.7 ± 2.2	75.7 ± 114.4	136 ± 139	36.2 ± 36.6
ANLL, CR, TdT(−)	1	110	2.0	55	177	67
Chronic leukemias						
CML, TdT(−)	2	1.1 (0.8–3.1)	0.0		1.3 (1.0–1.6)	0.3 (0.2–0.3)
CML, blastic, TdT(−)	3	1.5 (0.6–3.1)	0.0		1.8 (1.0–3.4)	0.3 (0.3–0.4)
CML, blastic, TdT(+)	4	5.9 ± 5.8	5.4 ± 3.9	0.8 ± 0.4	3.0 ± 1.6	−1.8 ± 4.3
CLL, TdT(−)	3	103 (35–210)	1.9 (1.2–2.8)	46.6 (29.4–74.5)	151.3 (38.2–135.3)	48.7 (13–72)
LSA-leukemia, TdT(−)	5	277 ± 157	4.9 ± 2.9	60.5 ± 13	413 ± 230	136 ± 89
HCL, TdT(−)	2	48.4 (39.8–57.0)	1.1 (0.9–1.2)	47.2 (46.8–47.5)	75 (67–83)	26.5 (26–27)
Controls, TdT(−)						
Solid tumors	3	670 (513–887)	19.9 (10.2–26.6)	44.2 (33.5–59.8)	906 (740–1,212)	236 (130–325)
Normal blood	7	185 ± 69	4.4 ± 1.8	42.9 ± 4.3	265 ± 77	80.9 ± 36.5

[a]For assay conditions and abbreviations, see Materials and Methods and legend to Table 1.

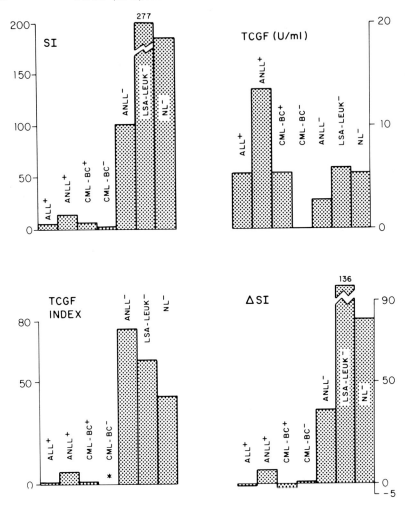

FIG. 2. Stimulation indices, TCGF production, TCGF response index, and response to exogenous TCGF (ΔS.I.) in patients with acute leukemias, CML in blast crisis, and in control lymphocytes. Experiments were carried out under standard conditions using PHA as mitogen. Results are expressed as mean value by clinical diagnosis and TdT phenotype. **A:** SI = stimulation index (cpm + PHA/cpm control). **B:** TCGF produced by 48 hr cultures (units/ml). **C:** TCGF index = S.I. observed in 72 hr cultures per unit/ml TCGF in 48 hr supernates. **D:** ΔSI = difference between S.I. in the presence of PHA and added TCGF (1 unit/ml) and the S.I. determined after culture with PHA alone. Index +/− refers to TdT(+) and TdT(−) phenotypes. ALL = acute lymphoblastic leukemia, ANLL = acute nonlymphoblastic leukemia, CML-BC = CML blast crisis, LAS-leukemia = lymphosarcoma cell leukemia, NL = normal controls. * Indicates no measurable TCGF production.

was in marked contrast to results obtained with control lymphocytes and in TdT(−) leukemias (ANLL, LSA leukemia, CLL, HCL), which exhibited significantly increased proliferation following costimulation with purified TCGF and PHA (Figs. 2–4). One case of "non-T, non-B" ALL exhibited no significant level of TdT activity [ALL, TdT(−); Tables 1 and 2] and also showed no evidence of factor production or response ["production(−)/response(−)"]. This TCGF pattern was also seen in 2 out of 2 cases of TdT(−) ANLL, in 2 out of 2 TdT(−) CML, and in 3 out of 3 TdT(−) CML in blast crisis, as well as in 1 case with TdT(−) LSA leukemia (Figs. 3 and 4). All other cases were TdT(−) and revealed an essentially normal pattern of TCGF production (Fig. 3).

Figure 2 details TCGF production and response parameters of blast cell populations, categorized by diagnosis and TdT phenotype. Figure 2A shows the characteristically low proliferative response to PHA in TdT(+) ALL, TdT(+) ANLL, TdT(+) CML-blast crisis, and in TdT(−) CML blast crisis compared to the average response seen in cases of TdT(−) ANLL, LSA leukemia, and in normal lymphocyte controls. However, TCGF production in TdT(+) ALL, ANLL, and CML-BC was similar or higher than in normals (Fig. 2B). As a result, this low proliferation, in comparison to the high amounts of TCGF produced, yielded remarkably low TCGF response index values in the TdT(+) phenotypes (Fig. 2C). Furthermore, proliferation in response to stimulation with PHA and human TCGF (purified from normal lymphocyte conditioned medium) resulted in decreased proliferation in the majority of cases, which was in contrast to the significantly increased response seen in TdT(−) ANLL, LSA-leukemia, and in control lymphocyte populations (Fig. 2D).

Figures 3 and 4 further detail the proliferative response to endogenously produced factor (TCGF index; F.I.) as well as response to costimulation with exogenous TCGF and PHA (ΔS.I.) for individual patients. Although all controls and the majority of the TdT(−) leukemic phenotypes showed a significant response to both endogenous and exogenously supplied TCGF, all TdT(+) phenotypes (with one exception) demonstrated very low F.I. as well as minimally stimulated or even decreased proliferation in response to added TCGF (Figs. 3 and 4). It was of interest that CML in chronic phase and in TdT(−) blast crisis was not found to produce detectable amounts of TCGF, while the TdT(+) phenotype of CML blast crisis showed the same pattern seen in other TdT(+) leukemias. Only two exceptions to these characteristic patterns of TdT expression and TCGF production were seen. One case of TdT(−) ANLL behaved in terms of TCGF production and response in a manner otherwise only seen in TdT(+) cases. Finally, one case of TdT(+) ANLL exhibited high TdT activity but a normal TCGF response pattern. Although technical errors cannot be completely ruled out, they appear unlikely in view of the consistency of all other results. No other clinical or morphological features were strikingly unique in these two cases.

We feel confident that the TCGF production and response data detailed above reflect, for the large majority, reactivities of the leukemic blast cell populations present in the peripheral blood, as opposed to responses of residual normal T cells. Our conviction is based primarily on the results of mixing experiments, in which normal lymphocytes were admixed in varying proportions with either CEM or MOLT-4 cells (two T cell leukemias adapted to standard *in vitro* culture) prior to use in identical TCGF production/response assays. As shown in Table 3, an admixture of only 50% cells derived from either leukemic T-cell line completely

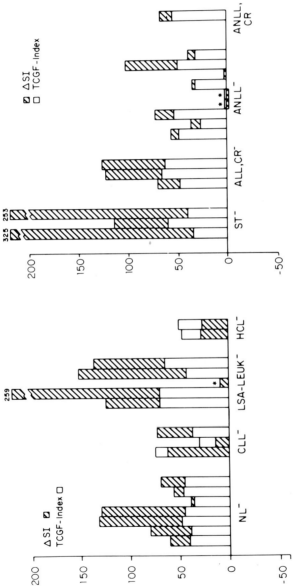

FIG. 3. Proliferation in 72 hr cultures in response to endogenously produced TCGF (TCGF index) and to added TCGF (ΔS.I.) in patients with TdT(−) phenotypes and in controls. Experiments were carried out under standard conditions using PHA as mitogen. Results are presented for each patient studied by diagnosis and TdT phenotype. CLL = chronic lymphocytic leukemia, HCL = hairy cell leukemia, CR = complete remission, ST = solid tumor. All other abbreviations are described in the legend to Fig. 2.

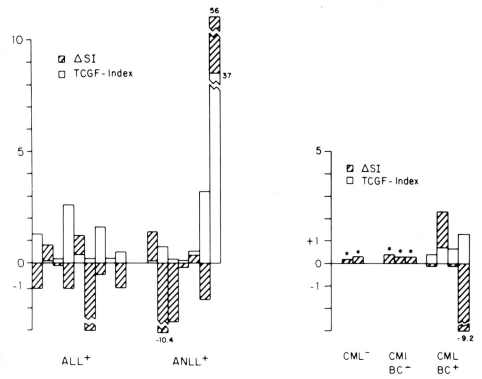

FIG. 4. Proliferation in 72 hr cultures in response to endogenously produced TCGF (TCGF index) and to added TCGF (ΔS.I.) in patients with TdT(+) acute leukemias and in CML. CML = CML, chronic phase; CML-BC = CML, in blast crisis. For other details see legends to Figs. 2 and 3.

suppressed mitogen induced stimulation and TCGF production by normal lymphocytes. Production/response patterns (factor response index values and ΔS.I.) even in 50/50% admixture populations were essentially identical to response mediated by the tumor cells alone. Since all patient blood samples assayed contained >80% leukemic blasts, it seemed reasonable to assume that the TCGF production and response pattern of the TdT(+) lymphoblastic leukemias detailed in this work represented leukemic as opposed to residual normal lymphocyte reactivity.

As mentioned earlier, the leukemic cell TCGF reactivity observed in each patient tested could be characterized by one of three response patterns, summarized in Tables 4 and 5. TCGF production and responses similar to those manifested by normal lymphocytes were observed only in one case of TdT(+) ANLL. Normal reactivity was typified by pronounced cellular proliferation and modest TCGF production in response to mitogen stimulation. Such values lead to calculation of relatively high endogenous TCGF indices (>25). PHA triggered cellular proliferation in either normal PBL or 20 TdT(−) leukemias was significantly augmented by costimulation with purified human TCGF (ΔS.I. values ranging from 30 to 196). The overwhelming majority of TdT(+) leukemic blast populations (19/20 samples)

TABLE 3. TCGF production and proliferation by mixed cultures of normal lymphocytes and human leukemic cells[a]

Proportions		+PHA			+PHA + TCGF		
Normal lymphocytes	Leukemic cells	Stimulation index (S.I.)	TCGF produced (units/ml)	TCGF index (F.I.)	Stimulation index (S.I.)	TCGF produced (units/ml)	TCGF index (F.I.)
Experiment 1 (MOLT-4)							
100%	0%	411.0	10.2	40.3	512	13.1	39.1
50%	50%	0.9	0		0.9	0	
25%	75%	0.6	0		1.0	0	
10%	90%	0.6	0		0.9	0	
0%	100%	0.6	0		1.00	0	
Experiment 2							
100%	0%	456.0	8.9	51.2	499	8.2	60.8
50%	50%	0.9	0		0.8	0	
25%	75%	0.7	0		0.7	0	
10%	90%	0.7	0		0.9	0	
0%	100%	0.6	0		0.8	0	

[a]Normal lymphocytes and leukemic cells were mixed to a final concentration of 10^6 cell/ml prior to stimulation. For other assay conditions and abbreviations, see Materials and Methods and legend to Table 1.

TABLE 4. *TCGF: phenotype and TdT activity in mononuclear blood cells from patients with leukemia*

TCGF, phenotype	TdT(+) (n/total)	Proliferative response (S. I.)	TCGF production (units/ml)	Endogenous TCGF response (F. I.)	Exogenous TCGF response (ΔS. I.)
ALL, type	19/20	<25	>1.0	<3.0	<20
Normal	1/21	>25	>0.5	>25	>30
Production(−)/ response(−)	0/8	<25	<0.2		<10

TABLE 5. *TCGF: phenotype and clinical diagnosis in patients with leukemias and in controls*

Clinical diagnosis	TCGF: phenotype		
	ALL, type	Normal (n/total)	Production(−)/ response(−)
Acute leukemias			
ALL, TdT +	9/9		
ALL, TdT −		1/1	
ALL, CR		3/3	
ANLL, TdT +	6/7	1/7	
ANLL, TdT −	1/9	6/9	2/9
ANLL, CR		1/1	
Chronic leukemias			
CML			2/2
CML-BC, TdT −			3/3
CML-BC, TdT +	4/4		
CLL		3/3	
LSA-leukemia		4/5	1/5
HCL		2/2	
Controls			
Solid tumors		3/3	
Normal controls		7/7	

tested mediated responses which were classified as typical of TdT(+) ALL. ALL-type reactivity was consistently characterized by poor mitogen-induced cellular proliferation in the face of significantly higher than normal TCGF production, leading to the calculation of extremely low endogenous TCGF indices. Most strikingly, addition of exogenous TCGF to PHA-stimulated cultures from TdT(+) leukemias resulted in little if any increase in cellular proliferation. In the majority of cases tested, such dual stimulation resulted in a significant diminution of cellular proliferation as opposed to cultures containing only PHA. Finally, a production(−)/response(−) pattern was observed in eight TdT(−) samples (predominantly CML). This phenotype was accompanied by poor mitogen-induced cellular proliferation and undetectable TCGF production, which precluded calculation of factor index values. As was the case with ALL-type samples, dual stimulation with TCGF and PHA of production(−)/response(−) leukemic blasts resulted in little if any increase in mitogen-induced cellular proliferation in this TCGF phenotype.

DISCUSSION

High levels of TdT activity in human leukemic blood cells have been documented to be associated with lymphoblastic leukemias or lymphoma in the vast majority of cases (19–25). These cells have been demonstrated to be in most instances of a pre-T or thymic T-cell phenotype (24,25) and occasionally of pre-B-cell type (24). However, there is still considerable controversy regarding the developmental counterpart, if any, of TdT(+) cells in blastic phases of other myeloproliferative or myelodysplastic disorders and in rare cases of AML. Pluripotential stem cells and "dedifferentiated" leukemic cells have been hypothesized to express TdT (31). However, our studies have failed to show TdT in murine pluripotential, myeloid, or erythroid stem cells (32). Further detailed analysis using multiple marker techniques of the cases of TdT(+) ANLL observed by us has shown TdT expression to be restricted to lymphoblastic cell populations in acute undifferentiated leukemias and has led to the concept of bi- or polyphenotypic leukemias (32,33; unpublished observations).

The patient population diagnosed as ANLL and analyzed in this study was preselected, in that predominantly acute undifferentiated leukemias (AUL; ref. 28) with nonspecific or equivocal morphology and cytochemistry were submitted for study. The group of AUL has previously been shown to express high levels of TdT activity in approximately one-half of the cases (28,29). Thus AUL appears to comprise a heterogeneous group of cases with markedly deranged morphology, making cell type identification impossible without marker studies. Several cases of biphenotypic leukemias (identified in this laboratory by multiple marker studies) carried a morphological diagnosis of AUL (32). Since the cell lineage associated with high levels of TdT in ANLL and blastic CML has remained controversial, we employed the analysis of TCGF production and response as new functional parameters to dissect leukemic cell lineage and function. TCGF production and response appear to be highly cell-lineage specific functions of T cells (1–18). Although other T-cell activating factors are known to be produced by other cell types, only TCGF can be measured in the microassay system used in our studies (CTLL proliferation). Since the target cell line employed in the standard TCGF assay is of murine origin, we also examined several of the supernatants using human TCGF-dependent lymphocyte cultures as test cells, yielding identical results (data not shown). Therefore, the production of TCGF as a "functional T cell marker" in 9 out of 9 cases of TdT(+) ALL, 6 out of 7 cases of TdT(+) ANLL, and 4 out of 4 cases of TdT(+) CML blast crisis (Table 5) strongly supports the hypothesis that these neoplasias are related to the T-cell lineage and confirms the significance of elevated TdT activity as a marker for immature cells of T-cell lineage.

The results obtained in this study suggest that the TCGF response pattern in TdT(+) phenotypes is due to the leukemic cell reactivity rather than the response of residual normal T lymphocytes. In the mixing experiment detailed in Table 3, addition of only 50% leukemic T lymphoblasts to normal blood lymphocytes completely suppressed TCGF production by normal T cells. In contrast to the patterns observed in TdT(+) phenotypes, TdT(−) phenotypes demonstrated either normal TCGF production and responses or a nonproducer/nonresponder pattern. It should be mentioned that the normal response patterns seen in TdT(−) leukemias could be due to increased TCGF production responses by residual normal T cells following mitogen sensitization in the presence of human Ia bearing leukemic cells. The admixture of Ia bearing cells was originally reported by Alvarez and his colleagues (34) as a method to boost TCGF production by PHA-stimulated normal human lymphocytes. Such an Ia-augmented costimulator effect is routinely observed with B lymphoblastoid cell lines (5,11,35). This may very well explain why TCGF production can be observed at all when TdT(−) and Ia-positive leukemic samples were tested, leading to maximum costimulation of residual normal T cells. The response pattern, however, was in all of these cases identical to that observed in normal controls. Although T lymphocytes in ALL have been shown to exhibit different stimulation kinetics in response to PHA as compared to normal controls (36), our TCGF patterns were not influenced by either variation in cell concentration, culture duration, or spontaneous incorporation (medium cpm). Normal, ALL-type, and nonresponder patterns were seen in cases with very high and low spontaneous proliferation. It is of interest that TCGF production by TdT(+) leukemias did not occur spontaneously but only in the presence of a ligand, a pattern similar to that of the normal TCGF producing peripheral T lymphocyte (1,16). Furthermore, the only mouse and human malignant T cell lines capable of producing TCGF also exhibit high levels of TdT activity (37; R. Mertelsmann and S. Gillis, manuscripts in preparation).

Normal peripheral T cells exhibit the phenotypes TdT(−)/TCGF production(+) and TdT(−)/TCGF response(+) (38,39). Studies in other systems have shown that immature T cells, or nude mouse pre-T cells (TdT not determined) do not produce TCGF but can respond to TCGF once activated by mitogen or antigen (12). Similarly, cortisone sensitive [i.e., TdT(+)] thymocytes do not produce TCGF but can respond to its proliferative effect once stimulated by ligand (10,11). Thus the most frequent TCGF phenotype observed in human TdT(+) leukemia [TdT(+)/TCGF producer] remains as yet without physiological equivalent. Circumstantial evidence, however, may further support a relationship between TdT expression and TCGF production, since both TdT(+) leukemic cells as well as TCGF production have been shown to be exquisitely sensitive to low doses of glucocorticoids (14,18). While an as yet unrecognized TdT(+), TCGF-producing pre-T type could be the target cell for leukemic transformation in lymphoblastic leukemias, the possibility of a leukemia-specific derangement of expression of cell markers and functions has to be explored. Although TdT(+) leukemic cells do not respond to exogenous TCGF by increased proliferation and show a low endogenous TCGF response index, it is possible that the producer cells in fact also respond to TCGF, leading to a self-stimulating and expanding cell compartment. This hypothesis would assume saturation of TCGF receptors by the high quantities of TCGF produced. This unphysiological response could be due to TCGF production by TCGF-receptor expressing cells or by expression of TCGF receptors on TCGF producer cells or on a related progenitor cell. Such a model would intimate that TCGF is an essential element of leukemic cell proliferation. Proof for such a hypothesis awaits more sensitive methods for detection of TCGF products (radioimmunoassay) and responsiveness (quantitative receptor assays using radiolabeled purified TCGF). Figure 5 details the possible pathogenetic defects of TCGF production and response in ALL.

TCGF PHYSIOLOGY AND HYPOTHETICAL DEFECTS IN ALL (---)

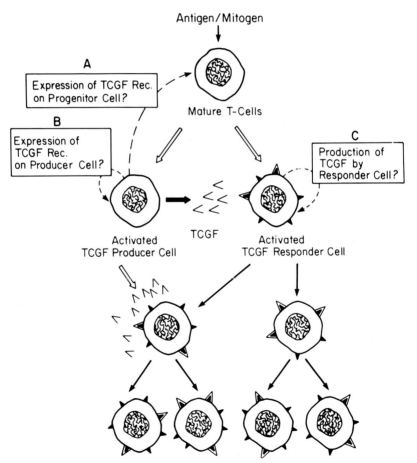

FIG. 5.   TCGF production and response by normal peripheral blood T cells and possible defects in acute lymphoblastic leukemia.

The significance of the slight decrease in proliferation observed after stimulation with exogenous "normal" TCGF in the majority of TdT(+) leukemic cases suggests the possibility of an atypical growth factor produced by the leukemic cells or, alternatively, a differentiation-inducing effect manifested by the TCGF itself. Further studies are necessary to prove or disprove the hypotheses suggested by the data. The significance of the two cases with "atypical" response patterns (Tables 1 and 2; Figs. 3 and 4), i.e., a TdT(+) leukemia with normal TCGF responses and a TdT(−) leukemia with ALL-type response, remains to be determined. The "pre-B, TdT(+)" phenotype recently described (24,40) could account for the TdT(+) leukemia with normal TCGF response patterns. Unfortunately, cytoplasmic Ig analysis was not performed in the cases studied.

Although only three cases of ALL in complete remission were studied, it appears that peripheral blood lymphocytes return to normal upon remission, not only with respect to TdT activity but with regard to TCGF production and response as well. It is of potential clinical interest that neither CML in chronic phase nor CML in TdT(−) blast crisis produced detectable amounts of TCGF, in contrast to all cases of TdT(+) blast crisis studied. Should this observation be consistent in studies on larger patient groups, it is conceivable that TCGF functional assays might prove to be valuable tools for cell lineage identification and early detection of lymphoblastic crisis in CML, with corresponding therapeutic implications (20).

This study demonstrates for the first time a consistent regulatory abnormality confined to a specific leukemic cell phenotype. The data obtained so far support the hypothesis that the expression of TdT in leukemic blasts is indicative of their T cell lineage in the majority of cases. Furthermore, the functional characterization of these malignant cells as TCGF producers suggests that the aberrant proliferation and lack of maturation observed in leukemic disorders may be associated with or be the result of a breakdown in regulator mediated control of proliferation. The application of this assay system to the analysis of other phenotypic and functional parameters should provide further insight into normal cell proliferation control and its possible derangements in human leukemia.

ACKNOWLEDGMENTS

We would like to acknowledge the expert technical assistance of Ms. Anne Gillis and Ms. Lorna Barnett. We appreciate the cooperation of the Tumor Procurement Service, MSKCC, and Drs. Arlin, Gee, Kempin, and Clarkson of the Hematology/Lymphoma Service, Memorial Hospital. We would like to thank Ms. Cynthia Garcia for the typing of the manuscript. This work was supported in part by grants CA-20194 and CA-08748, awarded by the National Cancer Institute, DHEW, grant 1-724 from the National Foundation, a grant from the Nationa Leukemia Association, Inc., and by the Gar Reichman Foundation. Steven Gillis is a Special Fellow of the Leukemia Society of America.

REFERENCES

1. Baker, P. E., Gillis, S., Ferm, M. M., and Smith, K. A. (1978): The effect of T cell growth factor on the generation of cytolytic T cells. *J. Immunol.*, 121:2168–2173.

2. Aarden, L. A., et al. (1979): Revised nomenclature for antigen-nonspecific T-cell proliferation and helper factors. *J. Immunol.*, 123:2928–2929.
3. Watson, J. (1979): Continuous proliferation of murine antigen-specific helper T lymphocytes in culture. *J. Exp. Med.*, 150:1510–1519.
4. Gillis, S., and Smith, K. A. (1977): Long-term culture of tumor-specific cytotoxic T-cells. *Nature*, 268:154–156.
5. Gillis, S., Baker, P. E., Ruscetti, F. W., and Smith, K. A. (1978): Long-term culture of human antigen-specific cytotoxic T-cell lines. *J. Exp. Med.*, 148:1093–1098.
6. Baker, P. E., Gillis, S., and Smith, K. A. (1979): Monoclonal cytotoxic T-cell lines. *J. Exp. Med.*, 149:273–278.
7. Ruscetti, R. W., Morgan, D. A., and Gallo, R. C. (1977): Functional and morphologic characterization of human T cells continuously grown *in vitro. J. Immunol.*, 119:131–138.
8. Morgan, D. A., and Ruscetti, F. W. (1976): Selective *in vitro* growth of T lymphocytes from normal human bone marrow. *Science*, 193:1007–1008.
9. Wagner, H., and Rollinghoff, M. (1978): T-T-cell interactions during *in vitro* cytotoxic allograft responses. I. Soluble products from activated Lyl + T-cells trigger autonomously antigen-primed Ly23 + T-cells to cell proliferation and cytolytic activity. *J. Exp. Med.*, 148:1523–1538.
10. Watson, J. D., Gillis, S., Marbrook, J., Mochizuki, D., and Smith, K. A. (1979): Biochemical and biological characterization of lymphocyte regulatory molecules. I. Purification of a class of murine lymphokines. *J. Exp. Med.*, 150:849–861.
11. Gillis, S., Smith, K. A., and Watson, J. D. (1980): Biochemical and biological characterization of lymphocyte regulatory molecules. II. Purification of a class of rat and human lymphokines. *J. Immunol.*, 124:1954–1962.
12. Gillis, S., Union, N. A., Baker, P. E., and Smith, K. A. (1979): The in vitro generation and sustained culture of nude mouse cytolytic T-lymphocytes. *J. Exp. Med.*, 149:1460–1476.
13. Wagner, H., Hardt, C., Heeg, K., Rollinghoff, M., and Pfizenmaier, K. (1980): T-cell derived helper factor allows in vivo induction of cytotoxic T-cells in nu/nu mice. *Nature*, 284:278–280.
14. Strausser, J. L., and Rosenberg, S. A. (1978): *In vitro* growth of cytotoxic human lymphocytes. I. Growth of cells sensitized *in vitro* to alloantigens. *J. Immunol.*, 121:1491–1495.
15. Tees, R., and Schrier, M. H. (1980): Selective reconstitution of nude mice with long-term cultured and cloned helper T-cells. *Nature*, 283:780–781.
16. Rosenberg, S. A., Spiess, P. J., and Schwarz, S. (1978): *In vitro* growth of murine T cells. I. Production of factors necessary for T cell growth. *J. Immunol.*, 121:1946–1950.
17. Gillis, S., Crabtree, G. R., and Smith, K. A. (1979): Glucocorticoid-induced inhibition of T-cell growth factor production. I. The effect on mitogen-induced lymphocyte proliferation. *J. Immunol.*, 123:1624–1632.
18. Gillis, S., Crabtree, G. R., and Smith, K. A. (1979): Glucocorticoid-induced inhibition of T-cell growth factor production. II. The effect on the in vitro generation of cytolytic T-cells. *J. Immunol.*, 123:1633–1638.
19. Bollum, F. J. (1979): Terminal deoxynucleotidyl transferase as a hematopoietic cell marker. *Blood*, 54:1203–1215.
20. Kung, P. C., Long, J. C., McCaffrey, R. P., Ratliff, R. L., Harrison, T. A., and Baltimore, D. (1978): Terminal deoxynucleotidyl transferase in the diagnosis of leukemia and malignant lymphoma. *Am. J. Med.*, 64:788–794.
21. Sarin, P. S., Anderson, P. N., and Gallo, R. C. (1976): Terminal deoxynucleotidyl transferase activities in human blood leukocytes and lymphoblast cell lines: high levels in lymphoblast cell lines and in blast cells of some patients with chronic myelogenous leukemia in acute phase. *Blood*, 47:11–20.
22. Mertelsmann, R., Mertelsmann, I., Koziner, B., Moore, M. A. S., and Clarkson, B. D. (1978): Improved biochemical assay for terminal deoxynucleotidyl transferase in human blood cells: results in 89 adult patients with lymphoid neoplasias and malignant lymphomas in leukemic phase. *Leuk. Res.*, 2:57–69.
23. Koziner, B., Filippa, D., Mertelsmann, R., Gupta, S., Clarkson, B. D., Good, R. A., and Siegal, R. P. (1977): Characterization of leukemic lymphomas by multiple differentiation markers of

mononuclear cells. Correlation with clinical features and conventional morphology. *Am. J. Med.*, 63:556–567.

24. Greaves, M. F., Verbi, W., Vogler, L., Cooper, M., Ellis, R., Ganeshaguru, K., Hoffbrand, V., Janossy, G., and Bollum, F. (1979): Antigen and enzymatic phenotypes of the pre-B subclass of acute lymphoblastic leukaemia. *Leuk. Res.*, 3:353–362.
25. Koziner, B., Mertelsmann, R., Siegal, F. P., and Filippa, D. A. (1978): Cell marker analysis in hematopoietic neoplasias. *Clin. Bull.*, 8:47–53.
26. Greaves, M., and Janossy, G. (1978): Patterns of gene expression and the cellular origins of human leukemias. *Biochem. Biophys. Acta*, 516:193–230.
27. Bennett, J. M., Catovsky, D., Daniel, M. T., Flandrin, G., Galton, D. A. G., Gralnick, H. R., and Sultan, C. (1976): Proposals for the classification of the acute leukaemias. *Br. J. Haematol.*, 33:451–458.
28. Mertelsmann, R., Cirrincione, C., To, L., Gee, T. S., McKenzie, S., Schauer, P., Friedman, A., Arlin, Z., Thaler, H., and Clarkson, B. (1980): Morphological classification, response to therapy and survival in 263 adult patients with acute non-lymphoblastic leukemia. *Blood*, 56:773–781.
29. Gordon, D. S., Hutton, J. J., Smalley, R. V., Meyer, L. M., and Vogler, W. R. (1978): Terminal deoxynucleotidyl transferase (TdT), cytochemistry, and membrane receptors in adult acute leukemia. *Blood*, 52:1079–1088.
30. Modak, M. J., Mertelsmann, R., Koziner, B., Pahwa, R., Moore, M. A. S., Clarkson, B. D., and Good, R. A. (1980): A micromethod for determination of terminal deoxynucleotidyl transferase (TdT) in the diagnostic evaluation of acute leukemias. *Can. Res. Clin. Oncol.*, 98:91–104.
31. Janossy, G., Hoffbrand, A. V., Greaves, M. F., Ganeshaguru, K., Pain, C., Bradstock, K. F., Pretice, H. G., Kay, H. E. M., and Lister, T. A. (1980): Terminal transferase enzyme assay and immunological membrane markers in the diagnosis of leukaemia: a multiparameter analysis of 300 cases. *Br. J. Haematol.*, 44:221–234.
32. Mertelsmann, R., Koziner, B., Filippa, D. A., Grossbard, E., Incefy, G., Moore, M. A. S., and Clarkson, B. D. (1979): Clinical significance of TdT, cell surface markers and CFU-c in 297 patients with hematopoietic neoplasias. In: *Modern Trends in Human Leukemia III*, edited by R. Neth, R. C. Gallo, P. Hofschneider, and K. Mannweiler, pp. 131–138. Springer-Verlag, New York.
33. Mertelsmann, R., Koziner, B., Ralph, P., Filippa, D., McKenzie, S., Arlin, Z. A., Gee, T. S., Moore, M. A. S., and Clarkson, B. D. (1978): Evidence for distinct lymphocytic and monocytic population in a patient with terminal transferase positive acute leukemia. *Blood*, 51:1051–1056.
34. Alvares, J. M., Delandazuri, O. M., Bonnard, G. D., and Herberman, R. B. (1978): Cytotoxic activities of cultured human T cells. *J. Immunol.*, 121:1270–1275.
35. Han, T., Dadey, B., and Minowada, J. (1979): Cultured human leukemic non-T/non-B lymphoblasts and their stimulating capacity in "one-way" mixed lymphocyte reaction. Suggestive evidence for early T-cell or B-cell precursors. *Cancer*, 44:136–140.
36. Fairchild, S. S., and Cohen, J. J. (1979): Delayed mitogenic responses to phytohemagglutinin in acute lymphoblastic leukemia. *Leuk. Res.*, 3:163–169.
37. Gillis, S., and Scheid, M. (1979): Identification and phenotypic characterization of T-cell growth factor producing T-lymphoma cell lines. *J. Supramol. Struct.*, 4:135–138.
38. Smith, K. A., Gillis, S., Baker, P. E., and McKenzie, D. (1979): T-cell growth factor-mediated T-cell proliferation. *Proc. N.Y. Acad. Sci.*, 332:423–432.
39. Bonnard, G. D., Yasaka, K., and Jacobson, D. (1979): Ligand-activated T-cell growth factor-induced proliferation: absorption of T-cell growth factor by activated T-cells. *J. Immunol.*, 123:2704–2708.
40. Vogler, L. B., Crist, W. M., Bockman, D. E., Pearl, E. R., Lawton, A. R., and Cooper, M. D. (1978): Pre-B-cell leukemia. A new phenotype of childhood lymphoblastic leukemia. *N. Engl. J. Med.*, 298:872–878.

Maturation Factors and Cancer,
edited by Malcolm A. S. Moore.
Raven Press, © New York 1982.

In Vitro Studies on Interleukin 1 and Tumor Cell Derived Immunosuppressive Peptides

*†Steven B. Mizel and **George J. Todaro

*Laboratory of Microbiology and Immunology, Cellular Immunology Section,
National Institute of Dental Research, NIH, Bethesda, Maryland 20205;
**Laboratory of Viral Carcinogenesis, National Cancer Institute,
National Institutes of Health, Bethesda, Maryland 20205*

The *in vivo* growth potential of immunogenic tumors is fundamentally related to the balance between host mediated concomitant antitumor immunity and tumor-mediated immunosuppression (1). A variety of immune cell types including macrophages, T and B cells, and natural killer cells have been shown to actively participate in the destruction of tumor cells. There is considerable evidence that the proliferation and functional maturation of lymphoid cells is regulated by soluble peptide mediators termed *monokines* (macrophage/monocyte-derived) and *lymphokines* (lymphocyte-derived) (2,4). Recent studies from several laboratories indicate that monokines and lymphokines may participate in cascade-type sequences (involving several classes or subclasses of macrophages, T cells, and B cells) that result in a marked amplification of an initial antigenic stimulus. The monokine interleukin 1 (formerly termed lymphocyte activating factor) (17) appears to play a primary role in the initiation of these cascade-type cellular interactions and thus may be of fundamental importance in the development of antitumor immunity. In our studies on interleukin 1, we have placed major emphasis on the purification and chemical characterization of the peptide. The results of these studies are summarized in this report.

In counterbalance to host-mediated antitumor immunity, tumor cells possess the ability to subvert immunoresponsiveness by any of several possible mechanisms. For example, tumor cells participate in the generation of suppressor T cells (7,10) and also induce the production of antibody-dependent blocking factors that specifically inhibit cell-mediated tumor cytotoxicity (11). Tumor cells may diminish host responses by releasing substances that directly depress immune cell function. The presence of immunosuppressive activities in the sera or ascites fluid of tumor-bearing humans and animals is well documented (12). Factors with a similar broad spectrum of immunosuppressive activities have also been isolated from tumor cells cultured *in vitro* (12,16). Our results with immunosuppressive peptides isolated

---

†Current address: Department of Microbiology, Cell Biology, Biochemistry, and Biophysics, The Pennsylvania State University, University Park, Pennsylvania 16802.

from *in vitro* cultures of human and murine tumor cells suggest that immunosuppressive factors may affect *in vitro* immune cell function by interfering with the events that occur during the initial phases of T cell activation. In view of the possible relevance of this mechanism of immunoparalysis to the situation in immunosuppressed tumor-bearing hosts, we will discuss in the second part of this review our findings on the chemical nature and biologic properties of the immunosuppressive factors that we have isolated from several murine and human tumor cell lines.

INTERLEUKIN 1

Interleukin 1 has been obtained from the culture fluid of human, rabbit, and mouse macrophages, as well as from murine macrophage cell lines that have been stimulated with any one of a variety of agents or treatments, including activated T cells, lipopolysaccharide, phorbol myristic acetate, or antigen-antibody complexes (see ref. 20 for a review of interleukin 1 sources and inducers). Although interleukin 1 was initially described as a thymocyte mitogenic factor (8), it appears to play a more general role in the functional maturation of T cells. The importance of interleukin 1 in the macrophage-dependent generation of helper (5) and cytotoxic T cells (6) is well established. Furthermore, interleukin 1 appears to be identical to (a) the endogenous pyrogen produced by macrophages (19,21) and (b) the macrophage product that stimulates synovial cells to produce collagenase and prostaglandins (15).

In our studies, we have focused on the $P388D_1$ murine macrophage cell line as a source of interleukin 1 (13–15,18). This cell line produces a species of interleukin 1 that is indistinguishable from the peptide produced by murine macrophages. In the course of our studies in the $P388D_1$ cell line derived interleukin 1, we have not only purified this monokine to apparent homogeneity (14a) but have also defined some of its important chemical features. Interleukin 1 is a single polypeptide chain of 12,000 to 16,000 molecular weight that is relatively resistant to the destruction of its biologic activity by proteolytic enzymes and denaturing agents such as urea, guanidine HCl, or sodium dodecyl sulfate (13). The biologically active form of interleukin 1 is not dependent on disulfide linkages, as evidenced by the insensitivity of interleukin 1 activity to incubation with 2-mercaptoethanol and iodoacetamide. However, interleukin 1 activity is destroyed by phenylglyoxal, a compound that covalently attaches to arginine residues (14). Phenylglyoxal not only abolishes the thymocyte mitogenic activity of interleukin 1 but also inhibits its ability to generate helper T cells (S. B. Mizel and J. J. Farrar, unpublished observations), to induce interleukin 2 (formerly termed T cell growth factor) production (8a), and to stimulate prostaglandin and collagenase production by human rheumatoid synovial cells (15). In contrast, histidine modification with diethyl pyrocarbonate had little if any effect on interleukin 1 activity (13).

Using culture fluid from phorbol myristic acetate-stimulated $P388D_1$ cells, a purification sequence of ammonium sulfate fractionation phenyl Sepharose hydrophobic chromatography, Ultrogel AcA54 gel filtration chromatography, and preparative isoelectrofocusing, we have purified interleukin 1 to apparent homogeneity (14a). The purified interleukin 1 is composed of two major and one minor charge species of identical molecular weight. We have designated the three species α, β, and γ, the α species being the dominant and most basic species. All three species are active in the concentration range of 10^{-11} to 10^{-10} M. The amino acid content of the interleukin 1α has been determined. The peptide, which has a weakly acidic pI of 4.9 to 5.1 (13), contains approximately 23 acidic residues (glutamic and aspartic acids) and only 8 basic residues (arginine and lysine). There are no prolines and only one methionine. It is also rich in serine (13.3 residues) and alanine (10.8 residues). Our recent studies on the purification of interleukin 1 clearly demonstrate that the compound can be produced and purified in sufficient quantities for future studies on its amino acid sequence and mode of action.

TUMOR CELL-DERIVED IMMUNOSUPPRESSIVE FACTORS

As previously mentioned, tumor cells can effectively challenge the host immune system by releasing factors that act directly or indirectly to suppress humoral and cellular immune reactions. Our recent studies have focused on the anaysis of the immunosuppressive factors released by human and murine tumor cells. Initially, we found that murine sarcoma virus (MuSV)-transformed 3T3 mouse fibroblasts spontaneously released very potent immunosuppressive factors that inhibited a broad spectrum of T cell-mediated *in vitro* immune responses, including antigen and mitogen-induced T cell proliferation (Table 1) as well as the generation of helper and cytotoxic T cells (16). The effect of the murine immunosuppressive factors was rapid in onset and of relatively long duration. For example, when mouse thymocytes were pulsed with the immunosuppressive factors for 4 hr, washed, and then incubated with interleukin 1 and phytohemagglutinin (PHA), the proliferation of these cells, as measured 72 hr later, was inhibited approximately 60% relative to cells incubated without the immunosuppressive factors (16). The inhibitory effect of these factors was not the result of cell death or the presence of interferon.

Chemical characterization studies revealed that the immunosuppressive activity obtained from the culture fluid of MuSV-3T3 cells was associated with two disulfide-containing peptides of molecular weight 12,000 and 8,000 (Fig. 1). The immunosuppressive factors were resolvable by gel filtration chromatography from the sarcoma growth factors (SGF) produced by these same cells (3).

More recently, we have tested two human tumor lines, a rhabdomyosarcoma (A673) and a lung carcinoma (9812), for the production of immunosuppressive activity. Our results indicate that these human tumors also produce very potent immunosuppressive factors which inhibit T cell activation and proliferation (Table 1). The human factors are also low molecular weight (10,000 MW), relatively basic disulfide-containing peptides.

Although our present knowledge of these immunosuppressive factors is based on *in vitro* analysis of their effects, we have conducted some preliminary *in vivo*

TABLE 1. *Inhibition of T cell proliferation by tumor cell-derived immunosuppressive factors*

Cell source of immunosuppressive factors[a]	T cell stimulants	ΔCPM ³H-TdR incorporation	Percent inhibition
Experiment 1			
None	PHA + interleukin 1[b]	43,809 ± 2,199	
MuSV-3T3 cells	PHA + interleukin 1	553 ± 104	99
Experiment 2			
None	Ovalbumin + interleukin 1[c]	34,959 ± 2,998	
MuSV-3T3 cells	Ovalbumin + interleukin 1	8,731 ± 1,588	75
Experiment 3			
None	PHA + interleukin 1[b]	37,092 ± 1,282	
Human lung carcinoma (9812)	PHA + interleukin 1	1,020 ± 76	97
Human rhabdomysarcoma (A693)	PHA + interleukin 1	2,167 ± 140	94

[a]The culture fluid of each cell line was extracted with 0.1% acetic acid and chromatographed on a Bio-gel P60 column (16). A pool of active fractions was used. Each pool of immunosuppressive factors was titrated in the thymocyte proliferation assay to determine the number of units of activity. One unit is equal to the concentration of factors required for 50% inhibition of mouse thymocyte proliferation.

[b]C3H/HeJ mouse thymocytes were incubated for 72 hr with interleukin 1 and PHA, with or without 125 units/ml murine or human tumor cell derived immunosuppressive factors.

[c]C57B1/6J ovalbumin-primed lymph node T cells were incubated for 72 hr with interleukin 1 + ovalbumin with or without 125 units/ml MuSV-3T3 immunosuppressive factors.

experiments. C57B1/6J mice were injected intravenously with 400 units of partially purified MuSV-3T3-derived immunosuppressive factors (1 unit producing 50% inhibition of *in vitro* murine thymocyte proliferation). Spleens were removed at 48 or 72 hr and the proliferative response to PHA or concanavalin A was assessed. As shown in Table 2, the immunosuppressive factors were also able to inhibit T cell proliferation when administered *in vivo*. Seventy-two hr after injecting the tumor products, the *in vitro* proliferation responses of the spleen cells from these mice were still maximally inhibited. These results are consistent with our results on *in vitro* thymocyte proliferation, which demonstrated the prolonged nature of the inhibitory effect of the immunosuppressive factors.

CONCLUSIONS

Although formal proofs of the *in vivo* relevance of monokines and lymphokines as well as tumor cell-derived immunosuppressive factors in antitumor immunity and tumor-mediated immunosuppression remain to be demonstrated, the results of *in vitro* studies support the hypothesis that the growth potential of immunogenic tumors may be critically related to the relative levels of these very potent and selective immunoregulatory substances. All of these substances—monokines, lymphokines, and immunosuppressive factors—have been detected in the sera of humans and animals under different experimental conditions. In conjuction with Dr. Steven Gillis (14a), we have recently demonstrated that interleukin 1 can induce

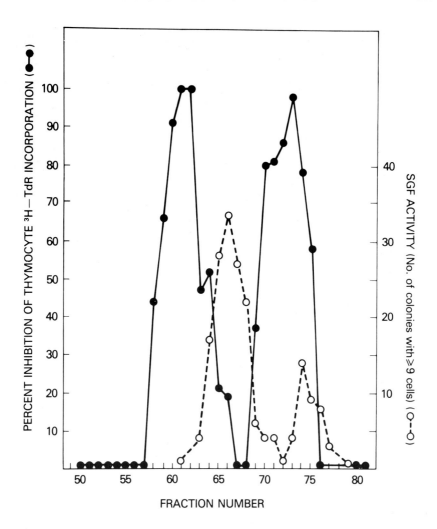

FIG. 1. Bio-gel P60 chromatography of MuSV-transformed 3T3 fibroblast derived immuno-suppressive peptides and sarcoma growth factors (16). Each column fraction was dialyzed against 1% acetic acid, lyophilized, and reconstituted for immunosuppressive factor (•———•) and sarcoma growth factor (○---○) assays. Immunosuppressive activity was determined with C3H/HeJ mouse thymocytes incubated with interleukin 1 + PHA in the presence or absence of the column fractions. SGF activity was determined on normal rat kidney fibroblasts cultured in soft agar (3).

the production and secretion of the mitogenic lymphokine, interleukin 2 (9), by several T cell lymphomas. These findings raise the interesting, albeit speculative, possibility that interleukin 1 may contribute both negatively (stimulation of T cell-dependent antitumor immunity) and positively (enhancement of interleukin 2 production for T-cell lymphoma growth) to the *in vivo* propagation of T cell lymphomas.

TABLE 2. In vivo *activity of MuSV-3T3 immunosuppressive factors*

Mice injected with immunosuppressive factors[a]	Time after injection of immunosuppressive factors (hr)[b]	In vitro T cell proliferation (ΔCPM ^{3}H-TdR incorporation)		Percent inhibition	
		+ PHA	+ Con A	+ PHA	+ Con A
−	48	8,653 ± 958	5,117 ± 776		
+		285 ± 25	384 ± 36	97	92
−	72	25,440 ± 1,119	12,478 ± 881		
+		339 ± 114	1,398 ± 507	99	89

[a]C57B1/6J mice were injected via the tail vein with 400 units of MuSV-3T3-derived immunosuppressive factors in phosphate buffered saline. Control mice received only buffer.
[a]After 48 or 72 hr, spleens were removed (2 mice/time point) and single cell suspensions were prepared. 1 × 10^5 cells were incubated in 200 μl of media with either 1 μg/ml PHA or 2 μg/ml Con A for 72 hr.

The recent finding of DeLarco and Todaro (3) that virus-transformed fibroblasts produce their own growth factors (SGF) is certainly consistent with the idea that interleukin 2 derived from a T cell tumor may enhance the growth of the same tumor T cells. The eventual availability of monoclonal antibodies should permit us to directly evaluate the functional importance of enhancing and suppressive peptides in the tumor-bearing host.

REFERENCES

1. Berendt, M. J., and North, R. J. (1980): T cell-mediated suppression of anti-tumor immunity. An explanation for progressive growth of an immunogenic tumor. *J. Exp. Med.*, 151:69–80.
2. Cohen, S., Pick, E., and Oppenheim, J. J., editors (1978): *Biology of the Lymphokines.* Academic Press, New York.
3. DeLarco, J. E., and Todaro, J. J. (1978): Growth factors from murine sarcoma virus-transformed cells. *Proc. Natl. Acad. Sci. U.S.A.*, 75:4001–4005.
4. deWeck, A. L., Kristensen, F., and Landy, M., editors (1980): *Biochemical Characterization of Lymphokin.* Academic Press, New York.
5. Farrar, J. J., and Koopman, W. J. (1978): Characterization of mitogenic factors and their effect on the antibody response *in vitro.* In: *Biology of the Lymphokines*, edited by S. Cohen, E. Pick, and J. J. Oppenheim, pp. 325–346. Academic Press, New York.
6. Farrar, W. L., Mizel, S. B., and Farrar, J. J. (1980): Participation of lymphocyte activating factor (interleukin 1) in the induction of cytotoxic T cell responses. *J. Immunol.*, 124:1371–1377.
7. Fujimoto, S., Greene, Mi. I., and Sehon, A. H. (1976): Regulation of the immune response to tumor antigens. II. The nature of the immunosuppressor cells in tumor-bearing hosts. *J. Immunol.*, 116:800–809.
8. Gery, I., Gershon, R. K., and Waksman, B. H. (1972): Potentiation of the lymphocyte response to mitogens. I. The responding cell. *J. Exp. Med.*, 136:128–142.
8a. Gillis, S., and Mizel, S. B. (1981): T cell lymphoma model for the analysis of interleukin 1-mediated T cell activation. *Proc. Natl. Acad. Sci. USA*, 78:1133–1137.
9. Gillis, S., Ferm, M. M., Ou, W., and Smith, K. A. (1978): T cell growth factor: parameters of production and a quantitative microassay for activity. *J. Immunol.*, 120:2027–2033.
10. Greene, M. I., and Perry, L. (1978): Regulation of the immune response to tumor antigen. VI. Differential specificities of suppressor T cells or their products and effector cells. *J. Immunol.*, 121:2362–2366.
11. Hellstrom, I., Sjögren, H. O., and Werner, G. (1971): Blocking of cell-mediated immunity by sera from patients with growing neoplasma. *Int. J. Cancer*, 7:226–237.
12. Kamo, I., and Friedman, H. (1977): Immunosuppression and the role of suppressive factors in cancer. In: *Advances in Cancer Research*, edited by G. Klein and S. Weinhouse, Vol. 25, pp. 271–321. Academic Press, New York.
13. Mizel, S. B. (1979): Physicochemical characterization of lymphocyte activating factor (LAF). *J. Immunol.*, 122:2167–2172.

14. Mizel, S. B. (1980): Studies in the purification and structure-function relationships of murine lymphocyte activating factor (interleukin 1). *Mol. Immunol.*, 17:571–577.

14a. Mizel, S. B., and Mizel, D. (1981): Purification to apparent homogeneity of murine interleukin 1. *J. Immunol.*, 126:834–837.

15. Mizel, S. B., Dayer, J. M., Krane, S. M., and Mergenhagen, S. E. (1981): Stimulation of rheumatoid synovial cell collagenase and prostaglandin production by partially purified lymphocyte activating factor (interleukin 1). *Proc. Natl. Acad. Sci. USA*, 78:2474–2477.

16. Mizel, S. B., DeLarco, J. E., Todaro, G. J., Farrar, W. L., and Hilfiker, M. L. (1980): *In vitro* production of immunosuppressive factors (ISF) by murine sarcoma virus transformed mouse fibroblasts. *Proc. Natl. Acad. Sci. U.S.A.*, 77:2205–2208.

17. Mizel, S. B., and Farrar, J. J. (1979): Revised nomenclature for antigen-nonspecific T cell proliferation and helper factors. *Cell. Immunol.*, 48:433–436.

18. Mizel, S. B., Oppenheim, J. J., and Rosenstreich, D. L. (1978): Characterization of lymphocyte activating factor (LAF) produced by a macrophage cell line, P388D$_1$. II. Biochemical characterization of LAF induced by activated T cells and LPS. *J. Immunol.*, 120:1504–1508.

19. Murphy, P. A., Simon, P. L., and Willoughby, W. F. (1980): Endogenous pyrogens made by rabbit peritoneal exudate cells are identical with lymphocyte activating factor made by rabbit alveolar macrophages. *J. Immunol.*, 124:2498–2501.

20. Oppenheim, J. J., Mizel, S. B., and Meltzer, M. S. (1978): Biological effects of lymphocyte and macrophage-derived mitogenic "amplification" factors. In: *Biology of the Lymphokines*, edited by S. Cohen, E. Pick, and J. J. Oppenheim, pp. 291–323. Academic Press, New York.

21. Rosenwasser, L. J., Dinarello, C. S., and Rosenthal, A. S. (1979): Adherent cell function in murine T lymphocyte antigen recognition. IV. Enhancement of murine T cell antigen recognition by human leukocytic pyrogen. *J. Exp. Med.*, 150:709–714.

Maturation Factors and Cancer,
edited by Malcolm A. S. Moore.
Raven Press, © New York 1982.

Factors Controlling B Lymphocyte Differentiation

Michael K. Hoffmann, Kathleen M. Gilbert, and Herbert F. Oettgen

Memorial Sloan-Kettering Cancer Center, New York, New York 10021

The activation of B lymphocytes in the initiation of the humoral immune response is regulated by a coordinated system of inductive and suppressive events. Essential components of B cell activation include signals that cause B cells to proliferate (clonal expansion) and signals that induce maturation (differentiation) of B cells. Antigen itself converts resting precursor B cells into dividing cells and thus makes them responsive to signals that cause their maturation into antibody forming cells. Maturation signals in the form of soluble helper factors are provided by helper cells. Helper cells have been identified as a subpopulation of T lymphocytes (helper T cells), and also as phagocytic, surface adherent cells (macrophages). The mediator released by macrophages is now called interleukin 1 (IL-1), formerly LAF, MP, BAF, BDF, and TRF-M (1). Its molecular weight is approximately 15,000 daltons (8). The mediator released by helper T cells is called T cell replacing factor (TRF) (4,9,18). Its molecular weight is 35,000 daltons (21). Interleukin 1 (IL-1) and TRF, when added to B cells in the appropriate sequence (together with antigen), induce maximal antibody production. These mediators represent important tools for the analysis of B cell activation in the humoral immune response (9).

SYNERGISM OF IL-1 AND TRF IN THE INDUCTION OF ANTIBODY FORMING B CELLS

Interleukin 1 is released by macrophages as a result of their interaction with antigen-stimulated T cells (2,6) or following incubation with lipopolysaccharides (LPS) derived from the cell wall of gram negative bacteria (8). IL-1 is also released by some established macrophage cell lines (8,16). TRF is released by antigen-stimulated helper T cells (18). Its release can also be induced with T cell mitogens (e.g., concacavalin A), an approach which has the advantage of stimulating greater numbers of T cells than specific antigens and thus permits production of TRF in larger quantities (21). The IL-1 used in the experiments described in this chapter was obtained from LPS-stimulated macrophages (8); TRF was prepared from culture supernatants of concanavalin A-stimulated T cells (21).

The helper activity of IL-1 and TRF was studied in cultures of mouse spleen cells, which were induced to produce antibody to red cell antigen according to the method of Mishell and Dutton (15). The experiment shown in Table 1 was performed with spleen cells derived from athymic nu/nu mice, which are deficient in helper T cells. Macrophages were removed by passing these spleen cells over Sephadex G-10 columns (14). The eluted cells did not respond to sensitization with sheep erythrocytes (SRBC) with the generation of antibody forming B cells, referred to here as plaque forming cells (PFC), since they were enumerated in hemolytic plaque assays (11,15). A substantial PFC response was induced when IL-1 or TRF was added alone. When both were added together, a synergistic effect was observed, which was most pronounced when IL-1 was added early in the response and TRF with a delay of 1 to 2 days. These results suggested the following concept (5): T cells provide a signal, TRF, necessary for the terminal differentiation of B cells into antibody secreting cells. Only a small fraction of precursor B cells is mature enough at any given time to respond to that signal. That fraction is increased in response to another signal, IL-1, which induces earlier stages of B cell differentiation.

TABLE 1. *Effect of time of addition of*
factors to cultures on the synergistic properties of TRF and IL-1[a]

Delay of addition of factors to cultures (hr)		Anti-SRBC PFC/culture in cultures of BALB/c nu/nu spleen cells		
TRF	IL-1	Unseparated	MΘ-depleted	MΘ-depleted + APC
None	None	10	25	30
None	0	1,900	1,800	2,900
None	24	2,250	875	3,000
None	48	1,375	375	1,050
0	None	2,175	120	1,600
0	0	1,150	7,250	9,250
0	24	3,100	7,000	11,500
0	48	6,500	1,050	3,500
24	None	2,575	110	2,400
24	0	3,950	15,750	13,500
24	24	8,300	11,500	18,000
24	48	6,000	3,750	6,000
48	None	980	90	450
48	0	12,000	16,500	17,500
48	24	12,250	14,000	12,000
48	48	9,750	1,550	3,000

[a]BALB/c nu/nu spleen cells (5 × 10⁶ cells/ml) were placed in culture either unseparated, MΘ-depleted (Sephadex G-10) (14), or MΘ-depleted and reconstituted with adherent peritoneal cells (APC, 5 × 10⁴/ml) and immunized with SRBC. PFC formation was determined on day 4. TRF (40 μl/ml) and IL-1 (100 μl/ml) were added to culture at time indicated.

FREQUENCY OF SRBC-REACTIVE PRECURSOR B CELLS
INTERACTING WITH HELPER T CELLS OR TRF

Precursor frequency assays were carried out using the procedure described by Hunter and Kettmann (10). C57BL/6 spleen cells were depleted of T cells and macrophages. The residual cells (primarily B cells) were plated at decreasing cell density in the presence of helper T cells, with or without IL-1 (Table 2). The cultures were immunized with SRBC, and antibody forming cells (PFC) were enumerated 4 days later. Cultures containing 3 or more PFC were scored as positive. The percentage of negative cultures was determined for each cell concentration, and the frequency of responding precursor B cells was computed on the basis of a Poisson distribution (5). The results, averaged from four experiments, are shown in Table 2. IL-1 was found to synergize with TRF as well as with helper T cells in increasing the frequency of responding B cells.

This finding is consistent with our notion that macrophages direct the maturation of immature B cells to mature cells capable of responding to T cell help. The concept assumes that macrophages and T cells influence different phases of the B cell response. This assumption was tested by treating B cells sequentially with the macrophage product, IL-1, and the T cell product, TRF.

TABLE 2. *The frequency of SRBC-reactive B cells responding to T cell help as increased by IL-1[a]*

	IL-1	SRBC reactive B cells per 10^7 culture cells
	−	1
	+	35.00 ± 13.37
TRF	−	34.50 ± 9.95
TRF	+	342.12 ± 95.67
T cells	−	29.14 ± 12.18
T cells	+	358.23 ± 86.35

[a]C57BL/6 spleen cells were passed over Sephadex G-10 columns (14) (for the removal of macrophages) and treated with monoclonal anti-Thy 1.2 serum and complement (for the removal of T cells). Monoclonal anti-Thy 1.2 serum was provided by Dr. U. Hammerling, Sloan-Kettering Institute. Cells were cultured under Mishell-Dutton conditions (15) in microcultures as adapted for the limiting dilution analysis by Hunter and Kettman (10). 10^5 SRBC-primed (0.2 ml 1% SRBC solution i.v., 8 days) spleen cells treated with 40 mg/ml mitomycin C for 30 min at 37°C were added per well as a source of helper T cells (10). TRF was added in a concentration of 3%, IL-1 5%. Anti-SRBC PFCs were determined in individual culture wells on day 4. A computer program based on the log of the fraction of cultures which failed to respond vs the number of cells cultured was used to calculate the frequency of SRBC-reactive B cells. The program was developed by Dr. John Hirst, Sloan-Kettering Institute. A total of at least 16 microcultures was assayed for each cell concentration in each experiment. The data are averages of four experiments.

RESPONSE OF B CELLS TO TRF AFTER PRETREATMENT WITH IL-1

B cell cultures were incubated with IL-1 for different periods of time (up to 40 hr), after which time IL-1 was removed. After 40 hr of culture, TRF was added and PFC responses were determined on day 4. This design allowed us to measure the time that was required for IL-1 to convert immature B cells into TRF-responsive B cells, and to determine whether IL-1 primed cells were responsive to TRF in the absence of IL-1. The results are shown in Table 3. The highest PFC responses were obtained when IL-1 was present during the entire culture period, but the majority of B cells had become responsive to TRF after incubation with IL-1 for 40 hr. TRF interacted with these B cells in the absence of IL-1.

The concept emerging from these experiments is shown in Fig. 1. It states that activation of B cells in the PFC response proceeds through two phases. The first phase is controlled by macrophages and mediated by IL-1. IL-1 induces differentiation of B cells and increases the numbers of B cells capable of responding to T cell help. Helper T cells (through TRF) control the second phase B cell activation associated with their conversion into antibody forming cells. This concept is consistent with earlier observations indicating that B cells become capable of cooperating with helper T cells relatively late in their development, at the time when they express receptors for complement on their surface (7), coinciding with the expression of SIgD (20). The assumption that IL-1 controls the functional differentiation of B cells (particularly in the early phases) is supported by the finding

TABLE 3. *Sequential treatment of spleen cells with IL-1 and TRF*

Treatment with IL-1 (hr)	TRF added after 40 hr	PFC per culture, day 4	
		Anti-SRBC	Anti-BRBC
0	−	0	0
6	−	265	104
24	−	670	240
40	−	1,200	630
96	−	1,550	945
0	+	90	62
6	+	2,950	970
24	+	9,250	1,600
40	+	12,200	4,100
96	+	13,600	4,850

[a]BALB/c nu/nu spleen cells were passed over Sephadex G-10 columns (14) and cultured for the time intervals indicated in the presence of IL-1, after which they were washed twice and reincubated with or without TRF. Only in two sets of cultures was IL-1 present for the entire culture period (96 hr), in which case it was freshly added after washing and reincubation of cells at 40 hr. SRBC and BRBC were added at the culture start and again upon reincubation of cells. Concentrations: IL-1 = 5%, TRF = 3%.

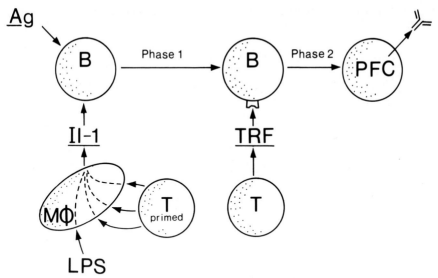

FIG. 1. IL-1- and TRF-controlled phases of B cell differentiation in the anti-SRBC IgM PFC response. For details see Discussion.

that IL-1 is a potent inducer of phenotypic B cell differentiation. It induces early (sIg, Ia) as well as late (complement receptors) appearing B cell surface markers (8). In contrast, TRF is inactive in this regard (unpublished data).

We should point out that this model of B cell maturation applies only to the immune response of spleen cells to antigens attached to red blood cells. The immune response to soluble antigens, such as KLH, appears to be more complex as it requires two distinct types of helper T cells (19). One helper cell is involved in the initiation of B cell proliferation and acts in an antigen-specific manner. Its activity cannot be replaced by TRF. The second type of helper cell is required for the response to soluble antigen as well as to RBC-bound antigen. Its activity can be replaced by TRF. The second helper T cell type can be distinguished from the first by its expression of Ia surface antigen (19). The major difference between PFC responses to soluble antigen and RBC-bound antigen appears to be that a special T cell that initiates the B cell response is required for the former, while RBC-bound antigen interacts with precursor B cells effectively without T cell help and depends on T cells only for the conversion of B cells into antibody secreting cells.

SYNERGISM OF IL-1 AND TRF IN THE SUPPRESSION OF ANTIBODY-FORMING B CELLS

The synergistic increase of antibody forming B cells is most pronounced if IL-1 is added early to the cultures and TRF is added 40 to 48 hr later. The question arose why TRF added early in the response is less effective than TRF added on day 2. Schimpl and Wecker attributed the phenomenon to degradation of TRF occurring before the majority of B cells were responsive to it (18). This assumption would be compatible with our model of B cell activation, suggesting that TRF added on day 0 is used up by the time it's required by IL-1-recruited B cells on day 2. To test this possibility, TRF was added to spleen cells from athymic mice (BALB/c nu/nu) on day 0 (along with antigen and IL-1) and then again on day 2 to replace TRF that could have been inactivated. As shown in Table 4, a second addition of TRF on day 2 did not restore the peak PFC response to the level induced by a single TRF addition on day 2. This observation indicates that the suboptimal antibody production associated with early addition of TRF cannot be attributed to degradation of TRF.

We next examined the possibility that the reduction in helper activity was due to suppressor cells generated by the early addition of TRF. BALB/c nu/nu spleen cells were incubated with TRF, IL-1, or a combination of both for 2 days following a protocol originally designed for the induction of suppressor T cells by Con A (3,17). The cells were washed and added in various concentrations to fresh athymic mouse spleen cells, which were stimulated to respond to SRBC by adding IL-1 on day 0 and TRF on day 2. Only spleen cell cultures that had been treated with both TRF and IL-1 inhibited the PFC response of fresh cultures (Fig. 2). Neither helper factor alone induced significant suppressor activity. Since the spleen cell cultures that exhibited suppressor activity had been carefully washed prior to their transfer,

TABLE 4. *Inability of late TRF addition to restore the PFC response induced by early TRF addition to levels induced by a single late addition[a]*

IL-1	TRF	Experiment	Day 4	Day 5
			Addition of factors to culture (hr)	Anti-SRBC PFC/culture
0	None	1	600	240
		2	690	543
		3	450	840
0	0	1	3,900	240
		2	15,300	3,390
		3	6,000	8,400
0	48	1	8,100	5,700
		2	27,000	29,700
		3	10,500	30,000
0	0 and 48	1	5,700	630
		2	11,400	9,000
		3	5,100	18,000

[a]BALB/c nu/nu spleen cells were cultured under Mishell-Dutton conditions (15) in tissue culture dishes (35 × 10 mm), and direct plaque-forming cells (11,15) were assayed on days 4 and 5. IL-1 (5%) and SRBC were added to cell cultures at the initiation of culture, and TRF (3%) was added at the times indicated.

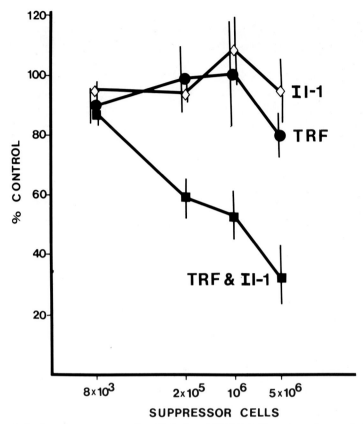

FIG. 2. Induction of suppressor cells with IL-1 and TRF. BALB/c nu/nu spleen cells (5 × 10⁶ cells/ml) were incubated with TRF (3%) (●), IL-1 (5%) (◇), or a combination of both (■) for 48 hr, following a protocol designed for induction of suppressor T cells by Con A (3,17). Following incubation, the cells were washed three times and added in the concentrations indicated to fresh BALB/c nu/nu spleen cells (5 × 10⁶ cells/ml) stimulated by the addition of SRBC and IL-1 (5%) at time 0 and TRF (3%) at 48 hr and incubated in tissue culture dishes (35 × 10 mm). Anti-SRBC PFCs were determined on day 4. The results (means of three experiments ± standard deviations) are expressed as percent of the response observed in cultures to which control cells incubated in medium alone were added.

their inhibitory activity appeared to reside in their cellular components and not in residual factors or their breakdown products.

The identity of the suppressor cells induced in this way was of considerable interest, since athymic mice are held to be deficient in mature T cells. The phenotype of these suppressor cells was examined through elimination experiments using antisera directed against both T cell and B cell surface markers. Following incubation with TRF and IL-1, athymic mouse spleen cells were treated with either normal mouse serum, anti-Thy 1, anti-Ia, or anti-IgG antisera and complement, and then added to fresh spleen cells stimulated with antigen and helper factors. Suppressor

activity was not affected by the removal of cells expressing Thy 1 antigen, but was
eliminated by removal of cells bearing the B cell markers Ia and IgG (Fig. 3).

   These experiments show that suppressor cells of B cell phenotype can be induced
by the combined addition of TRF and IL-1 to T cell deficient murine spleen cell
cultures. We propose that the reduction of the PFC response obtained by early
addition of TRF is due to the activation of such suppressor cells, which develop
before the majority of antigen-reactive B cells can differentiate into antibody-
secreting cells. It is of interest to note that, similar to antibody-forming B cells,

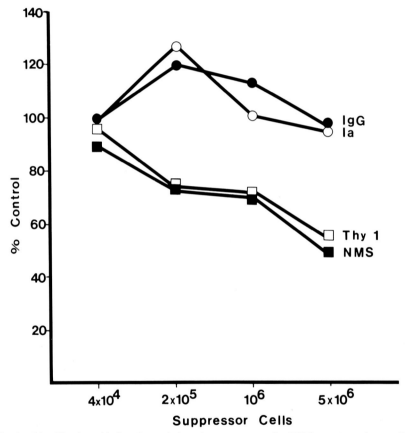

FIG. 3. Identification of helper factor induced suppressor cells. BALB/c nu/nu spleen cells (5
× 10^6 cells/ml) were incubated with TRF (3%) and IL-1 (5%) for 48 hr to induce suppressor
cells. Following incubation, the cells were washed three times and treated with the following
antisera and complement to eliminate cells expressing certain surface markers: NMS (■), anti-
Thy 1 (monoclonal) (□), anti-Ia (A.TH anti-A.TL) (○), or anti-IgG (rabbit antimouse IgG_1) (●). The
cells were washed three times and added in the concentrations indicated to fresh BALB/c nu/nu
spleen cells as described in Fig. 2. Anti-SRBC PFCs were determined on day 4. The results
(means of three experiments) are expressed as percent of the response observed in cultures
to which control cells treated with antisera and complement after incubation in medium alone
were added.

suppressor B cells require the synergistic activity of both IL-1 and TRF for maximal stimulation.

The existence of suppressor B cells has been demonstrated in several experimental systems, including LPS-induced suppression of delayed hypersensitivity (13) and antibody formation (12). In addition to polyclonal activation, suppressor B cells may also be induced in antigen specific responses (22,23). Recently, Zubler et al. reported that the suppression of the primary humoral responses to SRBC *in vitro* may be attributed to antigen reactive B lymphocytes (24,25). These studies of suppressor B cells in antigen specific immune reactions may provide a possible mechanism by which the helper factor-induced suppressor B cells described in this paper inhibit the antigen-dependent PFC response to SRBC.

In the model of B cell activation described here, antibody formation may be enhanced or suppressed by helper factors (IL-1 and TRF), depending on the sequence of helper factor addition. If TRF is added on day 2 or later, the predominant effect is inductive as TRF acts to stimulate a pool of IL-1 recruited B cells to produce antibody. If TRF is added prior to day 2, before the majority of B cells are responsive to TRF, the response is inhibited as TRF and IL-1 act together to induce suppressor cells. In this way, macrophages and T cells synergize to stimulate the antibody response while at the same time preventing excessive antibody formation by the generation of suppressor B cells.

ACKNOWLEDGMENTS

We wish to thank A. Micali and E. Williams for excellent technical assistance. The generosity of Dr. Chris Galanos in supplying highly purified LPS and of Dr. U. Hammerling in making available antisera is greatly appreciated. This work was supported by grants from the National Institutes of Health CA 17673-04, CA 16889, and CA 08748, and from the Cancer Research Institute.

REFERENCES

1. Aarden, L., et al. (1979): Revised nomenclature for antigen-nonspecific T cell proliferation and helper factors. *J. Immunol.*, 123:2928–2930.
2. Beller, D. I., Farr, A. J., and Unanus, E. R. (1978): Regulation of lymphocyte proliferation and differentiation by macrophages. *Fed. Proc.*, 37:91–104.
3. Dutton, R. W. (1972): Inhibitory and stimulatory effects of concanavalin A on the response of mouse spleen cell suspensions to antigen I. Characteristics of the inhibitory cell activity. *J. Exp. Med.*, 136:1445–1454.
4. Dutton, R. W., Falkoff, R., Hirst, J., Hoffmann, M., Kappler, J., Kettman, J., Lesley, J., and Vann, D. (1972): Is there evidence for a non-antigen specific diffusable chemical mediator from the thymus derived cells in the initiation of the immune response? In: *Progress in Immunology*, edited by B. Amos, pp. 355–391. Academic Press, New York.
5. Hoffmann, M. K. (1979): Control of B cell differentiation by macrophages. *Ann. N.Y. Acad. Sci.*, 332:557–564.
6. Hoffmann, M. K. (1980): Macrophages and T cells control distinct phases of B cell differentiation in the humoral immune response in vitro. *J. Immunol. (in press)*.
7. Hoffmann, M. K., Hammerling, U., Simon, M., and Oettgen, H. F. (1976): Macrophage requirements of CR⁻ and CR⁺ B lymphocytes for antibody production in vitro. *J. Immunol.*, 116:1447–1453.

8. Hoffmann, M. K., Koenig, S., Mittler, R. S., Oettgen, H. F., Ralph, P., and Hammerling, U. (1978): Macrophage factor controlling differentiation of B cells. *J. Immunol.*, 122:497–502.

9. Hoffmann, M. K., and Watson, J. (1979): Helper T cell replacing factors secreted by thymus-derived cells and by macrophages: cellular requirements for B cell activation and synergistic properties. *J. Immunol.*, 4:1371–1376.

10. Hunter, P., and Kettman, J. R. (1974): Mode of action of a supernatant activity from T cell culture that nonspecifically stimulates the humoral immune response. *Proc. Natl. Acad. Sci. U.S.A.*, 71:512–519.

11. Kettman, J., and Dutton, R. W. (1970): An *in vitro* primary immune response to 2,4,6 trinitrophenyl substituted erythrocytes: response against carrier and hapten. *J. Immunol.*, 104:1558–1569.

12. Koenig, S., and Hoffmann, M. K. (1979): Bacterial lipopolysaccharide activates suppressor B lymphocytes. *Proc. Natl. Acad. Sci. U.S.A.*, 76:4608–4646.

13. LaGrange, P. H., Mackaness, G. B., Miller, T. E., and Pardon, P. (1975): Effects of bacterial lipopolysaccharide on the induction and expression of cell-mediated immunity. I. Depression of the afferent arc. *J. Immunol.*, 114:442–453.

14. Ly, I. A., and Mishell, R. I. (1974): Separation of mouse spleen cells by passage through columns of Sephadex G-10. *J. Immunol. Methods*, 5:239–249.

15. Mishell, R. I., and Dutton, R. W. (1967): Immunization of dissociated spleen cell cultures from normal mice. *J. Exp. Med.*, 126:423–431.

16. Mizel, S. B. (1979): Physicochemical characterization of lymphocyte activating factor (LAF). *J. Immunol.*, 122:2167–2174.

17. Rich, R. R., and Pierce, C. V. (1973): Biological expression of lymphocyte activation. I. The effects of phytomitogens on antibody synthesis in vitro. *J. Exp. Med.*, 137:205–211.

18. Schimpl, A., and Wecker, E. (1972): Replacement of T cell function by a T cell product. *Nature (New Biol.)*, 237:15–24.

19. Sierkosz, J. E., Marrack, P., and Kappler, J. W. (1979): Functional analysis of T cells expressing Ia antigens. I. Demonstration of helper T cell heterogeneity. *J. Exp. Med.*, 150:1293–1304.

20. Sitia, R., Abbott, J., and Hammerling, U. (1979): Ontogeny of lymphocytes-B. 5. Lipopolysaccharide-induced changes of IgD expression on murine lymphocytes-B. *Eur. J. Immunol.*, 9:859–864.

21. Watson, J., Aarden, L. A., and Lefkovits, I. (1979): The purification and quantitation of helper T cell-replacing factors secreted by murine spleen cells activated by concanavalin A. *J. Immunol.*, 122:209–219.

22. Zan-Bar, I., Villeta, E. S., Assisi, F., and Strober, S. (1978): The relationship between surface immunoglobulin isotype and immune function of murine B lymphocytes III. Expression of a single predominant isotype on primed and unprimed B cells. *J. Exp. Med.*, 147:1374–1380.

23. Zembala, M., Asherson, G. L., Noworolski, G. L., and Mayhew, B. (1976): Contact sensitivity to picryl chloride: the occurrence of B suppressor cells in lymph nodes and spleen of immunized mice. *Cell. Immunol.*, 25:226–232.

24. Zubler, R. H., Benacerraf, B., and Germain, R. N. (1980): Feedback suppression of the immune response in vitro. II. IgVH-restricted antibody-dependent suppression. *J. Exp. Med.*, 151:681–694.

25. Zubler, R. H., Cantor, H., Benacerraf, B., and Germain, R. N. (1980): Feedback suppression of the immune response in vitro. I. Activity of antigen-stimulated B cells. *J. Exp. Med.*, 151:667–680.

Maturation Factors and Cancer,
edited by Malcolm A. S. Moore.
Raven Press, © New York 1982.

Differentiation Heterogeneity in Murine Hematopoietic Tumors

Noel L. Warner, Richard K. Cheney, Lewis L. Lanier,
Michael Daley, and Edwin Walker

Immunobiology Laboratories, Departments of Pathology and Medicine,
University of New Mexico School of Medicine, Albuquerque, New Mexico 87131

In virtually all hematopoietic cell lineages, it has become evident that the process of differentiation from the immature stem cell to the mature functional end cell is a complex process that involves many distinct stages. These may be distinguished by changes in functional properties, morphological properties, or by the expression of specific cell surface components, which presumably are involved in the given cells' particular function. This latter aspect has been considerably advanced in recent years by the combined approaches of two powerful analytical tools, namely, the use of hybridoma derived monoclonal antibodies (8,17), and flow cytometry (6,16). The latter technology further permits, through its flow sorting option, the isolation of cells of a defined differentiation state for assessment of their biological functions.

In the province of lymphoid and macrophage differentiation, these above considerations are further complicated by the existence of multiple subpopulations within both major lineages, each subpopulation in turn going through its own complex differentiation pathway. The simultaneous existence in most normal cell preparations of multiple lineages of cells at different stages renders the definition of each precise stage of differentiation exceedingly difficult. It is in this regard that tumors of hematopoeitic cell populations play an increasingly valuable role. Each tumor line is proposed to represent the clonal expansion of a cell derived from one particular lineage and subpopulation, arrested in differentiation at a particular stage (14). Based on this concept, the cells within a given tumor would thus be relatively homogeneous in both functional properties and in differentiation markers.

In this chapter, we wish to illustrate the use of tumor cell lines in defining stages of maturation arrest between tumors, and in addition, to demonstrate the intratumor heterogeneity that is superimposed upon this. With this background, it may then be possible to attempt to dissect whether apparent manipulation of the differentiation state within a tumor line involves a true change in the overall population, or a selection of a subpopulation within the tumor. To illustrate these approaches, we will use examples of studies with tumors of both mouse myeloid and B lymphocyte differentiation lineages.

RESULTS

Differentiation Heterogeneity Between Tumor Cell Lines

The analysis of differentiation states of cell populations can be readily assessed by quantitative evaluation of the expression of a wide variety of cell surface markers, preferably as defined by monoclonal antibodies and using flow cytometry. In such studies, the use of a single marker is seldom sufficient to precisely define differentiation stages; therefore, analysis of multiple components must be performed (23). In the case of B cell tumors, it has generally been concluded that there are at least four major stages of differentiation represented (5,15):

1. *Pre-B cells*, typified by intracellular synthesis of immunoglobulin (Ig) but lack of secretion or membrane expression of Ig
2. *Virgin B cells*, which express intact (L and H) membrane Ig, but fail to activate J chain synthesis, and hence secretion of polymeric IgM
3. *Activated B cells*, which synthesize J chains and secrete Ig
4. *Plasma cells*, of varying stages of maturity

On the basis of these properties alone, it is possible to classify B cell tumors into each of these groups. When such tumors are further studied by flow cytometry for the expression of other cell surface antigens, several general conclusions might be proposed. Our formulation of these following conclusions is based on data which are summarized in Table 1. A few specific examples, shown in Fig. 1, demonstrate the multiple differences between two specific tumors in the B cell lineage.

1. Certain cell surface markers *closely parallel* the categorization of tumors into the four groups noted above, which were in turn based solely on Ig status. For example, all pre-B tumors lack Ia antigens. However, B cell tumors of types II and III show variable to high levels of Ia; and plasma cell tumors are either negative or show only low surface density of Ia.

2. As will be discussed in the following section in more detail, certain tumors show marked *variability* among the cells within the tumor in the expression of a given surface component.

3. Particularly within groups II and III, there are still many marked differences in the presence or absence of various surface antigens between tumors (intertumor heterogeneity). For example, there is no apparent correlation between presence or absence of the markers defined by E2, ThB, F1, Lyt-1, and Qa-2/3 among tumors of this group. Whether each of these groupings (cell surface phenotypes) represents an analogous distinct normal B cell subpopulation remains to be evaluated (see Discussion).

4. Occasional surface antigens, previously thought to be restricted to other cell populations, have been found to be expressed on tumors of this series. Foremost among these is Lyt-1, which has now been found to be expressed on some (but not all) B cell tumors in both mouse (10) and man (12).

TABLE 1. Intertumor differentiation in B lymphomas and plasmacytomas[a]

	Surface Ig	Secreted Ig	Ia	Qa2,3	Thy1	Lyt1	Lyt2	ThB	E2	F1	T200
Group I: Pre-B lymphomas											
ABE-8	-	-	A-/E(C)-	-	-	-	-	-	-/sub+	++++	+++
Groups II and III: B lymphomas											
WEHI-5	μ,κ	ND	A+/E(C)+	ND	-	Trace	-	+	+	+	++++
WEHI-41	μ,κ	ND	A+/E(C)+	ND	-	ND	ND	-	-	-	+++
WEHI-55	μ,δ,κ	ND	A+/E(C)+	ND	-	+	-	+	±/+	-	++++
WEHI-231	μ,κ	-	A±/E(C)±	-	-	-	-	+++	+++	++++	++++
WEHI-259	μ,κ	ND	A+/E(C)+	ND	-	+	-	+++	+++	+	++++
WEHI-279.1/12	μ,κ	±	A±/E(C)±	-	-	-	-	+++	+++	+++	++++
2PK3	γ2,κ	+	A+/E(C)+	-	-	-	-	-	+	++	+++
UNM-22	μ,κ	ND	A+/E(C)+	ND	-	-	-	-	-	+	++++
UNM-27	μ,κ	ND	A+/E(C)+	ND	-	-	-	+	-	-	+++
UNM-30	μ,κ	ND	A+/E(C)+	ND	ND	ND	ND	+	-	+	++++
CH1	μ,λ	+	A+/E(C)+	-	-	-	-	+++	++	++++	++++
CH2	μ,λ	ND	A+/E(C)+	-	-	-	-	+++	-	-	++++
CH5	μ,κ	ND	A+/E(C)+	-	-	+	-	+	-	-	++++
Group IV: Plasmacytomas											
WEHI-2	-	+	A-/E(C)-	ND	-	ND	ND	±	-	±/+	++++
WEHI-37	-	+	A-/E(C)-	ND	-	-	-	-	-	+	++++
HPC-108	± (α,κ)	+	A+/E(C)-	-	-	-	-	-	-	+	-
HPC-213	-	+	A-/E(C)-	-	-	-	-	+++	-	-	++
MOPC-315	± (α,λ)	+	A-/E(C)-	-	-	-	-	±	-	-	++
MPC-11	± (γ2,κ)	+	A-/E(C)-	-	-	-	-	+	-	+	-
S107.J38	± (α,κ)	+	A-/E(C)-	ND	-	-	-	±	-	-	-

[a]Analysis performed using monoclonal antibodies (with the exception of Qa typing) and flow cytometry, as described in detail elsewhere (11). ND = not determined.

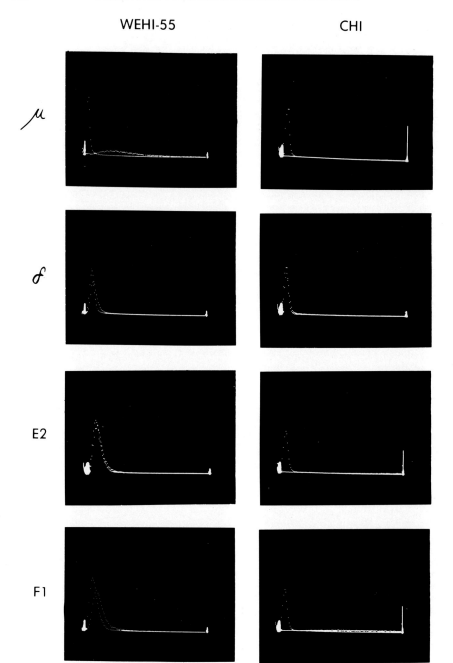

The major focus of these results, however, is to stress that the intertumor differences, which clearly exist, may represent distinct subpopulations or stages in B cell differentiation.

Analogous studies are in progress with tumors of the macrophage lineage. These, however, differ from the above studies in two main aspects. First, there are at present few available cell surface markers for defining stages of macrophage differentiation. Furthermore, the use of any such specific antibodies is seriously complicated by the presence of avid Fc receptors on many of these cells. Second, and in contrast with B and T cell tumors, there are, however, more available functional assays, which do not depend on knowledge of antigen specific reactivity. Some of our present data on the characterization of macrophage tumors are summarized in Table 2. The major point that we wish to draw from this chart is that in analogy to the study of B cell tumors, most tumors can be clearly distinguished either from each other, or at least into certain groups. That is, a clear *intertumor* heterogeneity is apparent.

In this particular instance, there is at present less precise knowledge of the counterpart normal differentiation lineage, at least in terms of whether these differences represent stages in a particular lineage or define distinct subpopulations. This is a most active area of current research, and one in which studies of macrophagelike cell lines, both in functional assays, and with newly developed monoclonal antibodies (20), may provide a most useful insight into normal macrophage differentiation.

Intratumor Heterogeneity

In general, the analysis of differentiation states of tumor cell lines has emphasized the differences *between* tumors and in turn has found a clear application in the characterization or classification of tumor types (14). However, in some instances, apparently confusing results have emerged in studying certain tumors, in that they did not readily appear to "fit" into predetermined stages or subpopulations. This

---

FIG. 1. B lymphoma intertumor heterogeneity. CH1 ascites and WEHI-55 cells were stained with optimal amounts of FITC goat antimouse μ, monoclonal antimouse δ (11-6.3 and 10-4.22 M.Ab.), monoclonal rat antimouse E2 (30-E2 M.Ab.), and monoclonal rat antimouse F1 (30-F1 M.Ab.) antibodies. For indirect immunofluorescence, FITC mouse (SJL) antirat Ig serum was used as the second stage. Fifteen × 10³ cells were analyzed using a FACS III system as described in detail elsewhere (9,10). In the above figures, the fluorescence histogram of the stained population was superimposed over the histogram of the autofluorescence control. All cells were analyzed at similar voltage and gain settings (*x* axis = fluorescence intensity, increasing left to right, linear scale, 128 channels; *y* axis = number of cells). Note the extreme *quantitative* difference in antigen expression between CH1 and WEHI-55 for surface μ, E2, and F1 antigen. The vertical line in fluorescence channel 128, for CH1 cells stained with anti-μ, anti-E2, and anti-F1 antibodies, indicates that a majority of the cells expressed extremely intense fluorescence and thus were accumulated in the last channel. WEHI-55 stains weakly for surface δ chain, whereas CH1 does not express δ chain. The expression of δ chain on the WEHI-55 has been confirmed by immunoprecipitation analysis (10).

TABLE 2. *Intermacrophage tumor heterogeneity*

| Cell line | Cell surface markers | | | Functional Properties | | | | | | |
| | Ia[a] | FcR[b] | CR[b] | Adherence[c] | Phagocytosis[d] | Chemi-luminescence[e] | Accessory cell function | | | Immune suppression[h] |
							M/D>SRBC1[f]	T cell proliferation[f]	IL-1[g]	
WEHI 3	+[i]	++	++[j]	+[j]	+[j]	−	+++	−	++++	−
HUCL-1	++	−	−	−	−	−	++++	±	++++	−
MW4	++	−	−	−	−	−	++++	±	++++	ND
PU5-1R	−	+++	+++	++	+++	++	±	ND	+++	±
P388.D1	−	+++	+++	++	++[j]	−	−	ND	+++	+++
J774	−	+++++	+++	−	++++	++	−	−	ND	++++
WEHI-274	−	+	±	−	−	++++	−	−	ND	−
WEHI-265	−	+	±	−	−	++++	−	−	ND	−
WEHI-5	++	ND	ND	−	−	−	−	++++	++++	ND

[a] Flow cytometry analysis of the expression of Ia antigens using ATH > ATL serum and monospecific anti-Ia.8 serum with fluorescenated goat antimouse IgG1, as previously described (23). In all cases in Table 2, the relative expression of a given surface marker or functional property across the group of cell lines described is expressed by the use of the symbol − for negative, ± for variable, and + through + + + + for increasing increments of positive response. The symbol ND means not done.

[b] Both Fc receptors and complement receptors were assessed using standard rosetting techniques described in designated chapters of ref. 18.

[c] No rigorous experimental quantitation of adherence was carried out. The description given here represents the consensus resulting from 3 years of weekly passage of cells and gross qualitative inspection of "stickiness."

[d] Phagocytosis was measured using uptake of FITC labeled latex beads and flow cytometry analysis described in ref. 22.

[e] Chemiluminescence measurements are described in ref. 22.

[f] Accessory cell function was measured by reconstituting macrophage depleted lymphocyte populations (by G-10 passage) with mitomycin treated, antigen pulsed macrophage and B cell tumor lines. The culture conditions for the Mishell-Dutton SRBC primary (35 mm cultures) and the ova primed T cell proliferation assay are exactly as described in the appropriate chapters of ref. 18.

[g] Interleukin-1 production was measured by the mitogen (Con A or PHA) enhanced thymocyte proliferation assay described in ref. 24.

[h] Described in ref. 4.

[i] Ia was detected on WEHI 3 only after treating the cell line with either TPA or LPS.

[j] Only a subpopulation of cells in culture demonstrated the presence of the property listed.

has perhaps particularly been noticeable within macrophage-like cell lines, in that within a given tumor, not all of the cells show the same properties, i.e., there is marked *intratumor* heterogeneity. Additionally, when a given tumor is studied at several different times after culture, apparently differing results may be obtained. These issues suggest that the concept of tumors as "frozen" stages in a differentiation lineage needs to be made more "elastic," at least for certain tumors. In this section, we would like to demonstrate several examples, and perhaps causes, of such intratumor heterogeneity. In the final section, the relationship of this intratumor heterogeneity to the ability to manipulate tumor differentiation will be considered in more detail.

One of the commonest examples of intratumor heterogeneity concerns different apparent levels in expression of a particular cell surface component. The commonest explanation for this simply relates to the fact that there are marked differences in cell volume within the tumor population. As shown in Fig. 2, the expression of Ia.8 antigen on the HUCL-1 macrophage cell line is considerably variable in amount. However when the cell volume is plotted against fluorescence intensity, a clear linear relationship is evident. Thus when the actual cell surface *density* of the particular component is determined, these data indicate that the apparent intratumor heterogeneity in amount of a particular surface component is not reflected in density heterogeneity.

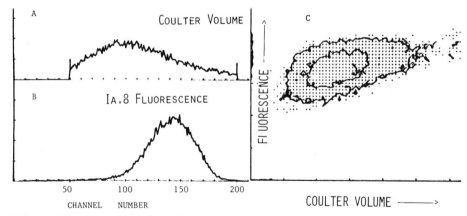

FIG. 2. Flow cytometry analysis of expression of Ia.8 antigen on HUCL-1 myeloid tumor cell lines. An aliquot of the HUCL-1 cells was stained with (A × B10A)F1 anti-B10.A(5R) antiserum (anti-Ia.8) followed by FITC conjugated goat antimouse IgG1. The cells were run in the Los Alamos flow cytometry system as previously described (23). Panel **A** shows the coulter volume profile for the cultured cells with windows set such that dead cells are excluded at the low volume range, and clumps to the right. Panel **B** shows the fluorescence profile using a three decade logarithmic amplifier over the 256 channels. A broad cell volume and fluorescence profile were observed. The correlation between these two profiles is shown in Panel **C** as a contour map of the coulter volume data expressed against the fluorescence data. Each point requires a minimum of 10 cells at the coordinates, with the outer contour being drawn around coordinates with a minimum of 15 cells, and the inner contour of 30 cells. A clear linear relationship is demonstrated between coulter volume and fluorescence, in that the larger cells have in general an average greater fluorescence intensity than smaller cells.

A related but separate aspect concerns variation in expression of components that occur in relation to cell cycle stages. Certain surface components and functions of cells are preferentially expressed at particular stages of the cell cycle (9). If these components or properties are also relatively transiently held by the cell once expressed, a distinct heterogeneity can be observed between cells in the population. Properties or cell surface components that demonstrate such cell cycle related heterogeneity are of essence variable, and do not represent stable "variants" in the population. This can be clearly demonstrated by sorting for cells within the population that differ in the particular property, and then reculturing such sorted cells. As shown in Fig. 3, the tumor line WEHI-3 consistently fails to show phagocytic activity in all cells of the population. When the highly phagocytic cells are separated from nonphagocytic cells (on the basis of uptake of fluorescent latex particles), and each population is recultured for a week, both redevelop the same intratumor heterogeneity in phagocytic activity. Both of these examples thus demonstrate intratumor heterogeneity, which is *not* representative of true heterogeneity in differentiation states within the population.

Of more relevance to our specific theme in this chapter are examples in which such differentiation heterogeneity does exist. In Table 3, we present data on the frequency of stem cells within several B cell/myeloma tumor populations, as assessed by ability to form colonies in soft agar. Although a property such as proliferation in agar is dependent on many factors extrinsic to the cell, we would emphasize that the results presented in this table are derived from an extensive series of earlier investigations on optimizing colony growth by these tumors. Therefore, they may indeed represent intrinsic differences between the tumor lines.

The essential point we wish to stress is that not all the cells within most tumor populations have the ability to form colonies in soft agar culture, which may indicate a true maturational heterogeneity within the tumor population. This conclusion can more firmly be drawn from studies in which attempts are made to enrich for several functional properties within the tumor population. A relatively simple approach to this is to separate cells on the basis of cell volume, using 1 g sedimentation velocity. As shown in Fig. 4, when cells of a given myeloma line are separated by this procedure, there is significant enrichment for colony forming capacity in certain fractions, whereas the more mature function of antibody secretion is enriched in other fractions. Studies of this type thus clearly demonstrate that these different functional properties are carried by *different* cells in the tumor population.

FIG. 3. Flow cytometry analysis of phagocytosis of fluorescent latex particles by the myelomonocytic leukemia WEHI-3. All cell samples were treated with fluoresceinated particles followed by trypsin treatment to remove surface adherent beads. WEHI-3 demonstrates a large proportion of negative cells and a population of cells varying in phagocytic activity. WEHI-3 cells were then sorted on the basis of phagocytic activity (negative or strongly positive) and recultured for 5 days. Each population was then retreated with the fluorescent particles. Panels **B** and **C** show the light scatter and fluorescence profiles of the originally positive (B) or negative (C) cells. Both populations have regenerated heterogeneity for phagocytic activity, suggesting that this property may be cell cycle related in this cell line.

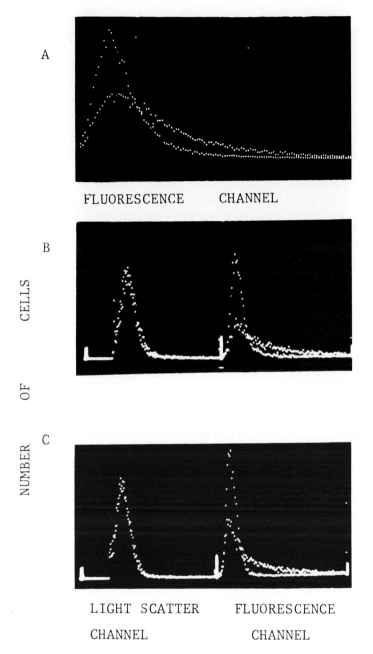

FLUORESCENCE CHANNEL

LIGHT SCATTER FLUORESCENCE
CHANNEL CHANNEL

TABLE 3. *Frequency of colony formation by B cell neoplasms*

Tumor line[a]	Type[b] (group)	Plating efficiency[c] (mean % soft agar colonies ± SEM)
HPC-213	Plasmacytoma (IV)	7.6 ± 7.3
HPC-209	Plasmacytoma (IV)	13.1 ± 6.8
HPC-108	Plasmacytoma (IV)	15.9 ± 4.1
2PK-3	B lymphoma (III)	16.4 ± 1.0
WEHI-231	B lymphoma (II)	23.6 ± 9.4
MPC-11	Plasmacytoma (IV)	25.1 ± 6.8
HPC-205	Plasmacytoma (IV)	34.9 ± 6.1
ABE-8	Pre-B lymphoma (I)	95.1

[a]Established tissue culture cell lines.

[b]Type and group from Table 1. All tumors are described in detail elsewhere (5,9,11,23).

[c]Percent of cells forming soft agar colonies after 7 days' culture in McCoy's 5a medium with fetal calf serum. Source of colony stimulating factor was serum from endotoxin treated mice, which was titrated for optimal colony inducing capacity. Details of these experiments will be submitted for publication elsewhere (3).

An approach to correlate functional heterogeneity with expression of cell surface markers of specific differentiation stages is to use flow sorting procedures to separate cells on the basis of quantitative expression of a particular surface component, and then to assess the functional properties of the sorted cells. An example of this approach is shown in Fig. 5, in which the plasmacytoma HPC-209 is separated on the basis of intensity of staining with anti-PCA-1 alloantiserum (21). The original population shows 43% of cells capable of forming colonies in soft agar, and this property is clearly enriched in the fraction showing low amounts of PCA-1 antigen expression.

Manipulation of Differentiation States Within Tumor Cell Lines

The essential point that we wished to demonstrate in the preceding section is that all the cells within a given tumor population need not be identical, even though the tumor population as a whole shows an arrest in differentiation. In this section, we now wish to illustrate the point that this internal heterogeneity within the tumor can be altered by specific treatment of the population with various agents.

One of the agents that has received considerable attention in relation to induction of myeloid differentiation with murine (13) and human (7,19) tumors is 12-O-tetradecanoyl phorbol-13-acetate (TPA). In most systems, this has been claimed to induce expression of a variety of macrophage associated properties. We have observed similar results with treatment of the myelomonocytic tumor WEHI-3, in that increased expression of Fc receptor density (Fig. 6) and new expression of Ia antigens (Fig. 7) occurred following 3 days' culture with 10^{-8} M TPA. The latter observation has considerable potential interest, since the parent WEHI-3 line has

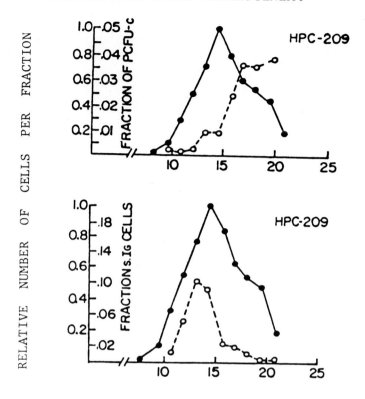

FIG. 4. Velocity sedimentation profile of secretory cells and stem cells (PCFU-C) of plasmacytoma HPC-209. The upper panel shows the sedimentation profile in a 1 g sedimentation system for the entire tumor population (solid line) and of the *in vitro* PCFU-stem cell frequency for the various fractions (dashed line). A clear enrichment of stem cell colony formation is observed in the fractions showing high sedimentation velocity (large cells). The lower panel shows the sedimentation profile for the entire population (solid line) and for the corresponding immunoglobulin secretory activity (dashed line) for the various fractions. Secretory assays were performed using the reverse plaque procedure with goat antimouse κ chain as the facilitating serum. In contrast to stem cell activity, the peak of Ig secretory activity is resident in the smaller cell fractions.

not been previously found to express Ia antigens, and yet it is capable of replacing at least certain macrophage functions in primary antibody response formation *in vitro* (E. Walker and N. L. Warner, manuscript in preparation).

In view of these results, we have also initiated studies on the effect of TPA on lymphoid tumors. In contrast to the results with WEHI-3, when the B lymphoma 2PK-3 was treated with TPA at similar concentrations, most surface markers studied did not show an increase in expression, but rather a decrease. The results for membrane Ig and several other properties are presented in Table 4 and Fig. 8. The

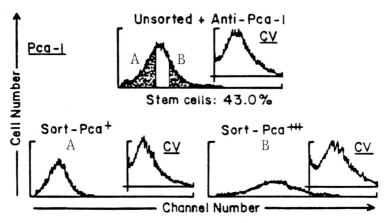

FIG. 5. Cell sorting of the stem cells of HPC-209 on the basis of PCA-1 expression. Cell sorting was performed on the FACS-III using the discriminating parameter of fluorescence intensity; 10^7 HPC-209 cells were labeled with anti-PCA-1 serum followed by FITC goat anti-mouse IgG1. The analysis of the relative fluorescence intensity and the coulter volume profiles (CV) are shown in the upper panel. Gain settings for sorting were established by peaking the autofluorescence control within the first 5 to 10 channels of the fluorescence distribution (total 128 channels). The gated channels used for the sorting were delineated by the shaded areas A and B. Reanalysis of these sorted cells is indicated in the lower two panels for the sorted low density PCA cells (A) and for the high density PCA cells (B). The coulter volume distribution of both of these sorted populations is shown in the insert. The stem cell frequency assay was then performed on the original population and on the sorted populations A and B. The stem cell frequency of the original fraction was 43.0%, for the low density PCA fraction 36.0%, and for the sorted high density PCA fraction 13.7%. This experiment therefore demonstrates that enrichment of stem cell activity can be achieved by sorting for low density PCA bearing cells.

consistent observation was that the population as a whole was altered toward the direction of more mature Ig secreting cells, in that surface densities if Ig, Ia, and Fc receptor were decreased. Furthermore, the population was considerably depleted of colony forming cells. When studied for reverse plaque formation, these cells showed considerably larger plaques, indicating possible increased Ig synthesis. However, the proportion of Ig secreting cells did not change.

DISCUSSION

Intertumor Heterogeneity

It has become reasonably well accepted that most hematopoietic tumors represent some degree of arrest in a particular differentiation lineage. The *majority* of cells within the tumor population are relatively homogeneous in maturational state, and as a *population* may be characterized as belonging to a particular group of tumors (14). This concept was illustrated in the first section of the results for both B lymphoid and macrophage tumor lines. Our studies in B cell tumors in this regard have been described in more detail elsewhere (11,23), and at present lead to the following general conclusions and issues.

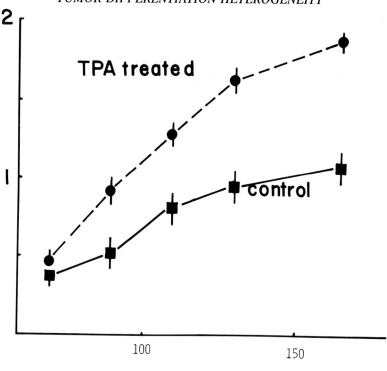

FIG. 6. Fc receptor analysis by flow cytometry of WEHI-3 myelomonocytic leukemia cells following treatment with TPA. In this study, cells from the same experiment as in Fig. 7 were treated with fluoresceinated labeled antigen antibody complexes as described previously (18). The flow cytometry data were reanalyzed for five separate subpopulations of cells based on cell volume. Populations falling in coulter channels 60–80, 80–100, 100–120, 120–140, and 140–180 were analyzed for mean fluorescence. The incremental fluorescence expressed as voltage units was determined for each of the gated populations in comparison to the autofluorescence control. These mean fluorescence values were then plotted against the mean coulter channel. The results clearly demonstrate an increase in fluorescence activity due to antigen antibody complex binding on the TPA treated cells.

First, there are at least four distinct groups of B cell tumors, as defined in Table 1, and most presently described B cell tumors can be placed within these categories. Second, this does not, however, infer that these four groups define the only *distinct* stages within B cell differentiation that are represented by tumor differentiation arrest. Indeed, several of the problems noted in the following sections might be resolved by the addition of further groups. Third, a major issue concerns the variability in cell surface phenotype between individual tumors within tumors of types II and III. In our extensive analysis of some 20 tumors, we have not observed any two which are identical in their reactivity with the various reagents used. At least three possible explanations might be proposed.

1. Each particular phenotype of a given tumor is indeed representative of a normal B cell subpopulation, and these subpopulations are in somewhat similar frequencies.

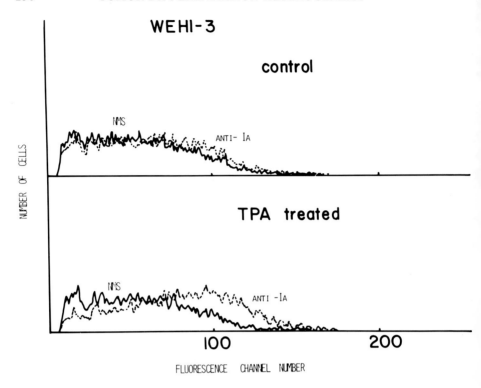

FIG. 7. Flow cytometry analysis of WEHI-3 myelomonocytic leukemia cells for Ia expression. WEHI-3 was cultured with 10^{-8} M TPA for 3 days, or with medium control. Aliquots of both cultures were treated with either normal mouse serum or anti-Ia.8 serum (as in Fig. 2) and FITC goat antimouse IgG1, and were analyzed by immunofluorescence as described in ref. 23, using the Los Alamos Scientific Laboratories flow systems. The x axis demonstrates the fluorescence intensity as channel number (using 3 decade logarithmic amplifier) plotted against the number of cells. In the control culture, there is a borderline shift of the cell population stained with anti-Ia serum as compared to the autofluorescence normal mouse serum treated control population. In contrast, the TPA treated population shows a clear shift in fluorescence intensity following anti-Ia staining. Whether only a subpopulation of cells is stained, or whether the entire population shows a significant shift remains to be determined.

Obviously, we should expect to soon detect some "repeats" in surface phenotypes as we study more tumors. It would also be of considerable relevance to attempt to determine whether we can detect normal B cells which express these individual phenotypes. If so, these might then be isolated and studied for functional properties.

2. Rather than considering these phenotypes as an absolute positive or negative, e.g., ThB$^+$ versus ThB$^-$, the true picture may be that our detection system is still not adequately sensitive. Therefore, many of the distinct phenotypic patterns are not true qualitative distinctions, but rather quantitative distinctions *within* a given subpopulation. For example, two tumors that are presently defined respectively as:

(1) MIg^{++}, ThB$^+$, F1$^-$ E2$^+$ Lyt-1$^-$, Qa-2$^-$
(2) MIg^{++}, ThB$^+$, F1$^+$ E2$^+$ Lyt-1$^-$, Qa-2$^-$

TABLE 4. *Influence of TPA on cultured 2PK-3 B cell lymphoma*

Property	Control 2PK-3	TPA treated 2PK-3[f]
Membrane Ig[a]	1.62 V	0.25 V
Membrane I-E[b]	1.33 V	0.71 V
Membrane FcR[c]	0.21 V	0.08 V
Stem cell assay (CFUc)[d]	21.4 ± 3.2	3.0 ± 1.7
Reverse plaque forming capacity[e]	30.0 ± 2.9	30.4 ± 2.4

[a]Flow cytometry analysis of membrane Ig assessed by binding of FITC sheep antimouse K chain. Results shown as incremental fluorescence signal in volts (V), calculated as previously described (23). Results show fivefold drop in M.Ig after TPA treatment.

[b]Flow cytometry analysis of membrane I-E as described previously (23). Results show twofold drop after TPA treatment.

[c]Membrane Fc receptor analysis by flow cytometry (23). Two-and-a-half-fold reduction after TPA treatment.

[d]Plating efficency of 2PK-3 cells in soft agar as assessed in Table 3. Results show mean of three experiments and demonstrate sevenfold reduction in CFUc.

[e]Ability of cells to secrete immunoglobulin as measured in a Staph A conjugated reverse plaque forming assay. Results show mean % of plaque forming cells from three assays.

[f]2PK-3 cells were cultured for three days in 1.6×10^{-8} M TPA in Dulbecco's modified eagles medium with fetal calf serum.

might not be representative of different groups, but rather differ only in that the first tumor *does* express the surface determinant detected by the F1 monoclonal, but in a density that is just under detectable limits.

3. The third general alternative is that only some of these surface marker phenotypes are truly representative of normal B cell subpopulations. Many of the tumors may "aberrantly" express gene products that are not expressed by their normal counterpart cell. A key example of this might be the expression of Lyt-1 antigen by certain B cell tumors, and this aspect is discussed in more detail elsewhere (10).

Finally, in several instances, it has not been particularly evident as to whether a given tumor belongs to, for example, category 3 or 4. This aspect is in essence the bridge into the next part of our discussion, which places emphasis on exactly *how homogeneous* are the individual component cells within a tumor. As clearly illustrated in the second section of the results, there is still considerable heterogeneity within certain tumor populations. This provides considerable difficulty in characterization, when the elements within a tumor span several of the categories.

Intratumor Heterogeneity

We have illustrated by use of biophysical cell separation (size), cell surface markers, and functional properties, that not all cells need be alike within a cloned tumor cell population. Two of the most frequent explanations for such intratumor heterogeneity relate to the fact that these are actively growing tumor cell lines and

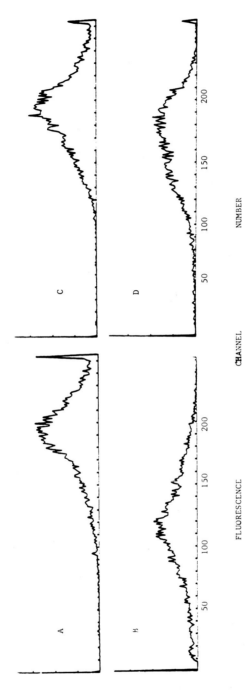

FIG. 8. Flow cytometry analysis of immunoglobulin and Ia expression by 2PK3 B lymphoma cells following culture with TPA. Cells were treated as for WEHI-3 cells in Fig. 6 anc were stained with fluorescein conjugated sheep antimouse κ chain antibody, or with anti-Ia.8, as described in fig. 1. Panels **A** and **B** show the control cells and TPA treated cells, respectively, stained with FITC anti-κ. Panels **C** and **D** show control and TPA treated cells, respectively, stained for Ia.8. In both instances, there is a clear reduction in fluorescence intensity of the TPA treated cells following staining for membrane Ig or Ia.

as such differ in volume and stages of cell cycle. As illustrated, both of these can directly contribute to some of the intratumor heterogeneity observed. These aspects have been discussed in more detail elsewhere (9,23), and will not be further considered herein. Neither of these aspects truly concerns heterogeneity within the population in a maturation sense.

Although many tumor cell lines that have been carried in established long term tissue culture can show up to 100% plating efficiencies in soft agar colony assays, this is not always the case. In the studies illustrated herein and to be described in more detail elsewhere (M. J. Daley and N. L. Warner, manuscripts in preparation), it has been observed that the stem cell fraction within several of the lymphoid tumor lines is a discrete subpopulation, which can be relatively selected by various procedures based on cell surface phenotypes or biophysical properties. In considering the possible relationship between the differentiated state and tumor stem cell activity (as defined by colony formation in soft agar), we would propose that there are three distinct alternatives, as outlined in Fig. 9.

1. The simplest possibility would be to propose that all cells in the tumor population are identical in all ways, both in terms of ability to form colonies and cell surface phenotype (Fig. 9, left). They differ only in relation to cell cycle related aspects. This is probably the case for some of the tumor lines we have studied. For example, with certain *myelomas*, 100% plating efficiency can be obtained, and all cells show similar cell surface densities of membrane Ig, plasma cell alloantigen, etc. These tumors may represent the accumulation of subsequent variant changes, the selection of certain component cells, or the end stage of the loss of normal regulatory controls. This situation, however, is clearly *not* the case for many of the tumors.

2. In this instance, it is proposed that all cells in the population express similar cell surface phenotypes, but that only a distinct subpopulation has a stem cell property (Fig. 9, center). Based on this concept, we therefore should not be able to select for stem cells, or for the more mature cells in the population, solely on the basis of expression of cell surface markers. Although our studies of the type illustrated in Fig. 5 are not yet complete, it has become apparent that at least in *some* tumors, this situation holds. That is, selection for high density expression of a cell surface component, which in *normal* differentiation is expressed only on the most mature cells in the lineage, does *not* selectively enrich for mature cells (e.g., Ig secreting) in the tumor population, nor does it selectively deplete for tumor stem cells. In contrast, for other tumors, this *is* the case.

3. This latter conclusion leads into the final possibility, which is that the intratumor heterogeneity which is present within a tumor is exactly that which is associated with the *normal* differentiation lineage (Fig. 9, right). That is, the stem cell compartment is distinct from the more mature elements in the population in terms of specific cell surface components that are selectively expressed at certain stages of differentiation.

In conclusion, we would at present propose that all three of these situations may exist for different tumors. Although some, and perhaps initially all, tumors behave

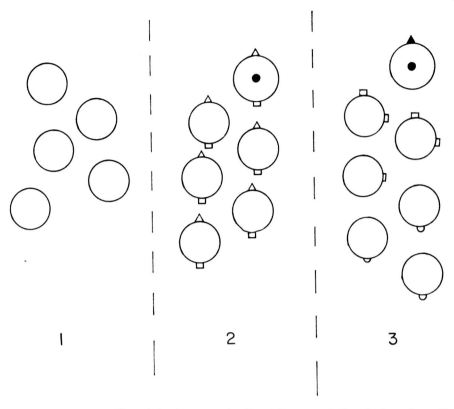

FIG. 9. Intratumor differentiation heterogeneity. Panel **1** represents the situation where all cells within a tumor population are identical in all parameters. Panel **2** indicates the possibility that all cells are identical in surface phenotypic markers (depicted by the triangle and square); the stem cell fraction (indicated by central dot) is present in a subpopulation of cells, which are, however, identical in surface phenotype to the nonstem cells in the population. Panel **3** illustrates the normal differentiation situation in which the stem cell activity is resident in cells that have a distinct surface phenotype from the other members of the population.

in a normal differentiation manner (Fig. 9, right), with subsequent changes and perhaps loss of growth regulation, many tumors progress into the two aberrant stages shown in Fig. 9 (center and left).

Induction of Differentiation

One of the most interesting aspects of tumor heterogeneity is whether this can be deliberately manipulated by experimental procedures. As such, this could have direct clinical relevance, if a true terminal maturation could be induced, providing this did not retain an aberrant stem cell function. We have illustrated the feasibility of this approach with a few selected examples with a myeloid and B cell tumor treated with TPA. Both results mirror the many other publications in this field (e.g., 2,7,13,19) in demonstrating that changes can occur in the tumor population as a result of such treatment. These changes could be interpreted as induction of differentiation; however, in view of the considerations noted above, we would propose that there are several possible explanations.

1. *Induction of differentiation*. Several studies have emphasized that the changes which can be observed in TPA treated tumors are multiple and involve the expression of phenotypic patterns that are truly those of a normal *mature* cell in the lineage under investigation. This "usual" explanation of induction of differentiation strictly implies that the change involves a true readout of a normal differentiation program at the genetic level. Namely, there is transcription, translation, and expression of gene products that were not perviously expressed by the tumor, and that these new products are indeed those associated with the next differentiation stage in the particular lineage. This event is also presumably occurring in a major population of cells within the tumor. If such treatments are to have clinical relevance, they also preferably involve maturation toward the nondividing cell stages.

2. *Membrane changes*. Since several of the agents used in this work have been reported to induce direct effects on cell membranes (25), it is possible that the apparent expression of a "new" surface marker only represents a membrane perturbation that results in better expression of a gene product than was already expressed, but possibly at an undetectable level. Thus according to this view, no new gene expression has occurred, and the term "induction of differentiation" would be strictly incorrect. In the studies we cite on the B lymphoma, although multiple changes were observed that are compatible with increased maturation, no increase in the *proportion* of Ig secreting cells was observed. The fact that the size of the reverse plaques was greater may only imply that membrane permeability has increased. We are presently attempting to determine whether there has been a true increase in biosynthetic activity of Ig in these cells.

3. *Selection*. The emphasis of our studies on intratumor heterogeneity is to stress that for many tumors, the cells within a tumor are not identical. Hence an alternative explanation of the effect of any agent on a tumor population may be to selectively eradicate (or promote growth) of a subset of cells within the tumor population. Thus the apparent change may be only due to selective amplification of a subset, possibly present at only a rare frequency, within the original tumor.

In all likelihood, it may develop that all these mechanisms are operative in different circumstances. The major point that we would like to stress, however, is that any consideration of differentiation induction of tumor populations should be made with cognizance of the various possibilities, and preferably be based on a detailed understanding of the complete differentiation status of the starting population. Such studies are accordingly likely to continue to yield extremely valuable information on an understanding of hematopoietic differentiation, possibly with direct relevance to the clinical intervention of tumor growth.

ACKNOWLEDGMENTS

The studies described in this chapter were funded by a research grant from the National Institutes of Health, CA 22105. Dr. Lanier is a fellow of the Damon

Runyan Walter Winchell fund. Excellent technical assistance in the performance of these studies was provided by Eva Barry, Tom Williams, and Jerome Zawadski. The flow cytometry studies performed at Los Alamos Scientific Laboratories were made possible by the expert assistance of Scott McLaughlin.

Note in proof: The reaction of the (A × B10.A) F_1 anti-B10A (5R) with HUCL-1 is not due to recognition of the Ia-8 determinant, but to another, as yet, undefined surface antigen (Walker, E. B., Lanier, L. L., and Warner, N. L. (1982): *J. Immunol.* 128:852–859.

REFERENCES

1. Burchiel, S., Leary, T., and Warner, N. L. *(submitted for publication)*.
2. Collins, J., Bodner, A., Ting, R., and Gallo, R. C. (1980): Induction of morphological and functional differentiation of human promyelocytic leukemia cells (HL-60) by compounds which induce differentiation of murine leukemia cells. *Int. J. Cancer*, 25:213–218.
3. Daley, M. J., and Warner, N. L. *(submitted for publication)*.
4. Giorgi, J. V., and Warner, N. L. (1981): In: *Immunosuppression in Human Disease*, edited by J. Goodwin. Marcel Dekker, New York.
5. Gutman, G. A., Warner, N. L., and Harris, A. W. (1981): Immunoglobulin production by murine B lymphoma cells. *Clin. Immunol. Immunopathol.*, 18:230–244.
6. Herzenberg, L. A., and Herzenberg, L. A. (1978): Analysis and separation using the fluorescence activated cell sorter (FACS). In: *Handbook of Experimental Immunology*, Vol. 2, edited by D. M. Weir, p. 22.1. Blackwell Scientific Publications, London.
7. Huberman, E., and Callahan, M. F. (1979): Induction of terminal differentiation in human promyelocytic leukemia cells by tumor promoting agents. *Proc. Natl. Acad. Sci. U.S.A.*, 76:1293–1297.
8. Kennett, R., McKearn, T. J., and Bechtol, K. B., editors (1980): *Monoclonal Antibodies*. Plenum Press, New York.
9. Lanier, L. L., and Warner, N. L. (1981): Cell cycle related heterogeneity of Ia antigen expression on a murine B lymphoma cell line: analysis by flow cytometry. *J. Immunol.*, 126:626–631.
10. Lanier, L. L., Warner, N. L., Ledbetter, J. A., and Herzenberg, L. A. (1981): Expression of Lyt-1 antigen on certain murine B cell lymphomas. *J. Exp. Med. (in press)*.
11. Lanier, L. L., Warner, N. L., Ledbetter, J. A., and Herzenberg, L. A. (1981): Quantitative immunoflorescent analysis of surface phenotypes of murine B cell lymphomas and plasmacytomas with monoclonal antibodies. *J. Immunol.*, 127:1691–1697.
12. Ledbetter, J. A., Evans, R. L., Lipinski, M., Cunningham-Rundles, C., Good, R. A., and Herzenberg, C. A. (1981): Evolutionary conservation of surface molecules that distinguish T lymphocyte helper/inducer and cytotoxic/suppressor subpopulations in mouse and man. *J. Exp. Med.* 153:310–323.
13. Lotem, J.,and Sachs, L. (1979): Regulation of normal differentiation of mouse and human myeloid leukemic cells by phorbol esters and the mechanism of tumor promotion. *Proc. Natl. Acad. Sci. U.S.A.*, 76:5158–5162.
14. Mathe, G., Seligmann, M., and Tubiana, M., editors (1978): *Lymphoid Neoplasias I. Classification, Categorization and Natural History. Recent Results in Cancer Research*, Vol. 64. Springer-Verlag, New York.
15. McHugh, Y., Yagi, M., and Koshland, M. E. (1981): The use of J and mu chain analyses to assign lymphoid cell lines to various stages in B cell differentiation. In: *B Lymphocytes in the Immune Response*, edited by I. Schur et al. Elsevier/North-Holland, New York.
16. Melamed, M. R., Mullaney, P. F., and Mendelsohn, M. M., editors (1979): *Flow Cytometry and Sorting*, John Wiley & Sons, New York.
17. Melchers, F., Potter, M., and Warner, N. L., editors (1978): *Lymphocyte Hybridomas. Contemporary Topics in Microbiology and Immunology*, Vol. 81. Springer-Verlag, New York.
18. Mishell, B., and Shiigi, S. M., editors (1980): *Selected Methods in Cellular Immunology*. W. H. Freeman, San Francisco.
19. Rovera, G., O'Brien, T., and Diamond, L. (1979): Induction of differentiation in human promyelocytic leukemia cells by tumor promoters. *Science*, 204:868–870.

20. Springer, T. A. (1980): Cell surface differentiation in the mouse. Characterization of "Jumping" and "Lineage" antigens using xenogeneic rat monoclonal antibodies. In: *Monoclonal Antibodies*, edited by R. H. Kennett, T. J. McKearn, and K. B. Bechtol, p. 185. Plenum Press, New York.
21. Takahashi, T., Old, L. J., Heu, E.-J., and Boyse, E. A. (1971): A new differentiation antigen of plasma cells. *Eur. J. Immunol.*, 1:487.
22. Walker, E., VanEpps, D., and Warner, N. L. (1981): Macrophage chemiluminiscence. In: *Manual of Macrophage Methodology*, edited by H. Herscowitz, p. 389. Marcel Dekker, New York.
23. Warner, N. L., Daley, M. J., Richey, J., and Spellman, C. W. (1979): Flow cytometry analysis of murine B cell lymphoma differentiation. *Immunol. Rev.*, 48:197–243.
24. Watson, J., Gillis, S., Marbrook, J., Mochizuke, D., and Smith, K. A. (1979): *J. Exp. Med.*, 150:849.
25. Weinstein, I. B., Lee, L.-S., Fisher, P. B., Mufson, A., and Yamasaki, H. (1979): Action of phorbol esters in cell culture: mimicry of transformation, altered differentiation, and effects on cell membranes. *J. Supramol. Struct.*, 12:195–208.

Maturation Factors and Cancer,
edited by Malcolm A. S. Moore.
Raven Press, © New York 1982.

Induction of Differentiated Functions Coupled with Growth Inhibition in Lymphocyte and Macrophage Tumor Cell Lines

*Peter Ralph, *Ilona Nakoinz, and **William C. Raschke

*Sloan-Kettering Institute for Cancer Research, Rye, New York 10580;
**The Salk Institute for Biological Studies, La Jolla, California 92037

LECTIN INDUCTION OF FACTOR PRODUCTION BY MURINE T LYMPHOMAS

A summary of our experience with induction or stimulation of differentiated functions in lymphoid cell lines coupled with growth inhibition or toxicity is shown in Table 1. Con A induced granulocyte/macrophage colony stimulating activity (G,M-CSA) in the EL4 line only at toxic concentrations (18). PHA at equally toxic doses did not induce factor production (Fig. 1). Both PHA and Con A induce or stimulate interleukin 2 (IL2) production in radiation-induced LBRM and Rauscher virus-induced RBL-3 lines at toxic concentrations (2,2a). We have recently found that megakaryocyte CSF and myeloid CSF are also induced by lectins in LBRM (Y.-P. Yung et al., unpublished data). It should be pointed out that these T lymphocytic-specific mitogens only stimulate a small fraction of T lymphoma lines tested, suggesting that the tumors belong to functionally different groups comparable to normal T-cell subsets. Similar concentrations (5–20 µg/ml) of Con A and PHA are toxic to most mouse and human hemic cell lines, including B lymphomas, erythroleukemia, and mastocytoma. Notable exceptions are murine and human plasmacytomas, which are relatively resistant (11,14). Thus the expression of a new product by a cancer cell line results from a specific interaction of lectins in addition to their toxicity.

INDUCTION OF IMMUNOGLOBULIN (Ig) AND Fc RECEPTORS IN MURINE PRE-B LYMPHOMAS

Many Abelson virus-induced lymphomas and chemically induced 70Z/2 and 70Z/3 lymphomas have the pre-B lymphocyte phenotype of surface Ig$^-$ (sIg$^-$) and cytoplasmic Ig$^+$ (cIg$^+$). Paige et al. showed that 70Z/2 and 70Z/3 could be induced

TABLE 1. *Induction of differentiated functions and growth inhibition in hemic cell lines*

Cell type	Species	Line	Inducer[a]	Function	Reference
T lymphocyte	Mouse	EL 4	Con A	G,M-CSF	18
				Mega-CSF,PF	25
Pre-B lymph-	Mouse	7OZ/3	LPS	sIg,Fc	9
ocyte			AM,BUDR	Fc receptor	20
		4 lines	LPS,DS,PMA	sIg	This chapter
B lymphocyte	Human	Many	PMA	Ig secretion	16
Macrophage	Mouse	PU5-1.8	LPS,BCG,Z	G,M-CSF	17
		4 lines	PMA,PPD	G,M-CSF	18
		6 lines	LPS,Z	Prostaglandin	8
		RAW 264	PMA	Plasminogen act.	4
		P388D1	LPS	Mega-CSF,PF	25
		J774	PMA,LPS	Tumor toxicity	21

[a]LPS, lipopolysaccharide; AM, actinomycin D; PMA, phorbol myristic acetate; DS, dextran sulfate; BCG, *Mycobacteria BCG;* Z, zymosan; PPD, mycobacterial purified protein derivative.

to express sIg by dextran sulfate (DS) and cytostatic concentrations of B-lymphocyte activator lipopolysaccharide (LPS) (Fig. 2 and refs. 9 and 20). Subsequent selection produced sublines of 7OZ/3 that showed sIg induction, but no growth inhibition, or neither effect, by LPS (20). Induction of surface μ heavy chain and Fc receptor probably involved expression of preformed protein molecules, since this was not blocked by inhibitors of RNA or protein synthesis (20). On the other hand, light chain induction is a true gene activation event, since the protein and mRNA are undetectable until triggering by LPS, as shown by Perry and Kelly (10) and Sakaguchi et al. (24). Surface Fc receptors were even induced by toxic concentrations of actinomycin D and BUdR (20). Other examples of sIg or Fc receptor induction in pre-B lines are given in Figs. 3 and 4, using LPS, DS, BUdR, or tumor promoter phorbol myristic acetate (PMA) at cytostatic or cytotoxic concentrations. In many of the cytostatic cases, the cells revert to normal growth and loss of surface markers within 2 days of removal of inducer with no evidence of cell death. The correlation of growth inhibition by B-lymphocyte mitogens and induction of sIg does not always hold, as seen with lines RAW307.1 and P388 (Fig. 4), which share similarities with the known pre-B lines but do not express Ig.

INDUCTION OF Ig SECRETION IN HUMAN B LYMPHOCYTES AND CELL LINES

The above examples with pre-B lines show induction of early steps in the maturation of B lymphocytes. We have found that PMA is a strong activator of human blood B cells, causing Ig secretion comparable to PWM in activity (16). For normal, resting B lymphocytes, PMA requires T cells to induce Ig secretion. In contrast, when human B-cell lines are incubated with PMA in the absence of other cell types, there is a 3- to 30-fold increase in Ig secretion measured by plaque-forming cells (PFC) using protein A-coupled RBC. Figure 5 shows results with line RPMI 1788, in which PFCs are increased 10-fold by incubation with cytostatic concentrations

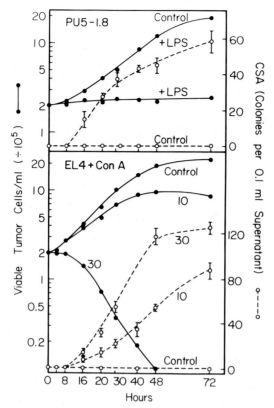

FIG. 1. Growth inhibition and induction of CSA production in a macrophage line by LPS and in a T lymphocyte line by Con A. EL4 cultures with Con A, 10 μg/ml (————) or 30 μg/ml (---), and PU5-1.8 cultures with LPS, 1 μg/ml, were initiated at 2 × 10⁵ cells/ml. At the times shown, viable cells in duplicate 2-ml cultures were counted, and the supernatant was assayed for CSA (colonies/7.5 × 10⁴ bone marrow cells/0.1 ml supernatant). Con A, 10 μg/ml, inhibited EL4 growth 58%, and 30 μg/ml was toxic. PHA was similarly toxic to EL4 but did not induce CSA. LPS inhibited PU5-1.8 growth more than 95% when measured at 48 hr.

of PMA. Six of 18 cell lines or clones studied showed up to 30-fold enhancement of PFC. Certain human and murine B-cell lines are 500 times more sensitive to growth inhibition by PMA than other lines (12). The dose of PMA required to stimulate Ig secretion in a line is generally correlated with growth inhibition of the line and cell death by day 4 or 5 of incubation.

FACTOR PRODUCTION AND TOXIC EFFECTOR FUNCTIONS IN MURINE MACROPHAGE TUMOR CELL LINES

In a study on production of G,M-CSF by the macrophage line PU5-1.8, we found that macrophage-activating agents LPS, the associated lipid A, zymosan, *Mycobacteria BCG*, mycobacterial extract PPD, and PMA were inducers for this factor at concentrations inhibiting PU5-1.8 growth (17). Other compounds inhibiting growth

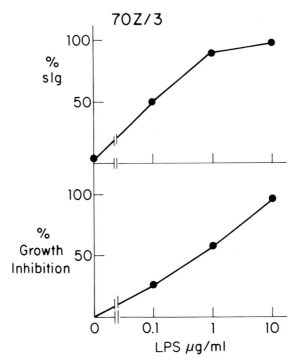

FIG. 2. Growth inhibition associated with induction of surface immunoglobulin (sIg) by LPS in pre-B lymphoma 70Z/3. Cultures were initiated at 10^5/ml with varying concentrations of LPS, and sIg by immunofluorescence and viable cell numbers were measured at day 2 (9). Controls increased 5 to $10 \times$ in cell numbers.

of the cell line, such as silica, cyclic AMP, or thymidine, or blocking growth by culturing without serum did not induce CSF, suggesting specific interactions of the effective agents. Induction of CSF was blocked by inhibitors of RNA and protein synthesis, showing that it involved expression of a new gene product.

Further analysis of a number of macrophage cell lines showed that most of them could be induced for CSF production by the same agents effective with PU5-1.8 (18). Induction was correlated with drug concentrations cytostatic for cell line growth. Other functions induced or augmented in these cell lines by growth-inhibiting agents include synthesis of prostaglandin (8), plasminogen activator (4), and megakaryocyte CSF (25), phagocytosis (6), antibody-dependent killing of RBC and tumor targets (15), and direct cytotoxicity to tumor targets (21).

A number of investigators in Japan, Israel, and Australia have shown similar correlations between induction of differentiated markers and growth inhibition using several relatively immature myeloid/macrophage cell lines. The results presented here suggest that even in mature, malignant macrophage tumors, signals pushing the cells to a more differentiated state also block proliferation.

A contrast to these conclusions is given by the monocytic line WEHI-3. We found that this constitutive producer of CSF appears to require its own CSF for

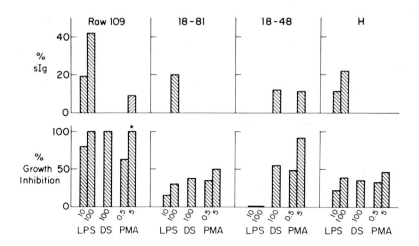

FIG. 3. Growth inhibition and induction of sIg in murine lymphomas. Abelson virus-induced cell lines RAW 109 (22), 18-81, and 18-48, and a subline (H) of 38C-13 (12) were cultured at 10^5 cells/ml plus 0, 10, 100 μg/ml LPS, 100 μg/ml DS, and 0.5 or 5 μg/ml PMA. sIg was assayed by protein-A rosettes (20) and cell numbers counted at day 2. PMA at 5 μg/ml was toxic to RAW 109 (∗) (less than 50% cells viable); in other conditions, cultures were greater than 90% viable.

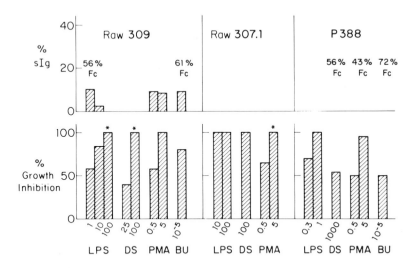

FIG. 4. Induction of sIg and Fc receptors in some murine lymphomas. Abelson virus-induced cell lines RAW 309, RAW 307.1 (22), and P388 were cultured at 10^5 cells/ml plus 0.3 to 100 μg/ml LPS, 25 to 1,000 μg/ml DS, and 0.5 or 5 μg/ml PMA or 10^{-5} M BUDR. At day 2, Fc receptors using EA-rabbit (% positive cells stated in figure) and sIg (bars) were assayed by rosetting (20). ∗ indicates toxic conditions.

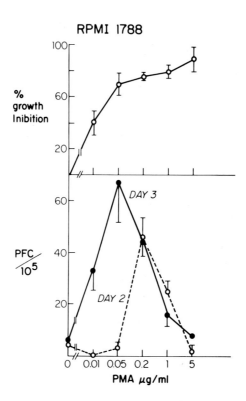

FIG. 5. PMA stimulation of Ig secretion by human B-cell line RPMI 1788. Cells were cultured 2 or 3 days with PMA, viable cells were counted, and average growth inhibition by PMA was calculated. Ig secretion was measured by plaque-forming cells (PFC), using protein A-RBC (16) per 10^5 cells recovered at day 2 (○) and day 3 (●). Cell numbers in control cultures increased 4.8-fold, and cell viability was greater than 90% at day 3.

growth. When CSF production was suppressed by lactoferrin derived from granulocytes, agar colony formation was inhibited. This effect could be reversed by exogenous CSF or by overriding the lactoferrin by LPS or other enhancers of CSF production by WEHI-3 (1).

EFFECT OF CORTICOSTEROIDS ON INDUCTION OF DIFFERENTIATED FUNCTIONS AND TOXICITY IN MACROPHAGE CELL LINES

In studying the stimulatory effects of macrophage activators on cell lines, we found that the simultaneous presence of hydrocortisone or dexamethasone could reverse these actions. This was true for induction of CSF and augmentation of phagocytosis and antibody-dependent lysis of RBC and tumor targets (19). In these examples, near physiological concentrations of the steroids also reversed the inhibition of growth caused by the activating agents. Steroids thus act like a growth requirement for macrophage lines in these conditions, whereas they are toxic at the same concentrations to most T- and early B-lymphocyte tumor lines (12).

Corticosteroids have positive (3) and negative (19) effects on generation of normal macrophages. Paradoxically, steroids induce macrophage markers in the immature myeloblast line M1 (23), while inhibiting some of the same characteristics in the mature tumor lines (13) (Table 2).

HOW CAN WE CATEGORIZE THE DIFFERENTIATION STATE AND POTENTIAL OF THE LYMPHOID TUMOR LINES DESCRIBED?

The lymphocytic and macrophage cell lines fall into two groups, based on their capacity to express new differentiation markers (Table 3).

Tumors Fixed in their State of Differentiation

Most thymomas and plasmacytomas appear to belong in this group. Thymomas are immature cells relative to peripheral T lymphocytes, and plasmacytomas represent the end cell stage of B lymphocytes. Both types are well differentiated in the sense of having many cell type-specific markers, and both are quite malignant as tumors. It may be that the thymomas can be differentiated further, as we learn

TABLE 2. *Corticosteroid abrogation of induction/stimulation and toxicity*

Line	Inducer	Function[a]	Reference
Steroid-resistant macrophages			
PU5-1.8	LPS, PPD	CSF, ADCC	19
RAW 264	LPS	ADCC	19
PU5-1.8	LPS, PPD	Phagocytosis	6
RAW 264	PMA	Plasminogen act.	4

[a]CSF, granulocyte/macrophage colony stimulating factor; ADCC, antibody-dependent cellular cytotoxicity.

TABLE 3. *Differentiation capacity of lymphoid tumor cell lines*

A. Fixed; "frozen"
   1. Immature; thymomas
   2. Mature; myelomas

B. Inducible; "poised"
   1. Reversible, Pre-B: sIgM, Fc
      Macrophage
   2. Irreversible/lethal? T cell: CSF
      B cell: Ig secretion

more about the physiological role of the thymic stromal cells. Some plasmacytoma lines show evidence of growth and functional regulation through specific interactions with the immune system (5).

Inducible Cell Lines

Reversible Inductive Systems

In these cell lines, there may be a very narrow spectrum of properties induced, in contrast to the range of molecules found, e.g., in the differentiating erythroleukemia, whose normal maturation pathway is an enucleated end cell. In some cases of murine pre-B lines, induction of sIg and Fc receptors occurs with no effect on cell growth and with no evidence for expression of later markers in B-lymphocyte differentiation. Even with cytostatic inducers of sIg and FcR, the effects are reversible, with normal growth and loss of induced markers several days after removing the inducer (9,20).

The rapidity of expression of induced B-cell markers (less than 24 hr) and the ability of BUdR and actinomycin to cause expression of FcR are remarkable. This suggests that many of these pre-B lines are "poised" at the threshold to sIg-positive maturation. Indeed, the LPS induction of μ-heavy chain and FcR on the cell surface is independent of RNA and protein synthesis, and these markers must be derived from pre-existing protein molecules. The expression of κ light chain is a true gene activation event correlated with κ mRNA synthesis.

Macrophage tumor lines show a longer time course for stimulation of ADCC and phagocytosis (2 days), and for induction of CSF (2–3 days), which is dependent on RNA and protein synthesis. The growth inhibition and induced functions disappear upon removal of the stimulatory agents.

Irreversible Induction and Cell Death

Several examples of induction result in the death of the cell. It may be that the particular inducing agents used, Con A for T-cell production of CSF and PMA for B-cell secretion of Ig, are toxic independently of stimulatory function. Other inducing agents, or pulsing protocols with toxic agents, may show only cytostatic or even nongrowth-inhibitory inductions. The induction of IgG in human IgM cell lines by coculture with normal T lymphocytes also results in death of the cells, at about day 7 (7). This is probably due to induction of T killers in the normal population, and attempts to overcome this problem by using purified T helper cells are under investigation.

CONCLUSIONS

It is evident that many tumors are not fixed, or autonomous, but have normal or paranormal growth hormone requirements and are responsive to differentiation or maturation signals with many similarities to their normal counterparts. Based on the studies of lymphoid lines, we expect many tumors will respond to the proper inducing agents to differentiate or express mature markers, and in many of the cases, the maturation will result in growth inhibition or death of the cell. The challenge will be to find optimal and physiological signaling agents with a more careful comparison to normal cell differentiation. We must then be prepared to see tumor cells evolve, in low frequency, to resistance to growth inhibition. This may occur by their becoming unresponsive to induction or by developing the ability to grow despite having the phenotype of end cells, with myeloma and macrophage tumors as examples.

ACKNOWLEDGMENTS

We thank M. A. S. Moore for advice and support. This work was funded by grants CA 24300, CA 21531, and CA 08748 from the National Institutes of Health, and the Gar Reichman Foundation.

REFERENCES

1. Broxmeyer, H. E., and Ralph, P. (1977): *In vitro* regulation of a mouse myelomonocytic leukemia line in culture. *Cancer Res.*, 37:3578–3587.
2. Farrar, J. J., Fuller-Farrar, J., Simon, P. L., Hilfiker, M. L., Stadler, B. M., and Farrar, W. L. (1980): Thymoma production of T cell growth factor (Interleukin 2). *J. Immunol.*, 125:2555–2558.
2a. Gillis, S., Scheid, M., and Watson, J. (1980): The isolation and phenotypic characterization of Interleukin-2 producing T cell lymphomas. *J. Immunol.*, 125:2570–2578.
3. Greenberger, J. S. (1978): Sensitivity of corticosteroid-dependent insulin-resistant lipogenesis in marrow preadipocytes of obese-diabetic mice. *Nature*, 275:752–755.
4. Hamilton, J. A., Ralph, P., and Moore, M. A. S. (1978): A macrophage tumor cell line and plasminogen activator: a model system for macrophage regulation of enzyme production. *J. Exp. Med.*, 148:811–816.
5. Activation and regulation of immunoglobulin synthesis in malignant B cells. (1979): *Immunol. Rev.*, 48: (whole issue).
6. Ito, M., Ralph, P., and Moore, M. A. S. (1979): *In vitro* stimulation of phagocytosis in a macrophage cell line measured by a convenient radio-labeled latex bead assay. *Cell. Immunol.*, 48: 48–56.
7. Kishimoto, T., Hirano, T., Kuritani, T., Yamamura, Y., Ralph, P., and Good, R. A. (1978): Induction of IgG production in human B lymphoblast cell lines with normal human T lymphocytes. *Nature*, 271:756–758.
8. Kurland, J. I., Pelus, L. M., Ralph, P., Bockman, R. S., and Moore, M. A. S. (1979): Induction of prostaglandin E synthesis in normal and neoplastic macrophages: role for colony-stimulating factor(s) distinct from effects on myeloid progenitor cell proliferation. *Proc. Natl. Acad. Sci. U.S.A.*, 76:2326–2330.
9. Paige, C. J., Kincade, P. W., and Ralph, P. (1978): Murine B cell leukemia line with inducible surface immunoglobulin expression. *J. Immunol.*, 121:641–647.
10. Perry, R. P., and Kelly, D. E. (1979): Immunoglobulin messenger RNAs in murine cell lines that have characteristics of immature B lymphocytes. *Cell*, 18:1333–1339.
11. Ralph, P. (1976): Differential toxicity of Con A and PHA on murine and human hematopoietic cell lines. In: *Concanavalin A as a Tool*, edited by H. Bittiger and H. P. Schnebli, pp. 613–621. John Wiley & Sons, New York.
12. Ralph, P. (1979): Functional subsets of human and murine B lymphocyte cell lines. *Immunol. Rev.*, 48:107–121.
13. Ralph, P. (1980): Functions of macrophage cell lines. In: *Mononuclear Phagocytes—Functional Aspects*, edited by R. van Furth, pp. 439–456. Martinus Nijhoff, The Hague.

14. Ralph, P., and Nakoinz, I. (1973): Inhibitory effects of lectins and lymphocyte mitogens on murine lymphomas and myelomas. *J. Natl. Cancer Inst.*, 51:883–890.
15. Ralph, P., and Nakoinz, I. (1977): Antibody-dependent killing of erythrocyte and tumor targets by monocyte related cell lines: enhancement by PPD and LPS. *J. Immunol.*, 119:950–954.
16. Ralph, P., and Kishimoto, T. (1980): Tumor promoter phorbol myristate induces immunoglobulin secretion correlated with growth cessation in human B lymphocyte cell lines. *J. Clin. Invest.*, 68:1093–1096.
17. Ralph, P., Broxmeyer, H., and Nakoinz, I. (1977): Immunostimulators induce granulocyte-macrophage colony-stimulating activity and block proliferation in a monocyte tumor cell line. *J. Exp. Med.*, 146:611–616.
18. Ralph, P., Broxmeyer, H., Nakoinz, I., and Moore, M. A. S. (1978): Induction of myeloid colony-stimulating activity (CSA) in murine monocyte tumor cell lines by macrophage activators, and in a T cell line by Con A. *Cancer Res.*, 38:1414–1419.
19. Ralph, P., Ito, M., Broxmeyer, H. E., and Nakoinz, I. (1978): Corticosteroids block newly-induced but not constitutive functions of macrophage cell lines: CSA production, latex phagocytosis, antibody-dependent lysis of RBC and tumor targets. *J. Immunol.*, 121:300–303.
20. Ralph, P., Paige, C. J., and Nakoinz, I. (1979): Mechanism of surface membrane expression in murine B lymphocyte cell lines. In: *T & B Lymphocytes: Recognition and Function*, edited by F. H. Bach, B. Bonavida, E. S. Vitetta, and C. F. Fox, pp. 143–154. Academic Press, New York.
21. Ralph, P., Nakoinz, I., Potter, J. E. R., and Moore, M. A. S. (1980): Activity of macrophage cell lines in spontaneous, LPS-, lymphokine- and antibody-dependent killing of tumor targets. In: *Genetic Control of Natural Resistance to Infection and Malignancy*, edited by E. Skamene, P. A. Kongsham, and M. Landy, pp. 519–529. Academic Press, New York.
22. Raschke, W. C., Baird, S., Nakoinz, I., and Ralph, P. (1978): Functional macrophage cell lines transformed by Abelson leukemia virus. *Cell*, 15:261–267.
23. Sachs, L. (1978): Control of normal cell differentiation and the phenotypic reversion of malignancy in myeloid leukemia. *Nature*, 274:535–539.
24. Sakaguchi, N., Kikutani, H., Kishimoto, T., Watanabe, T., and Yamamura, Y. (1980): Induction and regulation of immunoglobulin gene expressions in a murine pre-B cell line, 70Z/3. *J. Immunol.*, 125:2654–2659.
25. Williams, N., Jackson, H., Ralph, P., and Nakoinz, I. (1980): Cell interactions influencing murine marrow megakaryopoiesis: Nature of the potentiator cell in bone marrow. *Blood*, 57:157–163.

Maturation Factors and Cancer,
edited by Malcolm A. S. Moore.
Raven Press, © New York 1982.

Proliferation and Differentiation of Human Myeloid Leukemia Cell Lines *In Vitro*

Robert C. Gallo, Theodore R. Breitman, and Francis W. Ruscetti

Laboratory of Tumor Cell Biology, National Cancer Institute, Bethesda, Maryland 20205

Continually proliferating cell lines with appropriate markers for differentiation provide useful models for the study of the regulation of cell proliferation and differentiation. Murine myeloid and erythroid cell lines have been widely used for investigating the regulation of leukemic cell growth (15,23,49). These cell lines can be induced *in vitro* by a wide variety of compounds (30,33,49) to form morphologically and functionally mature cells of the myeloid/macrophage or erythroid lineages, respectively. The study of the interaction of these compounds with cultured cells not only may provide a better understanding of the nature of the leukemic phenotype but may also imply an alternative approach to the therapy of certain types of leukemias.

The study of the proliferation of human nonlymphoid leukemic cells has been restricted to colony assays (35), where because growth occurs for only short periods of time, there are severe experimental limitations. The first clearly human nonlymphoid leukemia cell line, K562, was established from the pleural effusion of a patient with chronic myelogenous leukemia (CML) in blast crisis (31). However, recent findings (2,48) show that these cells may be induced to differentiate along the erythyroid pathway. HL-60, the first human cell line with distinct myeloid features, was developed in our laboratory (9) from a patient with acute promyelocytic leukemia (APL). HL-60 shares some common features with the murine leukemic cell lines: leukemic derivation; clear commitment to myeloid differentiation; and capacity for terminal differentiation *in vitro* upon induction by certain agents (10,12,16). Subsequently, another myeloid cell line, KG-1, was developed (27), which is more immature than HL-60 and apparently does not differentiate in the presence of any presently known inducer (28). In this chapter, we report some features of these cell lines related to cell growth, phenotypic alterations, response to growth and/or differentiation inducing factors and their therapeutic implications.

MATERIALS AND METHODS

Culture Methods

HL-60, K-562, and KG-1 cells have been maintained in culture for over 3 years. Cell passages 25 to 200 were used in these experiments. The cells were grown in

RPMI-1640 or DME/V-12(1:1) supplemented with 10% heat inactivated fetal calf serum (FCS) or without serum (see below).

Differentiation Induction

Cells were suspended at 2.5×10^5 cells/ml with different concentrations of chemicals or biological "factors" and incubated for various periods under standard conditions. Differential cell counts were performed on 200 cells from Wright-Giemsa stained cytocentrifuge preparations. Nitroblue tetrazolium (NBT) reduction was assayed by resuspending the cells in 0.1% NBT and 100 ng/ml tetradecanoylphorbol acetate (TPA) and incubating 20 min at 37°C as previously described (11). The percentage of cells containing intracellular blue-black formazan deposits was then ascertained.

Cell Characterization

Surface Marker Characteristics

Erythrocyte rosette tests were performed by slight modifications of established techniques as detailed previously (21). The E-rosette assay utilized sheep erythrocytes. The EA and EAC-rosette tests were performed with both sheep and bovine erythrocytes. Tests for surface immunoglobulins IgG, IgM, and IgA utilized immunofluorescence as detailed elsewhere (21). Direct testing of HLA antigens was done by the standard two-stage microcytotoxicity method and by the method of Mittal et al. (37), with a panel of sera used to define HLA-A, -B, and -C locus antigens. Direct testing for human Ia-like antigens was done by complement dependent microcytotoxicity using rabbit and monkey antisera known to specifically detect Ia antigens (1).

Histochemical Assays

Published procedures for histochemical staining were followed for napthol ASD chloroacetate and α-naphthyl acetate (nonspecific) esterases (52), Sudan black B, myeloperoxidase (22), alkaline and acid phosphatases (22), and the periodic acid Schiff (PAS) reaction (22).

Ultrastructure

For electron microscopic analysis, cells were mixed in 2.5% gluteraldehyde, pH 7.2, in Sorenson's phosphate buffer, 300 mosmoles, for 1 hr at 25°C. The tissue was postfixed in 1% osmium tetroxide, pH 7.2, for 1 hr. Following dehydration in graded acetones, the cell pellets were embedded in Epon 812. Sections were cut on an LKB ultramicrotome and examined with a Siemens Elmiskop at 80 kV.

Chromosomal Analyses

Cells were incubated in the presence of colcemid, 20 ng/ml, for 1 hr at 37°C, then treated with 75 mM KCl for 20 to 30 min at room temperature, and fixed in three changes of methanol-acetic acid (3:1). Chromosomes were banded by the trypsin-Giemsa method; slides were treated with 0.01 to 0.3% trypsin in phosphate-buffered saline (Ca^{2+} and Mg^{2+}) for 3 to 6 min at room temperature and stained with 4% Giemsa stain in Sorenson's buffer at pH 6.7.

Functional Assays

Phagocytic capacity and response to chemotactic stimuli were performed as described (10,11).

Assays for Colony Formation

Colony formation was assayed in the soft gel system using either agar (35) or methylcellulose (47). Briefly, for methylcellulose, each 1 ml of culture contained 0.8% methylcellulose, 15% preselected FCS, alpha media, cells, and 10% stimulus when appropriate. For agar, the desired number of cells were suspended in Eagle's media, 20% FCS, 10% stimulus, and 0.3% agar. Cultures were incubated at 37°C in a fully humidified atmosphere of 10% CO_2 in air. Colony size (> 50 cells) and number were scored on the same plates on day 7 and 14. The morphology of individual cells in a colony was examined microscopically by removing and transferring each colony to a microscope slide and staining the slide with either Wright's-Giemsa, or peroxidase and nonspecific esterase. The following sources of colony-stimulating activity (CSA) were used: (a) conditioned medium from phytohemagglutinin (PHA) stimulated human lymphocytes (43) partially purified by ammonium sulfate precipitation and DEAE-Sepharose ion exchange chromatography; (b) partially purified human placental conditioned medium (CM) (40), a generous gift of Dr. N. Nicola, Melbourne, Australia; (c) serum-free CM from an SV-40 transformed human trophoblast cell line (7); and (d) CM from a cutaneous T-cell lymphoma cell line (CTCL) (19).

RESULTS

Growth Kinetics in Suspension Culture

K-562, HL-60, and KG-1 have been in continuous culture for over 3 years. After adapting to growth *in vitro*, they all have doubling times of 20 to 40 hr with high saturation densities. Maximum growth stimulation is achieved with 10 to 20% FCS. Recently, it was shown that HL-60 cells can be grown in a defined serum-free medium containing insulin and transferrin (4). In this medium, HL-60 proliferates at 80% of the maximal growth rate. Subsequently, we found that both K-562 and KG-1 grow as well in this defined media, while most other human leukemia cell lines, i.e., lymphoid cell lines, grow poorly or not at all. All the cell characteristics discussed here are the same whether the cells are grown with serum or with defined media.

Leukemic Phenotype

Cell lines derived from human blood, including those from patients with myeloid leukemia, are usually Epstein-Barr virus (EBV) genome-positive B lymphoblasts arising from contaminating normal B cells and not from the leukemic cells. In contrast, HL-60, K-562, and KG-1 are EBV negative and are representative of the patient's leukemic cells. The major karyotypic markers in the patient's fresh bone marrow are present in the metaphases of the cultured cells (9,27,31) (Table 1). HL-60 and K-562 also show other malignant characteristics, including tumorogenicity in nude mice and spontaneous colony formation in soft agar (16,17,26,31,32).

Cytological Features of Myeloid Cell Lines

Each of these cell lines represents a different stage of maturational arrest. K-562 is an undifferentiated blast with an intensely basophilic cytoplasm with no azurophilic granules. The rounded or indented nuclei have finely dispersed chromatin and varying numbers of prominent nucleoli. With the exception of acid phosphatase, all distinguishing cytochemical stains are negative.

The predominant KG-1 cell is a myeloblast with a biloped or kidney-shaped nucleus with several nucleoli. Most of the cells stain heavily with chloroacetate esterase, although only rare cells stain with peroxidase or Sudan black B. HL-60 cells resemble promyelocytes with large round nuclei, each containing two to four nucleoli and dispersed nuclear chromatin. The cytoplasm is basophilic with prominent azurophilic granules. Virtually 100% of the cells are histochemically positive for myeloid specific chloroacetate esterase, myeloperoxidase, and Sudan black

TABLE 1. *Properties of human myeloid leukemia cells grown* in vitro[a]

Characteristics	Leucocyte cultures		
	HL-60	KG-1	K-562
Disease source	APL	AML	CML/BC
Predominant cell	Promyelocyte	Myeloblast	Blast cell
Karyotype	Aneuploid	Hypodiploid	Ph[1]
Lymphocyte markers-EBV	None	None	None
Colony formation in agar			
Spontaneous	Yes	No	Yes
Induced by CSA	Yes	Yes	No
Differentiation in cultures			
Spontaneous	Yes	No	No
Induced by DMSO	Yes	No	No
Induced by hemin	No	No	Yes
Induced by retinoic acid	Yes	No	No

[a]Abbreviations: APL, acute promyelocytic leukemia; AML, acute myelogenous leukemia; CML/BC, chronic myelogenous leukemia in blast crisis; Ph[1], Philadelphia chromosome; EBV, Epstein-Barr virus; CSA, colony stimulating activity; DMSO, dimethylsulfoxide.

(9,17). Unlike K-562 and KG-1, HL-60 cells lack Ia antigens, which like their morphology, is illustrative of their more differentiated nature than either K-562 or KG-1. The distinct morphological and histochemical myeloid characteristics make HL-60 unique among human leukemic cell lines. A number of cell lines have been developed with leukemic characteristics of B cells, T cells, or null cells (36,41); none of these have the morphological or histochemical characteristics of HL-60.

Terminal Differentiation of HL-60 Cells: Induction by DMSO

A small percentage of the HL-60 cells (10–12% in early passages and 1–7% in later passages) spontaneously differentiate past promyelocytes to more mature myeloid cells, including myelocytes, metamyelocytes, and banded and segmented neutrophils (9). Dimethylsulfoxide (DMSO) markedly enhances the terminal differentiation of HL-60 cells (10). This terminal differentiation is analogous to that seen in cultured Friend mouse erythroleukemic cells, which consist predominantly of proerythroblasts that differentiate in the presence of DMSO to more mature erythroid cells producing hemoglobin.

Unlike the uninduced HL-60 cells, the DMSO-treated HL-60 cells display functional characteristics of mature granulocytes. These include the following: phagocytosis and killing of microorganisms (10,39); capacity to respond to chemoattractants (11,39); presence of complement receptors (11); increased hexose monophosphate shunt activity (39); increased release of packaged enzymes, including B-glucuronidase, lysozyme, and peroxidase (11,39); and capacity to generate superoxide anion (0_2) and reduction of NBT (11,39). However, at least two characteristics of normal mature granulocytes are not found or not fully developed in DMSO-treated HL cells. These are leukocyte alkaline phosphatase (LAP) as determined histochemically (17) and lactoferrin. The characteristics of uninduced and induced HL-60 cells are summarized in Table 2.

The ability of mature HL-60 cells to reduce NBT dye is of practical importance in assessing the response of HL-60 to various inducing agents. NBT, a water soluble dye, is converted to insoluble intracellular blue formazan by phagocytizing or TPA-treated neutrophils, a reaction mediated by superoxide (3,50). The percentage of HL-60 cells reducing this dye closely parallels the percentage of morphologically mature cells in the culture (11,12). Moreover, NBT reduction is one of the earliest differentiation markers expressed in maturing HL-60 cells (12). Thus this test is both a sensitive and an easily quantitated differentiation marker, eliminating observer subjectivity associated with morphological assessment alone.

Comparative Effect of Various Chemicals

A wide variety of compounds other than DMSO induce differentiation in both Friend cells (15,33) and HL-60 cells (10,12) (Table 3). These include a group of polar-planer compounds including DMSO (10,15), dimethylformamide (DMF), and hexamethylene bisacetamide (HMBA) (12,17,18,33). The optimal molar concentrations of these inducers in the HL-60 system are 40 to 60% less than those required

TABLE 2. *Characteristics of uninduced and induced HL-60 cells*

Characteristic	Uninduced HL-60	DMSO induced
Morphology	Promyelocytes	Granulocytes
Histochemistry	Specific myeloid	Specific myeloid
Karyotype	Aneuploid	Aneuploid
	(N = 45)	(N = 45)
Growth		
DNA synthesis	+	−
Proliferation in suspension	+	−
Colony formation in soft agar	+	−
Tumorigenic in nude mice	+	−
Functional		
Chemotaxis	−	+
Phagocytosis	−	+
NBT reduction	−	+
Bactericidal activity	−	+
Fc receptors	+	+
Complement receptors	−	+
Leukocyte alkaline phosphatase	−	−
Lactoferrin	−	−

in the Friend system, but the relative potency of these compounds in inducing differentiation is strikingly similar in both systems (12,33). The concentrations inducing maximum differentiation are only slightly below concentrations producing nonspecific cytotoxicity. Other types of compounds active in inducing HL-60 differentiation include butyric acid, hypoxanthine, and actinomycin D (12). Some compounds, including hemin, ouabain, and prostaglandin E_1, induce Friend cell differentiation but have no effect on HL-60 differentiation (12). The mechanism of action of these inducing agents is presently unknown, but the marked similarity in behavior of HL-60 cells and Friend cells in the presence of these compounds suggests that similar molecular mechanisms are involved in the induction of differentiation of these human myeloid and murine erythroid leukemic cells. Two compounds, hemin and sodium butyrate, induce differentiation of K-562 to more mature erythroid cells, which synthesize hemoglobin (2,48). None of the above mentioned compounds induce differentiation of KG-1.

Terminal Differentiation of HL-60 by Retinoic Acid

Terminal granulocytic differentiation of HL-60 has generally been shown with either nonphysiological compounds, e.g., DMSO, or physiological chemicals, e.g., hypoxanthine, at markedly greater than physiological concentrations. However, it was recently shown (6) that retinoic acid is a potent inducer of granulocytic differentiation of HL-60 at concentrations $1/10^3$ to $1/10^6$ the concentration of other inducers and at concentrations that are physiological (Fig. 1). After 6 days of incubation in 1 μM retinoic acid, over 90% of HL-60 cells resemble mature granulocytes. Differentiation of HL-60 in the presence of retinoic acid is time dependent

TABLE 3. *Effect of miscellaneous cell differentiation inducers of differentiation of HL-60 cells*

Compound	Concentration[a] (mM)	Viable cell count ($\times 10^5$/ml)	Mature myeloid cells[b] (%)	NBT reduction (%)
None		22	8	7
DMSO	180	11	75	80
HMBA	3	9	95	97
Hypoxanthine	5	4.2	86	90
Actinomycin D[c]	0.05	3.5	89	93
Butyrate	0.05	7.5	83	90
Hemin	0.1–1	10–20	5	6
Prostaglandin E₁	0.001–0.1	3.8–12	10	12
Ouabain	0.0001	20	6	6
Dexamethasone	0.1–0.001	23	7	10
Retinoic acid	0.001	10	94	95

[a]HL-60 cells were seeded at 2.5×10^5/ml in the indicated concentration of inducing agent and incubated under standard conditions. After 6 days, the cultured cells were assessed for viability, morphological, and functional (NBT reduction) differentiation.
[b]Myelocytes, metamyelocytes, and banded and segmented neutrophils.
[c]Medium changed at day 4 of 6 day incubation and replaced with fresh medium containing actinomycin D.

with the sequential appearance of maturing granulocytes easily measured (Fig. 2). At 8 days, 70% of the cell population has matured to banded and segmented neutrophils. Retinoic acid has no effect on Friend erythroleukemic cells, K-562 or KG-1.

The Effect of Retinoic Acid on Fresh Leukemic Cells

The findings with retinoic acid prompted an investigation of the sensitivity to this inducer of human myelocytic leukemic cells in short term primary suspension culture (5). Fresh leukemic cells from 21 patients were studied. These included AML (13 patients), APL (2 patients), acute myelomonocytic leukemia (2 patients), CML in a chronic phase (1 patient), and CML in blastic crisis (3 patients). Of these 21 specimens, only cells from the 2 patients with APL differentiated in response to retinoic acid. After an incubation period of 5 to 7 days in 1 μM retinoic acid, the cells from these 2 patients showed extensive morphological and functional maturation (5). Thus as with HL-60, it appears that retinoic acid specifically induces granulocytic differentiation of leukemic promyelocytes and has therapeutic utility in the treatment of APL.

These results clearly have clinical relevance. They indicate that some acute myeloid leukemias, i.e., those already showing a degree of significant maturation like APL, can be further induced to terminally differentiate. However, no one has yet shown that all cells can be induced to differentiate; i.e., after any given treatment of cells with inducer, it appears that a small number remain unaffected. Thus treatment with an inducer may be analogous to having one more effective chem-

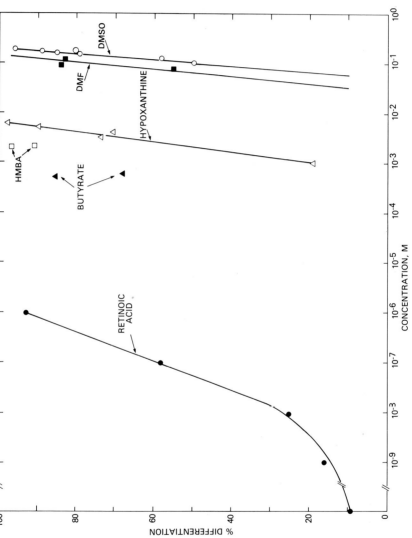

FIG. 1. Induction of differentiation in HL-60 cells by various inducers. Differentiation was determined by NBT reduction after 5 or 6 days growth in the indicated concentration of inducer. ○, dimethylsulfoxide; ■, dimethylformamide; △, hypoxanthine; □, hexamethylene bisacetamide; ▲, butyrate; ●, all-trans-retinoic acid.

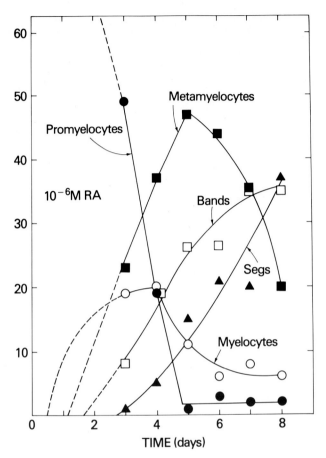

FIG. 2. Morphological differentiation of HL-60 cells induced by 1 μM retinoic acid. Numbers on ordinate are myeloid cell type as a percentage of total cells. ●, Promyelocytes; ○, myelocytes; □, metamyelocytes; ■, banded neutrophils; ▲, segmented neutrophils.

otherapeutic agent that works by a different mechanism. If so, it will be important to combine therapy with cytotoxic drugs which may kill noninducible cells. In this respect, we have found that the extent of retinoic acid induced differentiation of HL-60 is not affected by nongrowth or growth-inhibiting conditions, including (a) arabinosylcytosine, (b) hydroxyurea, (c) omission of arginine or lysine, and (d) omission of insulin or transferrin from the defined medium.

Colony Formation of Myeloid Leukemic Cell Lines: Response to CSA

The responsiveness of HL-60 and KG-1 to colony-stimulating activity (CSA), a possible regulator of *in vivo* proliferation and differentiation, was examined. These lines are stimulated to form colonies by conditioned media (CM) containing CSA from various sources (17,47) (Table 4). Moreover, two clones of SV-40 transformed

TABLE 4. *Effect of conditioned media derived from various sources and purified growth factors on colony formation by normal bone marrow cells and by HL-60*

Source of conditioned medium	Presence of known growth factor	CFU-C derived colonies, bone marrow colonies, 10^5 bone marrow cells/plate	HL-60 colonies, 10^4 cells/plate
Human placenta[a]	CSA	62 ± 8.7	550 ± 28.3
3a (trophoblast)[b]	CSA	71 ± 5.3	486 ± 19.7
3d (trophoblast)[b]	0	0	56 ± 5.0
HUT-102[c]	CSA	43 ± 3.3	386 ± 14.7
HUT-78[c]	0	0	50 ± 7.3
TCGF,[d] EGF,[d] NGF[d]	Not applicable	0	61 ± 7.7
None	Not applicable	0	49 ± 4.9

[a]Partially purified CSA from human placental CM (22).

[b]Serum-free CM from cloned human trophoblast cell lines transformed by simian virus 40 from the same placenta (16).

[c]CM from cell line developed from patients with cutaneous T-cell lymphomas (17).

[d]T-cell growth factor (TCGF), epidermal growth factor (EGF), and nerve growth factor (NGF) were used at concentrations from 1 ng/ml to 1 μg/ml.

human trophoblast cell lines identical in most parameters (7) but differing in that only one produces CSA, and these were also used in order to further determine that the stimulating effect was due to CSA. Only the CM from the line producing CSA was active. In addition, partially purified CSA from human placenta is active while other purified growth factors, including epidermal, nerve, and T-cell growth factors, are not. An examination of the morphology of individual colonies of HL-60 and KG-1 stimulated by CSA showed that the vast majority of the colonies consisted entirely of undifferentiated promyelocytes and myeloblasts (17,47). Only a rare colony contained cells which had all matured to some degree. Thus it seems that the effect of CSA on these myeloid cell lines favors the stimulation of proliferation over differentiation. Surprisingly, this is the case even with the HL-60 cells, which can be induced to terminally differentiate by a wide variety of presumably nonphysiologic compounds (12,18).

Studies on the colony formation of HL-60 and KG-1 were performed periodically over the extended culture life of the cells. The percentage of colony forming cells independent of CSA increased from 0.5 to 16% for HL-60 and from 0 to 2% for KG-1. The number of colony forming cells dependent on CSA declined over the same culture period (17). In addition, in the later passages, virtually none of the colonies stimulated by CSA showed any differentiation. Thus in these leukemic cell lines, it appears that there is a selective advantage for cells to become autonomous and independent of the action of CSA. Studies with individual clones isolated from HL-60 support these observations in that a clone that could differeniate in response to CSA could not be isolated. All clones displayed an increase in both colony size and number when stimulated with CSA (17).

Myeloid leukemic cells *in vivo* resemble these cell lines in one important respect. The leukemic population expands progressively even in the presence of normal or elevated levels of CSA in the patients (35). Responsiveness to CSA presumably develops following the commitment of marrow stem cells to the myeloid pathway when, presumably, specific receptors become functional. Since HL-60 and KG-1 respond to CSA, these myeloid leukemic cells are blocked in differentiation beyond that point. Thus at least some of the cells proliferate but do not differentiate in response to CSA. This has also been noted in studies using fresh AML cells. In a large study of 77 AML patients, bone marrow samples stimulated with CSA produced variable amounts of small colonies and clusters. However, maturation in all but 12% of the cases was greatly reduced and dysplastic (38). Thus it appears from these and our own studies that proliferation of leukemic cells after CSA stimulus is far easier to achieve than normal differentiation.

Phenotypic Macrophagelike Alteration of HL-60 by CSA

Conditioned media containing CSA also exerts an effect on HL-60 in suspension culture. When HL-60 cells are incubated with 20 to 50% CM containing CSA, the cells become morphologically altered and stop proliferating after 7 to 10 days. These morphological changes include diminished cytoplasmic basophilia, less prominent granules, and decreased nuclear-cytoplasmic ratios. The cells become strongly positive for nonspecific esterase, characteristic of monocytes and macrophages, and they have diminished amounts of myeloperoxidase (13,30). As a result, these cells have been called macrophages (13,30).

In our view, the nature of these CSA-treated cells is not so clear. Staining cells for both nonspecific esterase, specific for macrophages, and chloroacetate esterase, specific for the granulocytic cell lineage, has revealed that over 70% of these cells have both enzymes (unpublished results). In addition, these cells exhibit few, if any, functional characteristics associated with monocytes-macrophages such as adherence, phagocytosis of microorganisms, presence of Ia antigen, lymphocyte activating factor (LAF) and CSA productions. These CSA-treated cells may more properly represent intermediate myelomonocytic cells. Their characteristics are summarized in Table 5.

Phenotypic Macrophagelike Alterations of HL-60: Effect of TPA

Tumor promoters are a group of closely related membrane active compounds which, though not carcinogens themselves, promote tumor formation *in vivo* in the mouse two-stage carcinogenesis system (44). The most potent and widely studied of these compounds is TPA. This compound blocks both spontaneous and DMSO induced differentiation in certain clones of Friend erythroleukemic cells (45,53). Moreover, differentiation in various other cultured cells is blocked by TPA (8,25). These findings have led to the hypothesis that tumor promoters exert their effect

TABLE 5. *Characteristics of HL-60 cells growing in suspension cultures*

Characteristic	Untreated	DMSO-treated	TPA-treated	CSA-treated	Retinoic acid treated
Adherence to surface	−	−	+	−	−
Phagocytosis of bacteria	−	+	−	−	+
Response to chemotactic stimuli	−	+	−	−	+
Ingestion of latex beads	−	+	+	+	+
Nonspecific esterase	−	−	+	+	−
Chloroacetate esterase	+	+	+/−	+	+
Myeloperoxidase	+	+	+/−	+/−	+/−
NADase	−	−	+	NT[a]	+
Ia antigen	+/−	−	−	−	NT

[a]NT = not tested.

by blocking terminal differentiation *in vivo* and allowing unrestricted growth of more immature cells (51).

In contrast to other cell systems, TPA does not block differentiation of HL-60 but rather induces distinct phenotypic changes in these cells (30,46). These changes include some characteristics of macrophages such as adherence, ingestion of latex particles (not phagocytosis of bacteria), increased expression of nonspecific esterase and NADase (46), and morphological changes (loss of azurophilic granules, rounded or kidney-bean shaped nuclei) (46) (Table 5). The changes and degranulation of HL-60 cells could be a result of nonspecific membrane alterations by TPA. As is the case of CSA-treated cells, TPA-treated cells do not have a differentiated function that would definitively mark them as macrophages and not granulocytes, such as the presence of Ia, production of CSA and LAF, and the absence of myeloid specific enzymes (Table 5). Thus the "differentiation" of HL-60 cells induced by TPA might be a result of stimulation of their cell membranes, resulting in degranulation and activation of membrane-associated intracellular enzymes that are normally activated during membrane changes associated with phagocytosis (12,39). Similar effects on KG-1 by TPA have recently been reported (28). However, TPA can also induce certain clones of Friend cells and K-562 to adhere and to ingest latex particles (unpublished results).

Possible Use of HL-60 Cells as Test Indicators for Some Antileukemic Compounds

Since frank leukemic cells can sometimes be induced to terminally differentiate to nondividing functionally and morphologically normal cells, it seems prudent to consider that some antileukemic compounds might work this way and/or new compounds might be developed with this as their major effect rather than cell killing. This has, in fact, already been suggested from data in mouse myeloid leukemias. Obviously, the HL-60 system provides a system to test this, and some data with known antileukemic agents are presented here and published in detail elsewhere (12,18). As shown in Table 6, some compounds like daunomycin and actinomycin D do promote differentiation (12,18). On the other hand, it should be stressed that when *fresh* human leukemic cells are evaluated this way, most show no induction of differentiation. It seems to us then that the best use of this system, at the present time, with the objective of obtaining better treatment of these diseases, is to determine (a) the mechanism of differentiation in HL-60 cells and (b) why some cells respond and others do not.

Does HL-60 Produce its Own Growth Factor?

It is conceivable that the spontaneous colony formation in methylcellulose of HL-60 as well as the spontaneous myeloid differentiation of HL-60 noted in suspension (9) is a result of an endogenous production of these cells of CSA or a CSA-like growth factor by the HL-60 cells. The autonomy of these myeloid cell lines may well be driven by a growth factor similar to CSA or to a factor recently described which may specifically stimulate leukemic blast cell colony formation (47). However, CM from HL-60 does not have any CSA-like activity for normal or leukemic bone marrow samples, nor does it decrease or enhance the number of colonies in the presence of CSA. Moreover, CM from HL-60 had no effect on colony formation of HL-60 or KG-1 even after the CM was concentrated by ultrafiltration or fractionated by gel filtration.

DISCUSSION

The HL-60 human myeloid leukemic cells share with Friend mouse erythroid leukemic cells the capacity to be induced to terminally differentiate by various polar

TABLE 6. *Effect of standard chemotherapeutic agents on terminal differentiation of HL-60 cells*

Compound	Concentration (µg/ml)	Cell count (×10⁵/ml)	Mature[a] myeloid cells (%)
None		21	8
Adriamycin	0.0	6.4	23
Daunomycin	0.01	2.4	35
	0.005	8.8	19
Arabinosylcytosine	0.1	4.2	15
	0.05	8.2	15
Vincristine	0.005	8.8	18
Hydroxyurea	8	5.0	13
	4	11.6	8
6-Thioquanine	0.01	7.6	49
	0.005	16.7	35

[a]Myelocytes, metamyelocytes, and banded and segmented neutrophils. HL-60 cells were seeded at 2.5 × 10⁵/ml in growth media containing the indicated concentration of drug. After 6 days of incubation, morphological assessment of Wright-Giemsa stained cytospin preparations was performed.

planar compounds, as well as butyric acid, hypoxanthine, and actinomycin D. Therefore, despite karyotypic abnormalities, HL-60 cells contain the genetic information to code for most of the characteristics of normal functionally mature granulocytes. Why then was this information not expressed in the leukemic patient these cells were derived from? What is the cause and nature of the block in normal differentiation found in this particular patient and in other patients with leukemia as well as in Friend erythroleukemic cells? The similarity in response of Friend cells and HL-60 to various inducing agents which somehow overcome this block in differentiation suggests that the molecular basis for this block is similar in both systems. Friend disease itself is induced by a type-C oncornavirus, and most Friend cell lines produce replicating virus. We have not detected a replicating type-C virus in HL-60, KG-1, or K-562 by standard techniques, but this does not necessarily rule out a viral etiology for the block in differentiation of HL-60 cells, since in most *in vitro* systems, specific viral sequences rather than whole replicating virus are sufficient for transformation.

It is presently unclear whether the differentiation inducing agents active in both Friend and HL-60 cells have their primary site of action at the cell membrane or at nuclear chromatin. A histone derived polypeptide (HP) has been recently detected among the acid extractable chromosomal proteins of HL-60 (42). HP is related to histone H2a and is apparently a cleavage product of H2a. DMSO induced differentiation of HL-60 is accompanied by increased cleavage of H2a to HP. Whether the increased HP level directly leads to altering the transcription pattern of HL-60 genes, leading to terminal differentiation, or is merely another expression of the more differentiated phenotype is unknown. It is of interest that different levels of histone H2a are also found in clones of Friend cells having different capacities to differentiate (42). Isolation and purification of HP together with its quantitation in other cells and cell lines at various stages of differentiation should provide more clues in elucidating its potential role in differentiation.

The phenotypic alterations of HL-60 cells when treated with CSA or TPA and of KG-1 when treated with TPA are difficult to interpret. It could be that these cells have a myelo-monocytoid leukemic nature and the effects observed are peculiar to these cell lines. Alternatively, normal promyelocytes could still possess the ability to differentiate along the monocyte/macrophage pathway. A few experimental approaches suggest that monocytes can be derived from granulocytic progenitors (20,29,34). Staining techniques of normal bone marrow show transitional cells that have both myeloid and monocytoid-specific enzymes (29). In agar, single cells derived from bone marrow granulocyte colonies transform into macrophages in culture (34). Although a growth-promoting factor in HL-60 was not found, the monocytoid nature of these cells and their autonomous growth warrant a continued search for such a factor.

It has been proposed that CSA might be used therapeutically to induce differentiation in myeloid cells, thereby eliminating the capacity to proliferate (49). This approach has gained support from the work on the M1 mouse myeloid leukemic cell line, in which an impressive reduction in the capacity of the cells to produce leukemia *in vivo* was observed when they were treated with CSA prior to transplantation (14,24). However, in the HL-60 and KG-1 human myeloid leukemic cell lines studied here, the effect of human CSA greatly favors increased proliferation of colony forming cells over differentiation. Indeed, in later passages, a higher percentage of the colony forming cells have become independent of exogenously added CSA with little or no differentiation present in either type of colony (47). Until there is a better understanding of the proliferative and differentiative actions of CSA we feel the therapeutic potential of this molecule (or molecules) must be viewed with considerable caution.

The distinct and reproducible response of HL-60 cells to CSA suggests that these cells possess a receptor for this growth promoting factor. In this respect, HL-60 cells resemble the KG-1 cell line, which also shows an increased cloning efficiency in semisolid medium in the presence of CSA. The existence of these cell lines thus provides a unique opportunity for assessing CSA-receptor interaction and for isolating the specific receptor for this particular growth promoter. Moreover, compared to the previous use of human bone marrow, these cell lines should provide a more available and more reproducible assay system for human CSA. However, these studies could be hampered by the apparent molecular heterogeneity of human CSA and the difficulty of purifying this molecule (or molecules) in suffcient quantity.

REFERENCES

1. Anderson, J. K., and Metzgar, R. S. (1978): Detection and partial characterization of human T and B lymphocyte membrane antigens with antisera to HSB and SB cell lines. *J. Immunol.*, 120:262–269.
2. Anderson, L. C., Jokinen, M., and Gahmberg, C. G. (1979): Induction of erythroid differentiation in the human cell line-K-562. *Nature*, 278:364–366.
3. Baehner, R. L., Boxer, L. A., and David, J. (1976): The biochemical basis of nitroblue tetrazolium reduction in normal and chronic granulomatous disease polymorphonuclear leukocytes. *Blood*, 48:309–319.
4. Breitman, T. R., Collins, S. J., and Keene, B. R. (1980): Replacement of serum by insulin and transferrin supports growth and differentiation of the human promyelocytic cell line, HL-60. *Exp. Cell Res.*, 126:494–498.
5. Breitman, T. R., Collins, S. J., and Keene, B. R. (1980): Terminal differentiation of human promyelocytic leukemia cells in primary cultures in response to retinoic acid *(submitted for publication)*.
6. Breitman, T. R., Selonick, S. E., and Collins, S. J. (1980): Induction of differentiation of the human promyelocytic leukemia cell (HL-60) by retinoic acid. *Proc. Natl. Acad. Sci., U.S.A.*, 77:2936–2940.
7. Chou, J. Y. (1977): Human placental cells transformed by TSA mutants of simian virus 40: a model system for the study of placental functions. *Proc. Natl. Acad. Sci., U.S.A.*, 75:1409–1413.
8. Cohen, R., Racifici, M., Rubinstein, W., Biehl, J., and Holtzer, H. (1977): Effect of a tumor promoter on myogenesis. *Nature*, 66:538–540.
9. Collins, S. J., Gallo, R. C., and Gallagher, R. E. (1977): Continous growth and differentiation of human myeloid leukemic cells in suspension culture. *Nature*, 270:347–349.
10. Collins, S. J., Ruscetti, F. W., Gallagher, R. E., and Gallo, R. C. (1978): Terminal differentiation of human promyelocytic leukemia cells induced by dimethylsulfoxide and other polar compounds. *Proc. Natl. Acad. Sci. U.S.A.*, 75:2458–2462.
11. Collins, S. J., Ruscetti, F. W., Gallagher, R. E., and Gallo, R. C. (1979): Normal functional characteristics of cultured human promyelocytic leukemia cells after induction of differentiation by dimethylsulfoxide. *J. Exp. Med.*, 149:669–674.

12. Collins, S. J., Bodner, A., Ting, R., and Gallo, R. C. (1980): Induction of morphological and functional differentiation of human promyelocytic leukemia cells (HL-60) by compounds which induce differentiation of murine leukemia cells. *Int. J. Cancer*, 25:213–218.

13. Elias, L., Wogenrich, F. J., and Wallace, J. M. (1980): Altered pattern of differentiation and proliferation of HL-60 promyelocytic leukemia cells in the presence of leucocyte conditioned medium. *Leuk. Res.*, 4:301–307.

14. Fibach, E., and Sachs, L. (1975): Control of normal differentiation of myeloid leukemia cells. VII. Induction of differentiation to mature granulocytes in mass culture. *J. Cell. Physiol.*, 86:221–226.

15. Friend, D., Scher, W., Holland, J. G., and Sato, T. (1971): Hemoglobin synthesis in murine virus-induced leukemia cells *in vitro*: stimulation of erythroid differentiation by dimethylsulfoxide. *Proc. Natl. Acad. Sci. U.S.A.*, 68:378–382.

16. Gallagher, R., Collins, S., Trujillo, J., McCredie, K., Ahearn, M., Tsai, S., Metzgar, R., Aulakh, G., Ting, R., Ruscetti, F., and Gallo, R. (1979): Characterization of the continuous differentiating myeloid cell line (HL-60) from a patient with acute promyelocytic leukemia. *Blood*, 54:713–733.

17. Gallo, R., Ruscetti, F., Collins, S., and Gallagher, R. (1979): Human myeloid leukemia cells: studies on oncornaviral related information and *in vitro* growth and differentiation. In: *Hematopoietic Cell Differentiation*, edited by D. W. Golde, M. J. Cline, D. Metcalf, and C. F. Fox, pp. 335–354. Academic Press, New York.

18. Gallo, R. C., and Ruscetti, F. W. (1980): New human hematopoietic cell systems for the study of growth, differentiation and involved factors: some therapeutic implications. In: *Molecular Actions and Targets for Cancer Chemotherapeutic Agents*, edited by J. S. Lazo, J. R. Bertino, and J. Sartorelli. Academic Press, New York *(in press)*.

19. Gazdar, A. F., Carney, D. N., Bunn, P. A., Russell, E. K., Jaffe, E. S., Schechter, G. P., and Guccion, J. G. (1980): Mitogen requirement for the *in vitro* propagation of cutaneous T-cell lymphomas. *Blood*, 55:409–420.

20. Glasser, L. (1980): Phagocytosis in acute leukemia. *Cancer*, 45:1365–1369.

21. Glick, J. L. (1980): *Human Lymphoid Cell Culture: The Fundamentals*. Marcel Dekker, New York.

22. Hayhoe, F. G. J., Quaglino, D., and Doll, R. (1964): *Cytology and Cytochemistry of Acute Leukemias*. Her Majesty's Stationery Office, London.

23. Ichikawa, Y. (1969): Differentiation of a cell line of myeloid leukemia. *J. Cell. Physiol.*, 74:223–234.

24. Ichikawa, Y. (1970): Further studies on the differentiation of a cell line of myeloid leukemia. *J. Cell. Physiol.*, 76:175–181.

25. Ishii, D. N., Fibach, E., Yamaski, A., and Weinstein, I. B. (1978): Tumor promoters inhibit morphological differentiation in cultured mouse neuroblastoma cells. *Science*, 200:556–559.

26. Klein, E., Ben-Bassat, H., Neumann, H., Ralph, P., Zeuthen, J., Polliack, A., and Vanky, F. (1976): Properties of the K-562 cell line derived from a patient with chronic myeloid leukemia. *Int. J. Cancer*, 18:421–431.

27. Koeffler, H. P., and Golde, D. W. (1978): Acute myelogenous leukemia: a human cell line responsive to colony-stimulating activity. *Science*, 200:1153–1156.

28. Koeffler, H. P., Billing, R., Lusis, A. J., Sparkes, R., and Golde, D. W. (1980): An undifferentiated variant derived from the human acute myelogenous leukemia cell line (KG-1). *Blood*, 56:265–273.

29. Leder, L. D. (1967): The origin of blood monocytes and macrophages. *Blut*, 16:86–96.

30. Lotem, J., and Sachs, L. (1979): Regulation of normal differentiation in mouse and human myeloid leukemic cells by phorbal esterase and the mechanism of tumor promotion. *Proc. Natl. Acad. Sci. U.S.A.*, 76:5158–5162.

31. Lozzio, C. B., and Lozzio, B. B. (1975): Human chronic myelogenous leukemia cell line with positive Philadelphia chromosome. *Blood*, 45:321–328.

32. Lozzio, B. B., Machado, E. A., Lair, S. V., and Lozzio, C. B. (1979): Reproducible metastatic growth of K-562 human myelogenous leukemia cells in nude mice. *J. Natl. Cancer Inst.*, 63:294–298.

33. Marks, P. A., and Rifkind, R. A. (1978): Erythroleukemic differentiation. *Ann. Rev. Biochem.*, 47:419–448.

34. Metcalf, D. (1971): Transformation of granulocytes to macrophages in bone marrow colonies *in vitro*. *J. Cell. Physiol.*, 77:277–280.

35. Metcalf, D. (1977): *Hemopoietic Colonies: In Vitro Cloning of Normal and Leukemic Cells.* Springer-Verlag, New York.
36. Minawada, J., Ohnuma, T., and Moore, G. E. (1972): Rosette-forming human lymphoid cell lines. I. Establishment and evidence for origin of thymus-derived lymphocytes. *J. Natl. Cancer Inst.*, 49:891–895.
37. Mittal, K. K., Mickey, M. R., Singal, D. P., and Terasaki, P. T. (1968): Serotyping for homotransplantation IV III. Refinement of microdroplet lymphocyte cytotoxicity test. *Transplantation*, 6:913–920.
38. Moore, M. A. S., Williams, N., and Metcalf, D. (1973): *In vitro* colony formation by normal and leukemic human marrow cells: characterization of the colony forming cells. *J. Natl. Cancer Inst.*, 50:603–616.
39. Newburger, P. E., Chovaniec, M. E., Greenberger, J. S., and Cohen, H. J. (1979): Functional changes in human leukemic cell line (HL-70): model for myeloid differentiation. *J. Cell Biol.*, 82:315–322.
40. Nicola, N. A., Metcalf, D., Johnson, G. R., and Burgess, A. W. (1979): Separation of functionally distinct human granulocyte-macrophage colony stimulating factors. *Blood*, 54:614–621.
41. Nilsson, K., and Ponten, J. (1975): Classification and biological nature of established human hemopoietic cell lines. *Int. J. Cancer*, 15:321–341.
42. Pantazis, P., Sarin, P. S., and Gallo, R. C. (1979): Chromatin conformation during cell differentiation of human myeloid leukemia cells. *Cancer Lett.*, 8:117–124.
43. Prival, J. T., Paran, M., Gallo, R. C., and Wu, A. (1974): Colony-stimulating factors in the culture of human peripheral blood cells. *J. Natl. Cancer Inst.*, 53:1593–1598.
44. Raick, A. N. (1974): Cell differentiation and tumor promoting action in skin carcinogenesis. *Cancer Res.*, 34:2915–2935.
45. Rovera, G., O'Brien, T. G., and Diamond, L. (1977): Tumor promoters inhibit spontaneous differentiation of Friend erythroleukemic cells in culture. *Proc. Natl. Acad. Sci. U.S.A.*, 74:2894–2898.
46. Rovera, G., Santoli, D., and Damsky, C. (1979): Human promyelocytic leukemia cells in culture differentiate into macrophage-like cells when treated with a prorbol diester. *Proc. Natl. Acad. Sci. U.S.A.*, 76:2779–2783.
47. Ruscetti, F. W., Collins, S. J., Woods, A. M., and Gallo, R. C. (1980): Clonal analysis of the response of human myeloid leukemic cell lines to colony stimulating factor *(submitted for publication).*
48. Rutherford, T. R., Clegg, J. B., and Weatherall, D. J. (1979): K-562 human leukemic cells synthesize embryonic hemoglobin in response to hemin. *Nature*, 280:164–166.
49. Sachs, L. (1978): Control of normal cell differentiation and the phenotypic reversion of malignancy in myeloid leukemia. *Nature*, 274:535–539.
50. Segal, A. W. (1974): Nitrosoblue tetrazolium dye test. *Lancet*, 2:1248–1250.
51. Van Durren, B. L., and Sivak, A. (1968): Tumor-promoting agents from Croton *Tiglium* L and their mode of action. *Cancer Res.*, 28:2349–2356.
52. Yam, L. T., Li, C. Y., and Crosby, W. W. (1971): Cytochemical identification of monocytes and granulocytes. *Am. J. Pathol.*, 55:283–288.
53. Yamaski, H., Fibach, E., Nudel, V., Weinstein, I. B., Rikind, R. A., and Marks, P. A. (1977): Tumor promoters inhibit spontaneous and induced differentiation of murine erythroleukemia cells in culture. *Proc. Nat. Acad. Sci. U.S.A.*, 74:3451–3455.

Maturation Factors and Cancer,
edited by Malcolm A. S. Moore.
Raven Press, © New York 1982.

Induction of Differentiation of Human Myeloid Leukemic Cells by Phorbol Diesters

*B. Perussia, *D. Lebman, **G. Pegoraro, †B. Lange,
*C. Damsky, *D. Aden, *J. Vartikar, *G. Trinchieri,
and *G. Rovera

*The Wistar Institute, Philadelphia, Pennsylvania 19104; **Istituto di Medicina Interna,
University of Torino, Cso Polonia 14, Torino, Italy; †Children's Hospital,
Division of Oncology-Hematology, Philadelphia, Pennsylvania 19104*

Acute leukemias are probably the result of a block of differentiation at the level of immature progenitor cells or stem cells.[1] The ability of progenitor cells to proliferate and the lack of adequate feedback regulatory mechanisms generated by differentiated cells cause a progressive expansion of the pool of the malignant cells (13,39,40,51–53). It is not yet clear whether the genetic lesion that impairs the diffentiative program occurs only in the subpopulation of cells expressing the leukemic phenotype or whether the lesion is present but not expressed in a fraction of or all the multipotent stem cells (51–53). If the genetic lesion is present only in a subpopulation of cells, theoretically such populations could be selectively eliminated and multipotent normal stem cells allowed to recolonize the bone marrow.

After the pioneering work of Sachs (for a review, see ref. 61) and Friend and coworkers (24), it has become increasingly evident that the block in differentiation present in some types of leukemic cells could be more or less efficiently overcome *in vitro* through the use of appropriate chemical compounds. Under their stimulus, the leukemic cells undergo terminal differentiation: they become unable to further proliferate and begin to express markers typical of the differentiative state of either the myelomonocytic or erythroid cell lineage. The availability of human myeloid cell lines like HL60 and KG1 (14,31) and the finding that a variety of chemical compounds (15,16,30,32,36,37,57,58) can be used to overcome the block of differentiation in these lines have led to renewed interest in this phenomenon.

Among those agents affecting the process of terminal differentiation of leukemic cells are the phorbol diesters. Biologically active phorbol diesters are present in croton oil derived from the seed of *Croton tillium*. They are esters of the polycyclic alcohol phorbol with aliphatic or cyclic acids (8,29,66). Their biological activity

---

[1]Abbreviations used: TPA (12-0-tetradecanoyl-phorbol-13-acetate); PDD (phorbol-12,13- dideca-noate); Me$_2$SO (dimethyl sulfoxide); RA (retinoic acid).

is determined by the types of fatty acids esterified at positions 12 and 13 and by the presence of a primary allylic hydroxyl at C20 and the *trans* configuration of C4 and C10. When biological effects of phorbol diesters are tested, the possibility must be considered that esterases can rapidly hydrolyze the ester bonds at C12 and C13 to produce biologically inactive molecules both *in vivo* and in tissue culture (34,45).

Phorbol diesters have been known for many years to be tumor-promoting agents in mouse skin (4,5,41). These compounds are not carcinogenic or mutagenic per se, but when administered repeatedly to rodent skin that has been pretreated with a subthreshold dose of a carcinogen, they cause the appearance of a variety of benign papillomas followed by squamous cell carcinomas.

Studies on tumor promotion by phorbol diesters in target tissues other than the skin have not been as detailed. Mammary tumors in rats and forestomach tumors and some cases of leukemias have been reported to occur in mice and rats as a result of treatment with phorbol diesters (26,27). The parent compound phorbol itself has no biological activity in most of the model systems tested, but it can cause leukemias in certain strains of mice and rats (3,6) and promote mammary carcinogenesis in rats (3).

Recent studies on a variety of cell lines in tissue cultue have shown that phorbol diesters have remarkable pleiotypic effects (reviewed in refs. 19 and 67). These agents have been shown to reversibly inhibit differentiation *in vitro* in a variety of cell types and, in a few cases, to induce irreversible differentiation (reviewed in refs. 1 and 18).

We present here a summary of our studies of the past 2 years on the characteristics of the induction of differentiation by phorbol diesters in a myeloid leukemic cell line in culture. We also discuss the *in vitro* effects of phorbol diesters on primary cultures of nonlymphocytic leukemia cells and their *in vivo* effects on tumor growth using as a model system transplantable human leukemia cells.

EFFECT OF PHORBOL DIESTERS ON HL60 CELLS: EXPRESSION OF MARKERS OF DIFFERENTIATION AND ARREST OF CELLULAR PROLIFERATION

The HL60 cell line was derived by Collins et al. (14) from the peripheral blood of a patient with promyelocytic leukemia. When HL60 cells are treated in culture with a variety of chemical compounds, such as dimethyl sulfoxide (Me$_2$SO) and retinoic acid (RA), they differentiate into mature metamyelocytes and granulocytes (10,15,16,36,37). We and others (30,36,37,57,58) have reported that a number of biologically active phorbol diesters and the antileukemic drug mezerein (35) also induce differentiation of HL60 cells. Though TPA-treated HL60 cells were originally characterized according to morphological criteria as mature myeloid cells (30), Rovera and coworkers (57,58) and Lotem and Sachs (36) found them to be macrophage-like cells.

The addition of low concentrations of TPA (from 0.5 to 10 ng/ml) to HL60 cell suspension cultures typically causes a variety of rapid changes. The cells lose their

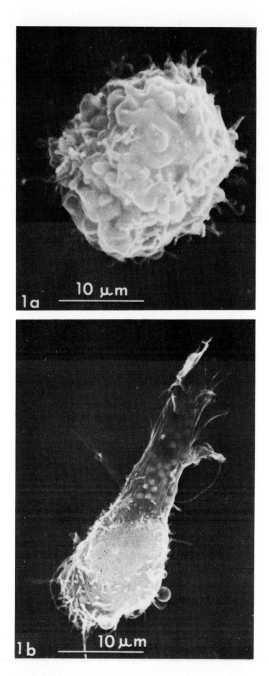

FIG. 1. Scanning electron microscopy of HL60 cells that are **(a)** nontreated and **(b)** treated with TPA for 2 days. Cells were examined using a JEOL 8SEM.

azurophilic granulations, become adherent to a plastic substrate, and show bipolar spreading (see Fig. 1). Proliferation is irreversibly arrested within 36 hr from the time of addition of TPA to the cultures. The cells develop the ability to phagocytize latex beads, IgG antibody-coated red blood cells, and serum-pretreated *Candida albicans* (30,37,57,58), and the percentage of cells bearing receptors for IgG and for complement (C3b) rapidly increases (36,58). Alpha-naphthyl acetate esterase, a marker of monocytes and macrophages (54,69) but not of myeloid elements, appears in almost all cells (see Fig. 2) after TPA treatment (58). This enzyme is also present in T lymphocytes and megakaryocytes, although its intracellular distribution and sensitivity to inhibition by sodium fluoride is different (50,69). Two other myeloid markers, chloroacetate esterase (present in small amounts in HL60; ref. 25) and peroxidase, drastically decrease or disappear entirely (56,58, and Perussia et al., unpublished observations).

Evidence for the TPA-induced terminal differentiation of HL60 cells upon TPA treatment to cells with many characteristics of monocytes/macrophages is summarized in Table 1. The changes in HL60 cells after TPA treatment are compared with those that occur after treatment with Me_2SO or retinoic acid (RA), two compounds that induce HL60 to differentiate along the myeloid lineage to metamyelocytes and granulocytes. The various markers whose expression changes after induction of differentiation of HL60 by TPA, Me_2SO, and RA have been grouped in three classes: (a) markers that are shared by the myeloid and the monocytic lineage, (b) markers detected in the myeloid but not in the monocytic lineage, and (c) markers detected in monocytic but not in granulocytic cells. Neither Me_2SO nor RA induce markers such as lactoferrin or alkaline phosphatase, which are truly unique to mature granulocytes. The markers induced by Me_2SO or RA are not specific since they also appear in monocytes/macrophages, and therefore the best evidence available so far that Me_2SO or RA induce myeloid differentiation is based on morphological grounds (disappearance of azurophylic granulations, appearance of hypersegmented nuclei). The markers induced by TPA that have been identified so far and which are specific for the monocytes and macrophages are, besides the α-naphthyl acetate esterase, some isozymes of acid phosphatase and the C3d receptors.

Lotem and Sachs (36) originally reported that C3b receptors increase after TPA treatment of HL60 cells. It is interesting to note that C3d receptors are also present after stimulation of differentiation of HL60 cells by TPA (see Table 2). While C3b receptors are found both on mature monocytes and mature granulocytes, C3d receptors are present on mature monocytes but not on mature granulocytes (56). C3d receptors, however, appear during the middle stages of myeloid differentiation in bands and young granulocytes (56), but at no time after induction with RA are C3d receptors detected (see Table 2).

FIG. 2. α-Naphthyl acetate esterase activity of HL60 cells that are **(a)** nontreated and **(b)** treated with TPA for 4 days. The assay was done using the method of Mueller et al. (47).

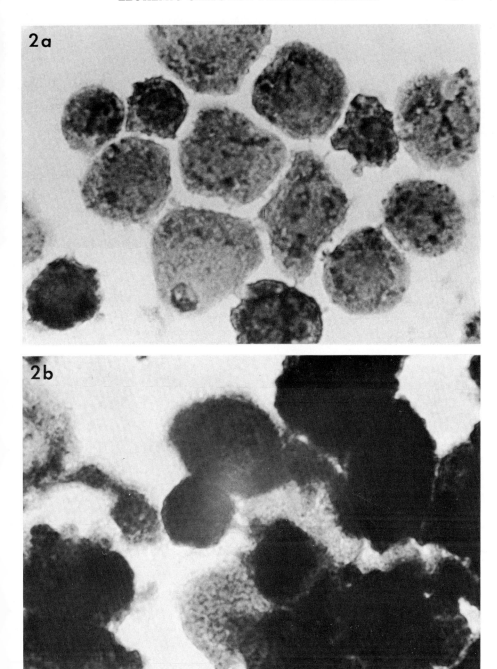

TABLE 1. *Surface, functional, and enzymatic markers in HL60 cells that are undifferentiated or induced to differentiate[a]*

Markers		No treatment	TPA treatment	Me₂SO or RA treatment	References
Present both in granulocytes and monocytes/macrophages	Lysozyme	+	+	+	58
	Peroxidase	+	−	−	58
	NBT reduction	−	+	+	32,44
	Acid phosphatase isozymes 1 and 4	−	++	+	67
	Fc(IgG) receptors	+	++	++	17,58
	C3b receptors	−	+	+	36
	Surface antigens[b]	−	+	+	48
Present in granulocytes or myeloid cells but not in monocytes/macrophages	Lactoferrin	−	NT	−	44
	Chloroacetate esterase	±	−	±	Unpublished data
Present in moncytes/macrophages but not in myeloid cells	HLA-DR locus antigens[c]	−	−	−	Unpublished data; this chapter
	C3d receptors	−	+	−	
	α-Naphthyl acetate esterase	±	++	±	58
	Acid phosphatase isozymes 3a, 3b	−	+	−	67
	Adhesion and bipolar spreading	−	+	−	30,58

[a]HL60 cells were treated with TPA (1.6 × 10⁻⁸ M) for 4 days or with Me₂SO (1.2%) or RA (1 × 10⁻⁷ M) for 5 days. NT = not tested.
[b]Detected by immunofluorescence and radioimmunoassay using monoclonal antibodies B9.8.1 and B13.4.1.
[c]RIA using monoclonal anti-DR antibodies D1.12 and B9.10.1. DR surface antigens are present in myeloblasts but disppear during myeloid differentiation at the level of promyelocytes.

TABLE 2. *Appearance of C3b and C3d complement receptors on HL60 cells after induction of differentiation*

	HL60	HL60 + TPA[a] day 3	HL60 + RA[b] day 5	Raji	Daudi
C3bR[c]	0–7[d]	19–35	21–31	31–69	0
C3dR[c]	0–2	3–13	0	47–95	6–43

[a]HL60 (3×10^5 cells/ml) were induced with TPA at a final concentration of 1.6×10^{-8} M.

[b]HL60 (2×10^5 cells/ml) were induced with RA at a final concentration of 10^{-7} M.

[c]EAC3b were prepared according to the method of Perussia et al. (47). EAC3d were prepared by incubating IgM antibody sensitized sheep E with normal mouse serum (7) for 90 min at 37°C, in order to allow decay of C3b to C3d; 95–98% of both granulocytes and monocytes bound EAC3b indicator cells, whereas only monocytes (95%) bound EAC3d indicator cells. Raji cells, which bear both C3b and C3d complement receptors, and Daudi cells, which bear only C3d complement receptors, were also used as controls for the specificity of the two indicator systems used.

[d]Data are given as the range of values of percent rosette-forming cells in three experiments.

In order to understand more about the function of some membrane molecules and the mechanism of action of inducing agents, we are currently investigating membrane changes that occur during the differentiation of myeloid cells. We are using in these studies two monoclonal antibodies (B13.4.1 and B9.8.1) reacting with different antigenic sites expressed on granulocytes and on monocytes (but not on eosinophils) (48). These antibodies were obtained by somatic cell hybridization technique by fusing mouse myeloma cells P3-X63 with spleen cells from mice immunized 3 days before with a single injection i.v. of human leukocytes, and both are of IgM class. The antigen recognized by B9.8.1 is expressed on normal bone marrow cells at the myelocyte stage, whereas the antigen recognized by B13.4.1 is expressed later at the level of metamyelocytes (48). Both of these surface antigens are induced by TPA and RA treatment of HL60 cells.

Figure 3 shows the time sequence of the events occurring in HL60 cells after induction of differentiation with TPA and the correlation between the expression of the surface antigens recognized by the two monoclonal antibodies and the appearance of other markers. These markers can be grouped into early, middle, and late events, depending on whether most of their expression is detected within 1, 2, or 3 days after TPA treatment. Early events include arrest of cellular proliferation, development of adhesiveness and bipolar spreading, phagocytic ability, and α-naphthyl-acetate esterase activity. Middle events include the appearance of C3b and Fc receptors, of acid phosphatase isozymes 3a and 3b, and of surface antigens recognized by the monoclonal antibody B13.4.1. Late marker events include appearance of C3d, receptors of acid phosphatase isozyme 4, and of surface antigen recognized by the monoclonal antibody B9.8.1.

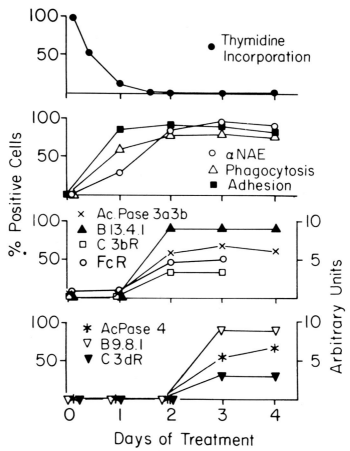

FIG. 3. Time sequence of arrest of proliferation and appearance of myelomonocytic markers in HL60 cells treated with TPA.

HLA-DR surface antigens are not detected in TPA-treated HL60 cells, suggesting that the DR genes, which are normally shut off during the myeloblast to promyelocyte transition, are not reactivated. It is not clear why the small fraction of myeloblasts present in the HL60 population (approximately 10%) does not express DR surface antigens (25, and our unpublished data), but the absence of DR surface antigens in TPA-treated cells does not imply that an important monocytic marker is deficient in these cells. Monocytes lacking DR surface antigens have been reported (21) and are thought to differ functionally from those bearing the antigens.

It is not known whether the various markers induced by TPA treatment of HL60 cells represent posttranslational activation of polypeptides that are already packaged in an inactive form within the promyelocytic cells or whether the induction is the result of new gene activation. It is possible that early changes such as adhesion and phagocytosis could be the result of posttranslational events; however, later events may or may not be related to true gene activation. The availability of monoclonal antibodies directed against surface antigens will certainly facilitate the identification of the mRNA coding for such molecules, and recombinant DNA techniques should be useful in determining whether gene expression also plays a role in some of the events occurring during myeloid and monocytic differentiation.

Among the earliest markers induced after TPA treatment of HL60 cells is the irreversible arrest of cell proliferation. The percentage of cells incorporating thymidine into DNA falls to 0 within 36 hr, and the cell number does not increase any further (60). Most of the treated HL60 cell population does not even require a round of DNA synthesis in order to differentiate (60). The arrest of cell proliferation, as well as the development of the other differentiation markers, can be achieved by pulse treatment of HL60 cells with TPA (59,60). Pulse induction with TPA followed by cloning of the cells in soft agar shows that cloning efficency drops from approximately 10% to 0, and no variant clones resistant to TPA can be easily isolated from a nonmutagenized cell population (unpublished observations). Thus the effect of TPA on cell proliferation of HL60 cells is different from that observed in other systems of induced differentiation. Arrest of cellular proliferation after Me$_2$SO treatment of HL60 cells or Friend erythroleukemia cells is a late event that occurs several days after treatment and it is preceded by the appearance of a variety of differentiation markers. Pulse induction has not been achieved in any other system; in fact, long-term contact of the inducing agent with the target cell is generally necessary (22,28).

Why pulse induction can be achieved after TPA treatment of HL60 cells is not very clear. One possibility is that some event triggers an irreversible cascade of events to cause the expression of the macrophagic differentiative program. The second possibility is that the high affinity of TPA for the target cells allows the intracellular accumulation of the phorbol diester at concentrations adequate for continuous induction. We favor the latter hypothesis in light of the observation that more efficient pulse induction is achieved by using a concentration of TPA approximately 1 log higher than the minimal active concentration (59).

EFFECT OF TPA ON OTHER MYELOID LEUKEMIC CELL LINES

Koeffler et al. (32) have reported that changes similar to those observed in the HL60 cells could also occur after TPA treatment in another established line of myeloid leukemia (KG1). The same authors reported that TPA had no effects on the human leukemia cell line K562 derived from a patient with chronic myeloid leukemia in acute phase (38). This finding contrasts with an earlier report of Huberman and Callahan that K562 cells differentiate into myelocytes after TPA treatment (30). As the potential of K562 cells for erythroid differentiation has been clearly demonstrated (2,61), this problem is of some interest, but the matter is somewhat complicated by the karyotypic instability of the cell line K562 available in different laboratories.

Results in our laboratory using a partially characterized clone of K562 cells, K562(S), which can be induced to synthesize embryonal and fetal hemoglobin by butyric acid and hemin (12), indicate that treatment of these cells with TPA results in specific changes. These changes include shutoff of hemoglobin synthesis, increased phagocytosis of latex beads, a higher percentage of cells that are positive for α-naphthyl acetate esterase, and a complete arrest of cellular proliferation. Except for adhesion, which is minimal in TPA-treated K562(S) cells, these changes correspond with the early marker events detected after TPA treatment of HL60 cells. However, the absence of both middle and late marker expression in TPA-treated K562(S) cells indicates that differentiation along the myelomonocytic lineage was incomplete. As discussed below in the *in vivo* experiments, the findings on the effect of TPA on K562(S) cells nevertheless suggest that arrest of cellular proliferation can occur in TPA-treated leukemic cells even in the absence of induction of other differentiated characteristics.

EFFECT OF TPA ON PRIMARY CULTURES OF HUMAN MYELOID LEUKEMIA

An important issue is whether the agents reported to induce *in vitro* differentiation in a few established human leukemic cell lines also induce leukemic cells freshly obtained from patients or whether successful induction is simply a function of cell line evolution or selection in culture. There is increasing consensus that primary cultures of acute and chronic myeloid leukemia cells treated with TPA *in vitro* differentiate, like the established HL60 and KG1 cell lines, into macrophagelike cells (46,59,64,65). Thus the effect of TPA is not limited to only a few established cell lines. Retinoic acid is the only other agent that appears to induce differentiation of primary cultures of promyelocytic leukemia cells specifically along the myeloid lineage into mature granulocytes (T. R. Breitman, personal communication). Therefore, TPA and retinoic acid are in this respect unique since no other agent has so far been reported to induce differentiation of primary myeloid cells in culture.

Table 3 shows the pattern of response of different types of human leukemias to TPA treatment in culture in an up-to-date number of cases (60 patients). Of the original 29 cases described in our preliminary report (46), 5 were from the Hematology-Oncology Department of the University of Pennsylvania; 10 from Children's Hospital of Philadelphia; and 14 from the Internal Medicine Institute of The University of Torino (Italy). The most recent group of cases (31 patients) were all diagnosed and tested for the appearance of markers after TPA treatment in culture at Internal Medicine Institute of the University of Torino. Both nontreated cases and cases in relapse were examined and no differences in patterns of response were observed. A consistent response to TPA treatment was apparent, with the two most common cases of human myeloid leukemia, i.e., acute myeloblastic and myelomonocytic leukemias, expressing the early markers of differentiation. Most of the early markers of differentiation were already present to various degrees in monocytic leukemias and did not increase further after TPA treatment. Promyelocytic leukemias did not consistently respond to TPA treatment.

Lymphoblastic leukemias did not develop markers of the myeloid lineage after TPA treatment. In one case of lymphoblastic leukemia reported in Table 3, phag-

TABLE 3. *Effect of TPA treatment on expression of early markers of monocytic differentiation in primary cultures of human leukemic cells[a]*

Cases of acute leukemia		Increased adhesion	Increased phagocytosis	Increased α-NAE
Undifferentiated	9	5	2	1
Myeloblastic	14	14	14	13
Promyelocytic	4	2	2	1
Myelomonocytic	14	13	13	9
Monocytic	7	4	3	3
Lymphoblastic	12	2	1	0

[a]A total of 60 cases if acute leukemia were examined. Relatively high levels of adhesion, α-NAE activity, and phagocytosis were observed in control cultures of myelomonocytic and monocytic leukemias. Some lymphoblastic leukemia cells had typical paranuclear α-NAE activity.

ocytosis and adhesion were induced by TPA treatment; however, this leukemia was classified as lymphoblastic essentially on the basis of morphology and the lack of other identifiable markers. Undifferentiated leukemias were heterogeneous; some responded to TPA treatment while others did not develop any macrophage differentiation markers. It is possible, therefore, that an examination of the response of poorly classified leukemias may help in understanding their potential for differentiation, and in turn, influence the choice of therapy (46).

It is not known whether the extent of changes induced by TPA treatment of primary cultures of acute myeloid leukemia cells is comparable to that observed in HL60 cells. For example, the available methods are inadequate to determine whether or not cellular proliferation consistently stops after TPA treatment of primary cultures of leukemic cells. In culture, the proliferation rate of leukemia cells decreases spontaneously and rapidly within a few days, and the growth fraction is already very low in nontreated cells and also quite variable. Clonal analysis of leukemic cells would determine the effect of the drug much more accurately, but this is not easily performed since leukemic colonies can be obtained only after PHA stimulation (11).

We have determined by autoradiography the percentage of cells in primary cultures of leukemia going through the S phase of the cell cycle before and after TPA treatment (59). As shown in Table 4, TPA reduces the proliferative capacity of myeloid leukemia cells, and in some cases, also of lymphoblastic leukemia and of undifferentiated leukemia. However, it is not clear from our data whether proliferation in TPA-treated cultures is completely arrested. Our assay was done within the first 24 hr of culture in order to detect a sizable amount of spontaneous proliferation in nontreated control cultures, but proliferation of TPA-treated HL60 ceases only after about 36 hr (60). Clonal analysis of PHA-stimulated leukemic cells (11) has shown that concentrations of TPA in the range of 10^{-8} to 10^{-9} M will prevent the formation of colonies of leukemic cells *in vitro*, suggesting that TPA treatment is indeed efficient in arresting cellular proliferation of leukemic cells. Clonal analysis

TABLE 4. *Inhibition of cellular proliferation in primary cultures of leukemia cells treated with TPA[a]*

		Labeling index after TPA treatment		
Cases of acute leukemias		Number of cases with >90% decrease	Number of cases with 40–80% decrease	Unchanged or increased
Myeloblastic	6	5	1	
Promyelocytic	1	1		
Acute lymphocytic	4	2		2
Chronic myeloid	7	4	3	
Monocytic	3	3		
Undifferentiated	3			1
Myelomonocytic	7	6	1	
Chronic myeloid in blastic crisis	2	1		1
Chronic lymphatic	1			1

[a]Primary cultures of leukemic cells were incubated with or without TPA for 3 days. After 24 hr ^{3}H thymidine (1 µCi/ml, specific activity 6.7 Ci/mmole) was added. After 72 hr, cells were collected and processed for autoradiography.

has also revealed that very low concentrations of TPA (in the range of 10^{-12} M) stimulate rather than inhibit cellular proliferation (11).

Since myeloid leukemia cells differentiate after TPA treatment, it was of interest to determine which cell types, among the various elements of the myeloid lineage, were the best responders. Svet-Moldawskii and coworkers (64,65) have reported that bone marrow cells from patients with chronic myeloid leukemia became transformed into macrophagelike cells when incubated in liquid culture with TPA. These macrophagelike cells survived in the culture for at least 2 weeks. We have investigated whether the effect of TPA is generalized on all the various cell types of the myeloid lineage present in such cultures of chronic myeloid leukemia cells or if TPA induction of differentiation is selective for a particular cell type. Peripheral blood cells of patients with chronic myeloid leukemia were fractionated into enriched subpopulations of myeloblasts, myelocytes, and metamyelocytes on albumin gradients. The myeloblasts were the best responders to the treatment with TPA *in vitro* and expressed all of the early markers of differentiation (46a). Other cell types failed to express some of the early markers, but most of the cells up to the myelocytic stage were able to develop at least some of the early markers. However, during the process of myeloid differentiation, the cells became progressively less sensitive to the effect of TPA in inducing macrophagelike differentiation and more committed to myeloid terminal differentiation; i.e., TPA-treated myelocytes and metamyelocytes still expressed chloroacetate esterase, a characteristic myeloid marker, and did not express α-naphthyl acetate esterase, the myelocytic/macrophage marker.

We should emphasize that the effect of TPA on differentiation of cells of the myeloid lineage is observed in normal elements as well as in leukemic cells. Svet-Moldawskii and coworkers (64,65) have observed that normal marrow cells also differentiate into macrophagelike cells when treated with TPA. They observed that in some cases colony formation (mostly macrophage) is induced after treatment of the cells with TPA without the need for colony-stimulating factors. Stuart and Hamilton (63) have reported essentially the same phenomenon using mouse bone marrow cells.

MECHANISM OF ACTION OF TPA ON HUMAN LEUKEMIC CELLS

Lotem and Sachs (36) suggested that the mechanism underlying TPA induction of HL60 cells to macrophages involves the sensitization of the myeloid cells to the macrophage stimulating factor (MGI) present in serum. Thus the mode of action of TPA would be indirect and mediated by the presence of this serum factor. The ability of HL60 cells to grow in synthetic (serum-free) medium (9) allows more direct testing of TPA's mode of action. When HL60 cells, grown for several generations in synthetic medium, are treated with 1.6×10^{-8} M TPA, most of the cells lyse and only a small fraction (less than 10%) become adherent and develop macrophage differentiation markers. The observation could be compatible with the interpretation that a serum factor is necessary for the complete expression of the phenotype of macrophagelike cells in TPA-induced differentiation. However, if cells growing in synthetic medium are shifted to serum-containing medium and treated with TPA, their survival and induced differentiation remain at the same low level. By contrast, if HL60 cells are maintained in medium with serum and then shifted to synthetic medium at the time of TPA addition, almost all the cells differentiate into macrophages.

For these reasons, we believe that TPA-induced differentiation involves a direct interaction of TPA with the target cells and does not require serum factors. The reason for increased lysis of HL60 cells in long-term culture in synthetic medium after TPA treatment could rest in an altered membrane composition secondary to growth in serum-deficient medium rather than the need for a serum factor.

The molecular basis of TPA action on HL60 cells is not well understood. At present, a specific receptor for TPA in HL60 cells has not been demonstrated, as it has in other cell types (20). It is possible that the lipophilicity of TPA binding to the cell membranes could by itself also modify the configuration of other receptors.

THE EFFECT OF TPA IN NUDE MICE BEARING HUMAN LEUKEMIC CELLS

TPA has been proposed repeatedly as a potential drug for the treatment of leukemias in experimental animals because of its ability to induce terminal differentiation (30,36,57). The arrest of cellular proliferation would selectively eliminate those myeloid cells that are extremely sensitive to the agent without impairing the proliferative capability of other cell types. TPA treatment in several other cell types actually results in a transient inhibition rather than induction of differentiation (1,18).

Toxicity of TPA is a major problem in terms of potential therapeutic applications. Figure 4 shows the toxicity of TPA, phorbol-12,13-didecanoate (PDD), and mezerein, the compounds most active in inducing differentiation of HL60 cells (57). The LD_{50} of TPA is approximately 5 μg per mouse, and PDD and mezerein are even more toxic. The highest nontoxic dose of TPA for the mouse is very close to the dose that effectively induces differentiation by pulse treatment of HL60 cells.

Mice treated with toxic doses of TPA, PDD, or mezerein die within the first 1 to 12 hr, suggesting that the toxicity of these agents is not related to alteration of the bone marrow elements. However, since TPA has been shown to stimulate CFUc and BFUe colony formation *in vitro* (23,63) and to stimulate cellular proliferation in some classes of T cells (55), possibly acting with an interleukinlike mechanism (55), long-term toxicity of low doses of TPA on bone marrow elements could be a problem. We have tested the effect of TPA treatment *in vitro* on the multipotent stem cells and have found no significant differences in the number and in the morphology of the colonies in the spleen of BALB/c mice when the cells were incubated *in vitro* with different TPA concentrations or for different periods of time, as compared to untreated controls (Fig. 5).

In order to test for the possible antileukemic action of TPA, PDD, and mezerein, we injected BALB/c nu/nu mice subcutaneously with 5×10^6 K562 cells as described by Lozzio and coworkers (38). Under these conditions, more than 95% of the animals developed tumors with histological characteristics of chloromas (65). K562 cells were used rather than HL60 because our HL60 cells were poorly tumorigenic. When the cells were pretreated *in vitro* with TPA at a concentration of 1.6×10^{-7} M for 1 hr (a dose comparable to the effective dose in HL60 cells), none of the animals developed tumors (see Table 5). Pulse treatment with TPA at 1.6×10^{-8} M for 1 hr *in vitro* caused the appearance of tumors in 40% of the cases. These data confirm the fact that pulse treatment of the K562 cells *in vitro* with adequate doses of TPA arrested proliferation and reduced cloning efficiency of the cells in agar to zero. However, when the animals were injected with nontreated

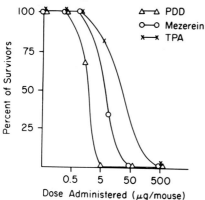

FIG. 4. Toxicity of TPA, PDD, and mezerein in the BALB/c mouse. Mice were injected i.v. with 0.5 ml of the chemical compounds diluted in normal RPMI medium containing 15% FCS. The chemical stocks were dissolved at a concentration of 1 mg/ml in acetone and stored at −20°C. Control animals received a 1% solution of acetone in medium.

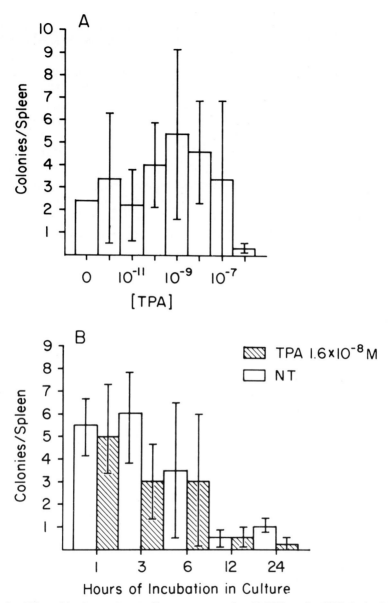

FIG. 5. Effect of *in vitro* treatment of bone marrow cells with TPA on the CFUs in the BALB/c mouse. Cells were incubated *in vitro* **(a)** with different concentrations of TPA for 1 hr and **(b)** with 1.6×10^{-8} M TPA for different lengths of time. One $\times 10^4$ cells were injected i.v. in mice irradiated 1 day earlier with 850 rads.

TABLE 5. *Effect of* in vitro *and* in vivo *treatment on tumorigenicity of K562(S) cells in nu/nu BALB/c mice*

Experimental conditions	In vitro pretreatment[a]	In vivo treatment[b]	Number of animals	Precent with tumors	Average tumor size[c]
Controls	No	No	15	95%	$13 \times 12 \times 12$
TPA (1×10^{-7}M)	Yes	No	10	0%	
TPA (1×10^{-8}M)	Yes	No	5	50%	$13 \times 11 \times 12$
TPA (0.5 μg/mouse)	No	Yes	15	95%	$16 \times 15 \times 14$
PDD (0.5 μg/mouse)	No	Yes	5	20%	$9 \times 9 \times 8$
Mezerein (1.5 μg/mouse)	No	Yes	5	20%	$8 \times 6 \times 6$

[a]Treated *in vitro* for 1 hr at 37°C. The cells were then washed twice and injected subcutaneously 5 × 10⁶ cells/ml.

[b]Treated *in vivo* by i.v. injection every 48 hr. The first injection was given 24 hr after the K562 cells (5 × 10⁶ cells) were injected subcutaneously.

[c]Tumor size (mm) was determined by caliper measurement, 30 days after the beginning of the experiment.

K562 cells, and TPA was applied every other day at a dose of 0.5 μg per mouse, tumor growth was not inhibited. PDD and mezerein, administered under the same regimen (see Table 5), were both effective in inhibiting tumorigenesis and tumor growth.

CONCLUSIONS

It has become increasingly clear that certain chemical compounds can be successfully used in culture to overcome the differentiation block in cells of myeloid leukemia. A number of agents have been shown to induce terminal differentiation in the HL60 and KG1 established cell lines (15,16,30,32,36,37,57,58). Studies on primary cultures of human myeloid leukemia cells have shown so far that TPA consistently induces several markers of differentiation in the great majority of human myeloid leukemias (46,58,64,65) and that retinoic acid induces differentiation in primary cultures of promyelocytic leukemia cells but probably not in other types of myeloid leukemias (T. R. Breitman, personal communication).

There are two major areas of interest that are opened by the studies on induced differentiation of established cell lines and primary cultures of human myeloid leukemia. One area concerns the detailed study of the molecular events that occur during the process of myelomonocytic differentiation in culture. The development of monoclonal antibodies (33) will be most valuable in identifying and characterizing surface membrane markers typical of the myelomonocytic lineage and of the different stages of differentiation of myeloid cells. Such surface markers can then be probed for possible functions, and the mechanisms controlling their expression investigated.

The second area involves the investigation in experimental animals of the therapeutic possibilities of induced differentiation of leukemic cells. The ability of TPA to induce differentiation of myeloid mouse cells (36) and even of avian myeloblastic leukemia (49) should provide models that are superior to the one we have tested. Of course, it is still only presumed that myeloid progenitor cells and not multipotent stem cells are affected by the genetic lesion coding for the leukemic phenotype. Proof to the contrary would preclude this type of therapy.

There are several possible objections to the use of TPA or related phorbol diesters as antileukemic drugs. These compounds are tumor promoters and leukemogenic in some strains of mice, and are also extremely toxic *in vivo*. Actually, TPA is a tumor promoter only when applied repeatedly over a long period of time and only if the experimental animal has been pretreated with a carcinogen. Such conditions would not exist in an experimental therapy aimed at quickly eliminating leukemic cells from the proliferative pool. Moreover, it is possible, using a variety of compounds, to dissociate the promoting capability of this compound from its ability to induce differentiation of myeloid cells (57). The fact that TPA or other phorbols are leukemogenic is noteworthy, but this has only been demonstrated in a particular strain of mice; these compounds have no leukemogenic effect on most of the other strains.

Toxicity of the phorbol diesters is a major problem, and it seems unlikely that using a dose lower than that required to induce all cells to differentiate *in vivo* by short contact with the inducing agent will be beneficial. Another problem is that hydrolases in the serum, the liver, and other tissues would quickly degrade the injected chemical compound into biologically noneffective molecules. In fact, it has been shown *in vivo* and *in vitro* that the metabolism of TPA occurs at variable rates in different tissues and in different species (34,35).

The fact that TPA *in vitro* probably has a selective effect on progenitor myeloid cells, sparing the multipotent stem cells, should also suggest the possibility of treating *in vitro* the leukemic marrow followed by a transplantation of the treated marrow into irradiated and chemotherapy-treated recipient leukemic animals. This last treatment should have cleared all the remaining leukemic cells from the recipients. In this case, if the disease does not involve the multipotent stem cells and just represents the overgrowth of a transformed clone of myeloid cells, then eradication of leukemic cells using highly selective agents which would arrest the proliferation of a well-defined lineage of cells is theoretically possible.

ACKNOWLEDGMENTS

We would like to thank Marina Hoffman for editorial assistance and Ann McNab for the typing of the manuscript. This work was supported by grants CA-10815, CA-20833, CA-21069, CA-21124, and CA-25875 from the National Cancer Institute, the W. W. Smith Memorial Fund, and the Rae-Uber Trust.

REFERENCES

1. Abrahm, J., and Rovera, G. (1980): The effect of tumor promoting phorbol diesters on terminal differentiation of cells in culture. *Mol. Cell. Biochem. (in press)*.
2. Andersson, L. C., Jokinen, M., and Gahmberg, C. G. (1979): Induction of erythroid differentiation in the human leukemia cell line K562. *Nature*, 278:364–365.

3. Armuth, V., and Berenblum, I. (1974): Promotion of mammary carcinogenesis and leukemogenic action by phorbol in virgin female Wistar rats. *Cancer Res.*, 34:2704–2707.

4. Berenblum, I. (1941): The cocarcinogenic action of croton resin. *Cancer Res.*, 11:44–50.

5. Berenblum, I. (1969): A re-evaluation of the concept of carcinogenesis. *Progr. Exp. Tumor Res.*, 11:21–30.

6. Berenblum, I., and Lonai, V. (1970): The leukemogenic action of phorbol. *Cancer Res.*, 30:2744–2748.

7. Bianco, C., Patrick, R., and Nussenzweig, V. (1970): A population of lymphocytes bearing a receptor for antigen-antibody-complement complexes. I. Separation and characterization. *J. Exp. Med.*, 132:702–720.

8. Boutwell, R. K. (1974): The function and mechanism of promoters of carcinogenesis. *CRC Crit. Rev. Toxicol.*, 2:419–443.

9. Breitman, T. R., Collins, S. J., and Keene, B. R. (1980): Replacement of serum by insulin and transferrin supports growth and differentiation of the human promyelocytic cell line HL60. *Exp. Cell Res.*, 126:494–498.

10. Breitman, T. R., Selonick, S. E., and Collins, S. J. (1980): Induction of differentiation of the human promyelocytic leukemia cell line (HL-60) by retinoic acid. *Proc. Natl. Acad. Sci. U.S.A.*, 77:2936–2940.

11. Chang, L. J. A., and McCulloch, E. A. (1981): Dose dependent effects of a tumor promoter on blast cell progenitors in human myeloblastic leukemia. *Blood*, 57: 361–367.

12. Cioe, L., McNab, A., Hubbell, H. R., Meo, P., Curtis, P., and Rovera, G. (1981): Differential expression of the globin genes in human leukemia K562(S) cells induced to differentiate by hemin or butyric acid. *Cancer Res.*, 41: 237–241.

13. Cline, M. J., and Golde, D. W. (1979): Controlling the production of blood cells. *Blood*, 53:157–165.

14. Collins, S. J., Gallo, R. C., and Gallagher, R. E. (1977): Continuous growth and differentiation of human myeloid leukemic cells in suspension culture. *Nature*, 270:347–349.

15. Collins, S. J., Ruscetti, F. W., Gallagher, R. E., and Gallo, R. C. (1978): Terminal differentiation of human promyelocytic leukemia cells induced by dimethyl sulfoxide and other polar compounds. *Proc. Natl. Acad. Sci. U.S.A.*, 75:2458–2462.

16. Collins, S. J., Bodner, A., Ting, R., and Gallo, R. C. (1980): Induction of morphological and functional differentiation of human promyelocytic cells, leukemia cells (HL60), by compounds which induce differentiation of murine leukemia cells. *Int. J. Cancer*, 24:213–218.

17. Crabtree, G. R. (1980): Fc receptors of a human promyelocytic leukemic cell line: evidence for two types of receptors defined by binding of the staphylococcal protein A-IgG1 complex. *J. Immunol.*, 125:448–453.

18. Diamond, L., O'Brien, T. G., and Rovera, G. (1978): Tumor promoters: effects on proliferation and differentiation of cells in culture. *Life Sci.*, 23:1979–1988.

19. Diamond, L., O'Brien, T. G., and Baird, W. M. (1980): Tumor promoters and the mechanisms of tumor promotion. *Adv. Cancer Res.*, 32:1–74.

20. Driedger, P. E., and Blumberg, P. M. (1980): Specific binding of phorbol ester tumor promoters. *Proc. Natl. Acad. Sci. U.S.A.*, 77:567–571.

21. Engleman, E. G., Charron, D. J., Benike, C. J., and Stewart, G. J. (1980): Ia antigen on peripheral blood mononuclear leukocytes in man. I. Expression, biosynthesis, and function of HLA-DR antigen on non-T cells. *J. Exp. Med.*, 152:99s–113s.

22. Fibach, E., Reuben, R. C., Rifkind, R. A., and Marks, P. A. (1977): Effect of hexamethylene bisacetamide on the commitment to differentiation of murine erythroleukemia cells. *Cancer Res.*, 37:440–444.

23. Fibach, E., Marks, P. A., and Rifkind, R. A. (1980): Tumor promoters enhance myeloid and erythroid colony formation by normal mouse hemopoietic cells. *Proc. Natl. Acad. Sci. U.S.A.*, 77:4125–4155.

24. Friend, C., Scher, W., Holland, J. G., and Sato, T. (1971): Hemoglobin synthesis in murine virus induced leukemia cells in vitro: stimulation of erythroid differentiation by DMSO. *Proc. Natl. Acad. Sci. U.S.A.*, 68:378–382.

25. Gallagher, R., Collins, S., Trujillo, J., McCredie, K., Ahearn, M., Tsai, S., Metzgar, R., Aulakh, G., Ting, R., Ruscetti, F., and Gallo, R. (1979): Characterization of the continuous differentiating myeloid cell line (HL-60) from a patient with acute promyelocytic leukemia. *Blood*, 54:713–733.

26. Goerttler, K., and Loehrke, H. (1976): Diaplacental carcinogenesis: Initiation with the carcinogens dimethylbenzanthracene (DMBA) and urethane during fetal life and postnatal promotion with the

phorbol ester TPA in a modified 2-stage Berenblum/Mottram experiment. *Virchows Arch. Pathol. Anat. Histol.*, 372:29–38.

27. Goerttler, K., and Loehrke, H. (1977): Diaplacental carcinogenesis: tumor localization and tumor incidence in NMRI mice after diaplacental initiation with DMBA and urethane and postnatal promotion with the phorbol ester TPA in a modified 2-stage Berenblum/Mottram experiment. *Virchows Arch. Pathol. Anat. Histol.*, 376:117–132.

28. Gusella, J., Geller, R., Clarke, B., Weeks, V., and Housman, D. (1976): Commitment to erythroid differentiation by Friend erythroid leukemia cells: a stochastic analysis. *Cell*, 9:221–229.

29. Hecker, E. (1971): *Methods Cancer Res.*, 6:439–484.

30. Huberman, E., and Callahan, M. F. (1979): Induction of terminal differentiation in human pro-myelocytic leukemia cells by tumor-promoting agents. *Proc. Natl. Acad. Sci. U.S.A.*, 76:1293–1297.

31. Koeffler, H. P., and Golde, D. W. (1978): Acute myelogenous leukemia: a human cell line responsive to colony-stimulating activity. *Science*, 200:1153–1154.

32. Koeffler, H. P., Bar-Eli, M., and Territo, M. (1979): Heterogeneity of human myeloid leukemia cell response to phorbol diester. *Blood*, 54(Suppl.1):174a.

33. Kohler, G., and Milstein, C. (1975): Continuous cultures of fused cells secreting antibody of predefined specificity. *Nature*, 256:495–497.

34. Kreibich, G., Witte, I., and Hecker, E. (1971): On the biochemical mechanism of tumorigenesis in mouse skin. IV. Methods for determination of the fate and distribution of phorbolester TPA. *Z. Krebsforsch*, 76:113–123.

35. Kupchan, S. M., and Baxter, R. L. (1975): Mezerein: antileukemic principle isolated from Daphne mezereum L. *Science*, 187:652–653.

36. Lotem, J., and Sachs, L. (1979): Regulation of normal differentiation in mouse and human myeloid leukemia cells by phorbol esters and the mechanism of tumor promotion. *Proc. Natl. Acad. Sci. U.S.A.*, 76:5158–5162.

37. Lotem, J., and Sachs, L. (1980): Potential pre-screening for therapeutic agents that induce differentiation in human myeloid leukemia cells. *Int. J. Cancer*, 25:561–564.

38. Lozzio, B. B., Lozzio, C. B., and Machado, E. (1976): Human myelogenous (Ph[1] +) leukemia cell line: transplantation into athymic mice. *J. Natl. Cancer Inst.*, 56:627–628.

39. Moore, M. A. S. (1977): Regulation of leukocyte differentiation and leukemia as a disorder of differentiation. In: *Recent Advances in Cancer Research: Cell Biology and Tumor Virology*, edited by R. C. Gallo, CRC, Cleveland.

40. Moore, M. A. S., Kurland, J., and Broxmeyer, H. E. (1978): Regulatory interactions in normal and leukemic myelopoiesis. In: *Differentiation of Normal and Neoplastic Hematopoietic Cells*, edited by Clarkson, B., Mark, W., and Till, S., pp. 393–404, Cold Spring Harbor Laboratory, Cold Spring Harbor, N.Y.

41. Mottram, J. C. (1944): A developing factor in experimental blastogenesis. *J. Pathol. Bacteriol.*, 56:391.

42. Mueller, J., Brun del Re, G., Buerki, H., Keller, H.-U., Hess, M. W., and Cottier, H. (1975): Nonspecific acid esterase activity: a criterion for differentiation of T and B lymphocytes in mouse lymph nodes. *Eur. J. Immunol.*, 5:270–274.

43. Nagasawa, K., and Mak, T. W. (1980): Phorbol esters induce differentiation in human malignant T lymphoblasts. *Proc. Natl. Acad. Sci. U.S.A.*, 77:2964–2968.

44. Newburger, P. E., Chovaniec, M. E., Greenberger, J. S., and Cohen, H. J. (1979): Functional changes in human leukemic cell line HL60. A model for myeloid differentiation. *J. Cell Biol.*, 82:315–322.

45. O'Brien, T. G., and Diamond, L. (1978): Metabolism of tritium-labeled 12-0-tetradecanoyl-phorbol-13-acetate by cells in culture. *Cancer Res.*, 38:2562–2566.

46. Pegoraro, L., Abrahm, J., Cooper, R. A., Levis, A., Lange, B., Meo, P., and Rovera, G. (1980): Differentiation of human leukemias in response to 12-0-tetradecanoyl-phorbol-13-acetate in vitro. *Blood*, 55:859–862.

46a. Pegoraro, L., et al. (*submitted for publication*).

47. Perussia, B., Casali, P., Joppolo, G., and Borzini, P. (1976): Complement receptors (C3b, C4b/C3d) unbalance on CLL lymphocytes. *Boll. 1st Sieroter Milanese*, 55:235.

48. Perussia, B., Lebman, D., Ip, S., Rovera, G., and Trinchieri, A. (1981): Terminal differentiation surface antigens on myelomocytic cells are expressed on human promyelocytic leukemic cells (HL60) treated with chemical inducers. *Blood*, 58:836.

49. Pessano, S., Gazzolo, L., and Moscovici, C. (1979): The effect of a tumor promoter on avian leukemic cells. *Microbiologica*, 2:379–392.
50. Pinkus, G. S., Hargreaves, H. K., McLeod, J. A., Nadler, L. M., Rosenthal, D. S., and Said, J. W. (1979): α-Naphthyl acetate esterase activity—a cytochemical marker for T lymphocytes. *Am. J. Pathol.*, 97:42.
51. Quesenberry, P., and Levitt, L. (1979): Hematopoietic stem cells. *N. Engl. J. Med.*, 301:755–760.
52. Quesenberry, P., and Levitt, L. (1979): Hematopoietic stem cells. *N. Engl. J. Med.*, 301:819–823.
53. Quesenberry, P., and Levitt, L. (1979): Hematopoietic stem cells. *N. Engl. J. Med.*, 301:868–872.
54. Radzun, H. J., Parwaresch, M. R., Kulenkampff, Ch., Staudinger, M., and Stein, H. (1980): Lysosomal acid esterase: activity and isoenzymes in separated normal human blood cells. *Blood*, 55:891–897.
55. Rosenstreich, D. L., and Mizel, S. B. (1979): Signal requirements for T lymphocyte activation. I. Replacement of macrophage function with phorbol myristic acetate. *J. Immunol.*, 123:1749–1754.
56. Ross, G. D., Jarowski, C. I., Rabellino, E. M., and Winchester, R. J. (1978): The sequential appearance of Ia-like antigens and two different complement receptors during the maturation of human neutrophils. *J. Exp. Med.*, 147:730–744.
57. Rovera, G., O'Brien, T. G., and Diamond, L. (1979): Induction of differentiation in human promyelocytic leukemia cells by tumor promoters. *Science*, 204:868–870.
58. Rovera, G., Santoli, D., and Damsky, C. (1979): Human promyelocytic leukemia cells in culture differentiate into macrophage-like cells when treated with phorbol diesters. *Proc. Natl. Acad. Sci. U.S.A.*, 76:2779–2783.
59. Rovera, G., Santoli, D., Meo, P., Pegoraro, L., Levis, A., Lange, B., Abrahm, J., and Cooper, R. A. (1980): Induced differentiation of human leukemias by phorbol esters, In: *In Vivo and In Vitro Erythropoiesis: The Friend System*, edited by G. Rossi, pp. 585–592. Elsevier/North-Holland, New York.
60. Rovera, G., Olashaw, N., and Meo, P. (1980): Terminal differentiation in human promyelocytic leukemic cells in the absence of DNA synthesis. *Nature (in press)*.
61. Rutherford, T. R., Clegg, J. B., and Weatherall, D. J. (1979): K562 human leukemic cells synthesize embryonic hemoglobin in response to hemin. *Nature*, 280:164–165.
62. Sachs, L. (1978): Control of normal cell differentiation and the phenotypic reversion of malignancy in myeloid leukemia. *Nature*, 274:535–539.
63. Stuart, R. K., and Hamilton, J. (1980): Tumor-promoting phorbol esters stimulate hematopoietic colony formation in vitro. *Science*, 208:402–404.
64. Svet-Moldavskii, G. I., Holland, J. F., Svet-Moldavskaia, I. A., and Clarkson, B. D. (1979): Differentiation of cells of normal and leukemic human bone marrow in tissue culture induced by tumor promoter. *Dokl. Akad. Nauk. SSSR*, 249(3):720–722.
65. Svet-Moldavskii, G. I., Svet-Moldavskaia, I. A., Zinzar, S. N., Mann, P. E., and Vergara, C. (1980): Effect of 12-0-tetradecanoyl-phorbol-13-acetate (TPA) on human bone marrow cultures. *AACR Abstracts*, p. 109.
66. Van Duuren, B. L. (1969): Tumor promoting agents in two stage carcinogenesis. *Prog. Exp. Tumor Res.*, 11:31–68.
67. Vorbrodt, A., Meo, P., and Rovera, G. (1979): Regulation of acid phosphatase activity in human promyelocytic leukemic cells induced to differentiate in culture. *J. Cell Biol.*, 83:303–307.
68. Weinstein, I. B., Wigler, M., and Pietropaolo, C. (1977): In: *Origins of Human Cancer*, edited by H. H. Hiatt, J. D. Watson, and J. A. Winsten, pp. 751–772. Cold Spring Harbor Laboratory, Cold Spring Harbor, N.Y.
69. Yam, L. T., Li, C. Y., and Crosby, W. M. (1971): Cytochemical identification of monocytes and granulocytes. *Am. J. Clin. Pathol.*, 55:283.

Maturation Factors and Cancer,
edited by Malcolm A. S. Moore.
Raven Press, © New York 1982.

Self-Renewal of Leukemic Blast Progenitors as a Target for Therapeutic Intervention

R. N. Buick, C. A. Izaguirre, and E. A. McCulloch

Ontario Cancer Institute, Toronto, Ontario M4X 1K9, Canada

In the last decade, methods have been developed that allow study of the normal and leukemic cell renewal system of man by assessing in culture the clonogenicity of stem and other progenitor cells (for a review, see ref. 19). The biological behavior of any cell renewal system is governed in great part by the process of stem cell self-renewal (20). It is the purpose of this chapter to review the available information on the process of self-renewal in human leukemic clones and to draw attention to the fact that this process is an important target to be considered in the design of clinical protocols.

COLONY ASSAYS FOR LEUKEMIC PROGENITORS

A necessary requirement for measurement of leukemic stem cell self-renewal is that one must have a system which allows clonal expansion from leukemic stem cells. A number of such systems have been proposed in recent years for acute myeloblastic leukemia (AML). All rely on colony growth in semisolid (agar) or viscous (methylcellulose) medium under the influence of specific stimulators. It is striking that a requirement has been seen for PHA in a number of systems; leukemic colony growth has been facilitated by preincubation with PHA (6), by culturing in suspension over agar with PHA in both phases (11), or by continuous feeding with conditioned medium from PHA-treated cells (16).

The colony assay around which this study is conducted is also based on stimulation by PHA-LCM (1,12). The characteristics of this assay have been reported; briefly, colonies are grown in methylcellulose from peripheral blood blast populations depleted of T cells (15). The cells of origin of the colonies are believed to be part of the blast population since (a) a highly significant correlation was found between concentrations of morphologically identifiable blast cells in the peripheral blood and colony formation at diagnosis (1), (b) chromosomal abnormalities identified in the marrow or peripheral blood of certain patients were also found in metaphases within colonies (8), and (c) the cells were identified morphologically as blasts by light and electron microscopy (13) and did not express any lymphoid markers (12). An equivalent assay for clonogenic cells in acute lymphoblastic leukemia has proven more elusive. However, very recently, reports have been made of colony assays capable of detecting progenitors of normal and malignant lymphoid cells. The data in this paper derive from a clonogenic assay with three requirements: (a) depletion of T lymphocytes from the cells to be cultured, (b) addition of homologous irradiated T lymphocytes, and (c) a conditioned medium obtained from PHA-stimulated purified T lymphocytes (PHA-TCM). PHA-TCM contains a factor (or factors) required for colony formation by B lymphocytes or cALL blasts. It also contains a T-cell growth factor and CSA activity for CFU-GM. However, cell separation procedures render the assay specific for non-T-lymphocytes or blasts (9). Using this assay, colony formation has been obtained from normal B lymphocytes and malignant B lymphocytes (B-ALL, non-Hodgkin's lymphoma of B-cell origin, Burkitt's lymphoma, hairy cell leukemia of B-cell type, and multiple myeloma) (10).

The results of these initial studies are consistent with the view that a minority subpopulation of leukemic blasts in AML or ALL have sufficient proliferative capacity to be clonogenic and in fact that these cells represent the population (or part of it) maintaining the tumor *in situ*. As such, these cells should display the biological characteristics of self-renewal.

MEASUREMENT OF SELF-RENEWAL CAPACITY

Self-renewal during colony formation can be considered to have taken place when one can demonstrate cell(s) within a colony capable of yielding new colonies when replated under identical conditions. For the assessment of self-renewal of blast progenitors, cells are pooled from many colonies, mechanically rendered into a single cell suspension, and replated. If the number of colonies contributing to the pooled cell suspension is sufficiently large, the value of secondary plating efficiency (PE2) is a measure of the progenitor's property of self-renewal (as opposed to the initial plating efficiency, PE1, which is a minimum estimate of progenitor frequency).

Experiments designed to manipulate the self-renewal capacity are performed in the following manner. Primary plating is carried out in the presence of (or under the influence of) an agent or cellular manipulation. Surviving colonies are pooled and then replated for measurement of PE2. A comparison can then be made between survivors of a given manipulation and control, untreated cells. These measurements therefore rely on the ability to measure self-renewal (PE2) independently of primary colony growth (PE1), even though primary growth is necessary for expression of self-renewal capacity. We have demonstrated that PE2 and PE1 are not correlated.

CHARACTERISTICS OF PE2 FOR AML BLAST PROGENITORS

Secondary colony growth has satisfied certain conditions which allow us to equate PE2 with the process of self-renewal. For example, the colonies obtained by replating dispersed primary colonies are indistinguishable from primary colonies in size, colony morphology (2), cellular markers (peroxidase, lack of lymphoid surface markers), and optimum PHA-LCM concentration (2). The extent of renewal capacity is limited. We have succeeded in transferring single colonies three times but never a fourth (2). Of course, we cannot estimate the extent to which physical damage limits the ability to be clonogenic on repeated transfers. The time at which transfer is made is extremely important, with 5 to 7 days in primary culture being optimal. The clonogenicity in the PE2 assay is linear with respect to cell number in the operative range (2). PE2 is heterogenous with respect to cell size, consistent with the theory that blast cells form a lineage undergoing progressive loss of self-renewal capacity (4). Table 1 shows the basic characteristics of PE2 measurement.

CLINICAL CORRELATES OF PE2 FOR AML

Of considerable interest is the status of PE2 in relation to disease state. Marked patient-to-patient variation is found; however, in the limited experience so far available, we have found that PE2 is a stable characteristic. When comparing PE2 of leukemic blasts from seven patients at presentation and subsequent to treatment, the values are similar (14). PE2 therefore seems to be a heritable characteristic of the clone rather than reflecting its physiology.

On a theoretical basis, self-renewal capacity might be expected to be related to the inherent aggressiveness of leukemic clones. We have performed measurements of PE2 on 44 evaluable, previously untreated patients. In this nonselected group, 47.7% remission induction was achieved, and there was a highly significant correlation between low PE2 and successful remission induction ($0.001 < P < 0.01$, $n = 44$, rank sum test) (3). Other variables such as age, presenting blasts, and platelet count have been implicated as prognostically important (7,18). None of these factors, however, is correlated with PE2, indicating that the effect of PE2 on remission induction is not acting through another identifiable variable.

We are in the process of analyzing data related to a multivariate analysis of prognostic factors, including laboratory-derived factors such as PE2. Preliminary data indicate that PE2 is an important parameter in outcome determination, ranking with age as one of the two most important variables.

MANIPULATION OF PE2

The prognostic importance of PE2 indicates the importance of self-renewal as a target for attempted manipulation. A leukemic clone with reduced renewal capacity should be less dangerous to the patient. Accordingly, we have attempted to deter-

TABLE 1. *Characteristics of PE2 assay for AML blast progenitors*

1. Secondary colonies indistinguishable from primary colonies (size, colony morphology, cell markers) (2,14)
2. Same optimum PHA-LCM concentration as for PE1 (2)
3. Self-renewal is limited (three passages maximum) (2)
4. Optimal time of transfer is 6–7 days (2)
5. Progenitors with renewal capacity are heterogeneous with respect to cell size; consistent with a blast lineage (4)
6. PE2 is relatively stable through disease states, although PE1 is not (14)

mine whether exposure to cytotoxic drugs used in chemotherapy causes a change in self-renewal capacity. Adriamycin, cytosine arabinoside, and methane sulphon-amide, N-[(4-19-acridinylamino)-3-methoxyphenyl] (m-AMSA) were selected for study due to their role in the therapy of AML (3). The dose response curves for the effect of the drugs on primary colony formation were measured, and surviving colonies at a variety of doses were pooled (for each individual dose) and replated for measurement of PE2. Primary colonies at all levels of survival to adriamycin had an apparently equal probability of self-renewal during development. However, for cytosine arabinoside, a frequent finding was that a decrease in self-renewal could be seen in colonies surviving 10^{-6} to 10^{-7} M drug. For m-AMSA, the reverse situation was apparent; clonogenic cells surviving m-AMSA treatment had a higher (two- to three-fold) probability of renewal during clonal expansion.

By far the most dramatic changes in self-renewal capacity of AML progenitors has been brought about by agents thought to act at the level of control of differentiation. Chang and McCulloch (5) described increased PE2 in surviving colonies after treatment with tumor promotors, and Taetle et al. (17) described an inhibition of PE2 by low doses of human fibroblast interferon. A summary of factors influencing PE2 values is shown in Table 2.

PE2 FOR ALL BLAST PROGENITORS

PE2 measurements for cALL progenitors are very preliminary. Initial replating experiments conducted on primary colonies of cALL blasts indicate that PE2 can be measured and that it displays considerable patient-to-patient heterogeneity. This is consistent with a model of lymphopoiesis in cALL consisting of a small sub-population of self-renewing cells maintaining a large blast population with little proliferative capacity.

IMPLICATIONS FOR THERAPY

The experience with a large series of AML patients (3) confirms our initial claims (2) as to the prognostic indication of the leukemic progenitors. Our data show that

TABLE 2. *Manipulation of PE2 of AML blast progenitors*

Manipulation	Effect on PE2	Reference
Basic culture conditions	No effect	(3)
Treatment with cytotoxic agents		
Adriamycin	No effect	(3)
Cytosine arabinoside	Decreased	(3)
m-AMSA	Increased	(3)
Treatment with hemopoietic differentiation modifiers		
Tumor promoters	Increased	(5)
Interferon (human fibroblast)	Decreased	(17)

low secondary plating efficiency is significantly associated with remission induction ($0.01 < P < 0.001$) using a rank sum test. The strength of this correlation leads us to propose that this culture parameter may prove to be a very important additional prognostic indicator to those already described.

As a corollary to those clinical observations, it is clear that the self-renewal capacity of the clonogenic cells is an important target for intervention. Since patients with low self-renewal do best clinically, is it possible to devise ways of reducing the self-renewal capacity in those patients with aggressive disease? We have attempted to investigate this possibility in two areas: fortuitous change in self-renewal caused by cytotoxic drugs used for cytoreduction or designed intervention based on interaction of noncytotoxic agents with the process.

An analysis of three cytotoxic drugs in terms of their effect on primary growth and self-renewal capacity indicates that significant effects on self-renewal cannot be brought about with usual doses of chemotherapeutic drugs. However, some obvious generalities can be made. From the point of view of the future selection of agents useful in the treatment of AML, it would be advantageous to choose compounds with a dual role; cytoreduction and inhibition of self-renewal. m-AMSA (3) consistently allows increased self-renewal in survivors of treatment, whereas on a molar basis, it seems as efficient as adriamycin in terms of cytoreduction. On a theoretical basis, these characteristics would be consistent with a drug which was efficient in remission induction, but which would not be associated with lengthy remissions.

The possibility also exists for manipulation of self-renewal by more physiological agents. As a preliminary step to these studies, attempts to manipulate PE2 by simple alteration of culture conditions have been strikingly unsuccessful. For example, primary colonies growing with low efficiency in medium deficient in PHA-LCM have identical PE2 to colonies grown in optimum conditions. Clearly, the capacity for renewal is expressed even in situations where primary colony growth is limited by deficiency of growth factors. However, some studies have indicated that self-renewal can be manipulated by agents which are thought to act at levels other than cytotoxicity.

In terms of designing intervention at the biological level, our knowledge of the self-renewal process must be extended. From our initial attempts to alter PE2 by simple alterations to the culture medium and by sampling at different times during an individual patient's disease course, we know that the renewal process is not easily manipulated. Since, in conventional thinking, the cell's alternative to self-renewal is differentiation, it is possible that agents known to induce hemopoietic differentiation may be the same agents we are seeking as self-renewal inhibitors.

ACKNOWLEDGMENTS

We acknowledge the grant support of the National Leukemia Association (R. N. Buick), National Cancer Institute of Canada, Medical Research Council, and the Ontario Cancer Treatment and Research Foundation (E. A. McCulloch). C. Izaguirre is a research fellow of the National Cancer Institute of Canada.

REFERENCES

1. Buick, R. N., Till, J. E., and McCulloch, E. A. (1977): Colony assay for proliferative blast cells circulating in myeloblastic leukaemia. *Lancet*, 1:862–863.
2. Buick, R. N., Minden, M. D., and McCulloch, E. A. (1979): Self-renewal in culture of proliferative blast progenitor cells in acute myeloblastic leukemia. *Blood*, 54:95–104.
3. Buick, R. N., Chang, L. J.-A., Messner, H. A., Curtis, J. E., and McCulloch, E. A. (1981): Self-renewal capacity of leukemic blast progenitors. *Cancer Res.*, 41:4849–4852.
4. Chang, L. J.-A., Till, J. E., and McCulloch, E. A. (1980): The cellular basis of self-renewal in culture by human acute myeloblastic leukemia blast cell progenitors. *J. Cell. Physiol.*, 102:217–222.
5. Chang, L. J.-A., and McCulloch, E. A. (1981): Dose dependent effects of a tumor promotor on blast cell progenitors in human myeloblastic leukemia. *Blood*, 57:361–367.
6. Dicke, K. A., Spitzer, G., and Ahearn, M. J. (1976): Colony formation *in vitro* by leukemic cells in acute myelogenous leukaemia with phytohaemagglutinin as stimulating factor. *Nature*, 259:129–130.
7. Gehan, E. A., Smith, T. L., Freireich, E. J., Body, G., Rodriguez, V., Speer, J., and McRedie, K. (1976): Prognostic factors in acute leukemia. *Semin. Oncol.*, 3:271.
8. Izaguirre, C. A., and McCulloch, E. A. (1978): Cytogenetic analysis of leukemic clones (abstract). *Blood*, 54(Suppl 1):287.
9. Izaguirre, C. A., Curtis, J. E., Messner, H. A., and McCulloch, E. A. (1980): A colony assay for blast cell progenitors in non-B non-T (common) acute lymphoblastic leukemia. *Blood*, 57:823–829.
10. Izaguirre, C. A., Minden, M. D., Howatson, A. F., and McCulloch, E. A. (1980): Colony formation by normal and malignant human B lymphocytes. *Br. J. Cancer*, 42:430–437.
11. Lowenberg, G., and Hagemeijer, J. (1978): Attempts at improving colony methods for human leukemic cells. *J. Supramol. Struct.*, 2:182.
12. McCulloch, E. A., Buick, R. N., and Till, J. E. (1978): Cellular differentiation in the myeloblastic leukemias of man. In: *Cell Differentiation and Neoplasia*, edited by G. F. Saunders, pp. 211–221. Raven Press, New York.
13. McCulloch, E. A., Howatson, A. F., Buick, R. N., Minden, M., and Izaguirre, C. A. (1979): Acute myeloblastic leukemia considered as a clonal hemopathy. *Blood Cells*, 5:261–282.
14. McCulloch, E. A., Buick, R. N., Curtis, J. E., Messner, H. A., and Senn, J. S. (1980): The heritable nature of clonal characteristics in acute myeloblastic leukemia. *Blood*, 58:105–109.
15. Minden, M. D., Buick, R. N., and McCulloch, E. A. (1979): Separation of blast cell and T-lymphocyte progenitors in the blood of patients with acute myeloblastic leukemia. *Blood*, 54:186–195.
16. Park, C., Savin, M. A., Hoogstraten, B., Amare, M., and Hathaway, P. (1977): Improved growth of the *in vitro* colonies in human acute leukemia with the feeding culture method. *Cancer Res.*, 37:4594–4601.
17. Taetle, R., Buick, R. N., and McCulloch, E. A. (1980): Effect of interferon on colony formation in culture by blast cell progenitors in acute myeloblastic leukemia. *Blood*, 56:549–552.
18. Till, J. E., Lan, S., Buick, R. N., Sousan, P., Curtis, J. E., and McCulloch, E. A. (1978): Approaches to the evaluation of human hematopoietic stem-cell function. In: *Differentiation of Normal and Neoplastic Cells*, edited by B. Clarkson, P. A. Marks, and J. E. Till, pp. 81–92. Cold Spring Harbor Laboratory, Cold Spring Harbor, N.Y.
19. Till, J. E., and McCulloch, E. A. (1980): Hemopoietic stem cell differentiation. *Biochim. Biophys. Acta*, 605:431–459.
20. Steel, G. G. (1977): *Growth Kinetics of Tumours*. Clarendon Press, Oxford.

Maturation Factors and Cancer,
edited by Malcolm A. S. Moore.
Raven Press, © New York 1982.

Regulatory Factors in Hemopoiesis: Recognition and Restriction

G. B. Price, J. S. Senn, and R. M. Gorczynski

Ontario Cancer Institute, Toronto, Ontario, M4X 1K9 Canada, and Department of Medicine, Sunnybrook Medical Centre, University of Toronto, Toronto, Ontario, Canada

Investigations of the past 8 years (20) seemed to point to an existence of relationships between hemopoietic growth factors for myeloid and lymphoid cell differentiation. We decided that the genetic control afforded by the use of the mouse system, as a model, might highlight critical features of interactions between human regulatory growth factors and their target populations. As previously summarized (18,20), the properties of human hemopoietic growth factors and certain growth factors in mouse macrophage supernatant fluids appear similar. Among these properties, the membrane association, β_2-microglobulin (β_2m) antigenic determinants, and apparently similar functional activities were perhaps the more influential in the design and execution of studies reported here.

METHODS

Mice

All mice were kept five to a cage and allowed food and water *ad libitum*. Mice were typically used at 10 weeks of age. All mouse strains were obtained from Jackson Laboratories, Bar Harbor, Maine, except B10.A(2R) and B10.AQR, which were a gift from Dr. M. Feldmann (I.C.R.F., London, England).

Cell Preparation

Cell suspensions of bone marrow and spleen were prepared as previously described (13). All peritoneal cell donors were exsanguinated and 5 ml sterile PBS was injected into the peritoneal cavity. Peritoneal cells were washed, treated with antibrain θ serum and complement to remove any resident T cells, and used as described. Irradiated cells were prepared by exposure of cells, chilled on ice, to 1,500 rads at a dose rate of 100 rads/min by ^{137}Cs gamma radiation.

Cultures

Cells were cultured in α-MEM supplemented with 5×10^{-5} M 2-mercaptoethanol (2-ME) and 10% fetal calf serum (αF_{10}). Since certain functions of macrophages *in vitro* may be replaced by addition of 2-ME (4), 2-ME was used throughout all cultures. All lymphocyte cultures were performed in glass culture tubes (12 × 75 mm; John's Glass, Ontario, Canada) as previously described (8).

When macrophages were tested for their ability to reconstitute lymphocyte responses, the modulation of induction of cytotoxic T lymphocytes *in vitro* was investigated. One million macrophage-depleted responder spleen cells were cultured in 1.0 ml with 5×10^5 irradiated anti-θ treated macrophage-depleted (C3H/HeJ × C57B1/6J) F_1 (designated C3B6F$_1$) spleen cells as stimulator. Cells were tested in triplicate for their cytotoxicity in a 4 hr ^{51}Cr-release test with 1×10^4 ConA-stimulated ^{51}Cr-labeled C3B6F$_1$ spleen cell blasts (13).

When different macrophage preparations were to be analyzed for antigen-presentation function, 5×10^5 cells were incubated for 90 min at 37°C in 0.1 ml α F_{10} with the appropriate antigen at 10 times the limiting concentration, 10^{-2} μg/ml in most cases. After washing three times with 5 ml PBS, the cells were aliquoted to each of six cultures of whole spleen cells (4×10^6 cells per tube in 2 ml α F_{10}). One set of three received no further antigen, and the others received an optimal concentration of antigen to ensure that a failure to induce a response with antigen-pulsed cells was not because of the nonspecific inhibition by the macrophages in the spleen cells but was a result of failure in effective antigen presentation by the macrophage population being tested (10).

Bone Marrow Cultures

Bone marrow cells from femurs of mice were suspended in 0.8% methylcellulose, 20% F.C.S., and 2×10^5 cells/ml with a standard concentration (20% v/v) of L-cell conditioned medium (2). Beginning after 7 days of incubation, and at weekly intervals thereafter, macrophage colonies (28) from the various cultures were harvested, washed twice in 10 ml PBS, and irradiated with 2,000 rads. These cells were then used as a source of accessory cells in the assays described above.

RESULTS

Heterogeneity and Properties of Macrophage Regulatory Factors

Heterogeneity in production of different molecular weight species of factors was observed after velocity sedimentation of peritoneal macrophages (Table 1). The 10 to 15 mm/hr subpopulation of macrophages was able to produce a factor of apparent molecular weight 15,000 in addition to factors of 30,000 to 45,000 and 70,000 to 90,000 MW, which were also produced by the 2 to 7 mm/hr subpopulation of macrophages (9). All factors were capable of inducing cytotoxic T lymphocytes and stimulation of CFU-C (13,18).

From our experience in the description of human granulocyte colony stimulating activities (CSA), we observed:

1. CSAs are membrane-associated (21,22,29,30)

TABLE 1. *Induction of cytotoxic T lymphocytes and stimulation of CFU-C by factors from macrophage culture supernatant fluids*

Source of stimulating factors			
Macrophage source[a] (sedimentation velocity)	Apparent molecular weight[b]	% specific cytotoxicity[c]	CFU-C[d]
2 to 7 mm/hr	30,000–45,000	21.6	
	70,000–90,000	24.9	
10 to 15 mm/hr	15,000	23.4	145
	30,000–45,000	24.6	175
	70,000–90,000	31.4	197
None		8.4	0
L cell conditioned medium			231

[a]Peritoneal exudate cells were prepared as previously described (12) and then sedimented at unit gravity (16).
[b]Apparent molecular weight was estimated by Sephadex G100 gel filtration (9).
[c]Arithmetic mean of cytotoxicity represented by 15% of the recovered cells per culture to 1×10^4 ^{51}Cr-labelled targets. Cultures initially received 1×10^6 spleen cells and 5×10^5 irradiated stimulator cells.
[d]Cultures of mouse bone marrow cells were established as described in Methods. Arithmetic mean of two cultures is given.

TABLE 2. *Induction of cytotoxic T lymphocytes and mouse CFU-C by human urinary β_2-microglobulin*

Stimulator source	% Specific cytotoxicity[a]	CFU-C[a]
Human urinary β_2m[b]		
1.0×10^{-7}M	18.4	26
3.0×10^{-8}M	31.4	19
1.0×10^{-8}M	24.2	10
3.0×10^{-9}M	9.4	5
None	8.4	0
Mouse macrophage factor[a] (15,000 MW)	33.4	46

[a]See footnotes to Table 1.
[b]Human β_2m (Cedarlane Laboratories Ltd.) (18).

2. CSAs bear antigenic determinants which cross-react with anti-HLA sera or anti-β_2-microglobulin (19,24,30)
3. Two purified preparations of human urinary β_2-microglobulin promoted growth of granulocyte colonies (20).

As was reported by us (18), the similarity of physiochemical properties of mouse macrophage supernatant factors to human counterparts suggested that β_2-microglobulin might also substitute for and promote cytotoxic T lymphocytes or CFU-C. As shown again in Table 2, 1×10^{-8} M human urinary β_2-microglobulin stimulated both cytotoxic T lymphocytes and CFU-C (18).

The congenic recombinant inbred strains of mice for the major histocompatibility complex (MHC) afforded us the opportunity to examine the processes of recognition and stimulation by these macrophage factors (13). As shown in Table 3, B10.SgN and B10.BR factors of 70–90K and 30–45K, although competent to stimulate homologous cells, exhibited apparent restriction when tested on the other MHC congenic cell sources for induction of cytotoxic T lymphocytes. Although a few similar variations in stimulation of CFU-C were observed, a pattern of MHC restriction has not yet been recognized. The 15K molecules of macrophage supernatant have never shown any coherent pattern of restriction. The low molecular factor of less than 15K generally promoted only a low level of CFU-C activity, although it apparently stimulated cytotoxic T lymphocytes in a non-MHC restricted manner. A mixture of B10.SgN and B10.BR factors proved that the restriction resided with stimulatory factors and not as a result of active inhibition, and it further documented that there was no apparent interference between the factors from the two different congenic strains.

As demonstrated in Table 4, the H-2K/D loci seem to be the source of incompatibility or restriction of the 70 to 90K macrophage factors. Further, Table 5 demonstrates that (30–45K) molecular weight macrophage factors showed activity only when responder cells and cells used as source of factor were compatible at the genes located in the IA/IB region. Additional experiments using an antiserum to Ia antigen have been performed and have demonstrated anti-Ia-mediated inhibition of the 30 to 45K factor activity but not activity derived from 70 to 90K factors (13).

TABLE 3. *MHC restriction of macrophage supernatant factors*

Source of factors[a]	Apparent molecular weight[b]	Stimulation of cytotoxicity in[b]		CFU-C in[b]	
		B10	B10.BR	B10	B10.BR
B10.SgN	Unfractionated	25.9	24.0	96	153
	70–90K	21.6	0.3	100	121
	30–45K	24.8	5.9	48	62
	15K	21.6	20.4	23	69
	15K	22.9	23.8	8	7
B10.BR	Unfractionated	21.7	24.8	101	135
	70–90K	8.6	25.9	61	96
	30–45K	7.4	23.8	42	80
	15K	24.4	23.8	80	71
	15K	21.6	22.9	5	0
B10 + B10.BR	70–90K	27.4	24.9		
	30–45K	26.3	25.2		
None		5.8	4.7	0	0

[a]Macrophage supernatants and the G100 fractions thereof were prepared as described in Methods. The concentration used in the test was optimal for homologous cells; in general, there was little difference in titration curves of activity on homologous or heterologous cells, where a factor is active on a heterologous cell source.
[b]See footnotes to Table 1.

TABLE 4. *Genes involved in restriction by (70–90K) factors*

Source of factors[a]	B10.AQR, % specific cytotoxicity[a]	CFU-C[a]	B10.A(2R), % specific cytotoxicity	CFU-C
B10.AQR (qkkdddd)	38.0	249	4.2	170
B10.A(2R) (kkkdddb)	7.6		29	122
No factor	6.4	0	4.9	0

[a]See footnotes to Table 1.

TABLE 5. *Genes involved in restriction by (30–45K) factors*

Source of factors[a]	B10.AQR % Specific cytotoxicity[a]	CFU-C[a]	B10.A(2R) % Specific cytotoxicity	CFU-C	B10.A(5R) % Specific cytotoxicity	CFU-C
B10.AQR (qkkdddd)[b]	33.9	127	36.9	61	4.1	56
B10.A(2R) (kkkdddb)	30.1		33.6	3	3.9	31
B10.A(5R) (bbbdddd)	6.3	129	7.6	41	33.9	53
No factor	4.1	0	6.0	0	5.1	0

[a]See footnotes to Table 1.
[b]Parentheses enclose the MHC haplotype of recombinant inbred strains.

Heterogeneity of Macrophage Populations in Antigen Presentation

The peritoneal macrophage population was divided into three subpopulations based upon sedimentation velocity. As demonstrated in Table 6, the 4 to 7 mm/hr and 10 to 14 mm/hr population presents TNP-dextran$_{1299}$ successfully, but the 7 to 10 mm/hr population appears incompetent. The 10 to 14 mm/hr population seemed competent to present most of the antigens tested. The TNP-coupled bacteriophage T$_4$ antigen was presented fairly adequately by all subpopulations; the most dramatic heterogeneity in presentation of antigen was observed with TNP-dextran$_{1299}$ and TNP-levan (10,11).

Heterogeneity of Macrophage Progenitors (CFU-C)

Figure 1 illustrates that bone marrow cells after culture to produce macrophage colonies will demonstrate heterogeneity with regard to presentation of TNP-levan or TNP-dextran$_{1355}$. Thus after 14 days culture, different progenitor populations (lower panel) produced macrophages of restricted competence for presentation of

TABLE 6. *Ability of macrophage subpopulations to present different carbohydrate groups in immunogenic form*

Macrophage subpopulations[a] (sedimentation velocity)	Anitgens used for pulse[b]	Anti-TNP-PFC/ culture[c]
4–7 mm/hr	TNP-Dextran$_{1355}$	184 ± 26[d]
	TNP-Dextran$_{1299}$	196 ± 19
	TNP-Levan	93 ± 14
	TNP-T$_4$	158 ± 18
	None	8 ± 3
7–10 mm/hr	TNP-Dextran$_{1355}$	168 ± 23
	TNP-Dextran$_{1299}$	19 ± 4
	TNP-Levan	12 ± 4
	TNP-T$_4$	104 ± 16
	None	11 ± 3
10–14 mm/hr	TNP-Dextran$_{1355}$	214 ± 31
	TNP-Dextran$_{1299}$	211 ± 33
	TNP-Levan	229 ± 29
	TNP-T$_4$	216 ± 32
	None	11 ± 3
None	TNP-T$_4$ + TNP-T$_4$ in cultures	258 ± 39

[a]See footnotes to Table 1.
[b]TNP-dextran$_{1355}$, TNP-dextran$_{1299}$, TNP-levan, and TNP-T$_4$ were prepared as described elsewhere (10,11).
[c]Anti-TNP specific plaque forming cells using TNP-coupled SRBC (24a) (per 10^6 cells cultured; see Methods).
[d]Arithmetic mean of three cultures ± SEM.

TNP-carbohydrate coupled antigens. (Compare presentation of antigen of macrophages derived from CFU-C of sedimentation velocity 2 to 9 and 10 to 14 mm/hr).

Although not presented here, we have also shown that if macrophages are left in culture from 7 to 28 days, the competence of a given subpopulation of macrophages derived from CFU-C to present TNP-coupled carbohydrate antigen is changed (10). This heterogeneity of macrophages derived from CFU-C may arise from changes in the activity of a given cell at various times in its life history (a programme) or may reflect the development of novel and heterogeneous cell types continuously within the colony.

Generally speaking, the heterogeneity uncovered with TNP-coupled carbohydrate antigens was not seen with TNP-coupled protein antigens (T$_4$ and KLH). However, as reported by Gorczynski et al. (10), a heterogeneity of macrophages was in evidence using hapten-protein conjugated antigens in optimally stimulated spleen cell cultures after the addition of extraneous macrophages derived from CFU-C colonies if we examined the qualitative patterns of antibody production (assessed by relative avidities of anti-TNP antibody in a plaque assay).

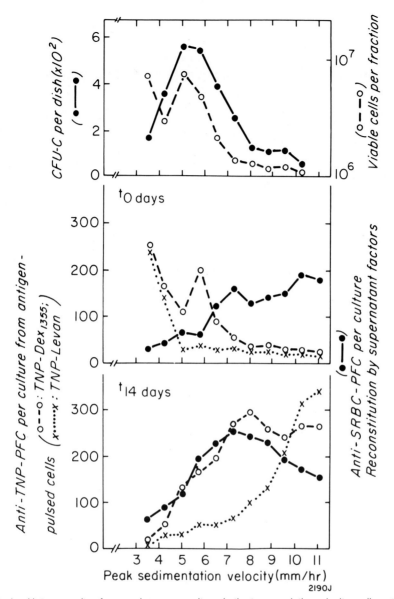

FIG. 1. Heterogeneity of macrophage progenitors. In the top panel, the velocity sedimentation profile of viable C3B6F$_1$ bone marrow cells is given (○––○). The profile of CFU-C macrophage colonies per constant volume of each fraction is also shown. In the middle panel, the abilities of different populations of macrophages and bone marrow cells on the day of velocity sedimentation (t_0) to present antigen for stimulation of antibody producing cells, plaque forming cells (PFC) are shown; (●———●), anti-SRBC PFC; (○––○), anti-TNP-dextran$_{1355}$; (× ··· ×), anti-TNP-levan. In the lower panel, the antigen presenting abilities of different populations of CFU-C and their macrophage progeny at day 14 of culture (t_{14}) are shown.

Modification of Human Hemopoietic Factor Production by Disease and Immunostimulatory Reagents

Analysis of the heterogeneity (molecular weight) of purified factors produced by leukocytes of patients in various disease states is provided in Table 7. As previously reported (20,26,27,30), patients with untreated acute leukemia, chronic leukemia, or acute leukemia in relapse generally produce a single molecular weight species of 36,500 MW. Patients with nonmalignant disorders typically show all three HMW-CSA moieties after fractionation (23). However, membrane fractionation of leukocytes from either leukemia patients or normal volunteers after solubilization in detergent (sodium dodecyl sulphate) gave three apparent moieties (20,22). In two leukemia patients expressing a single moiety, addition of the T lymphocyte mitogen PHA to the culture medium (14) seemed to potentiate release of three moieties. In two other leukemia patients, another immunostimulant, levamisole, was apparently successful in allowing release of three moieties into medium (25). With one patient given levamisole for 5 days, culture of leukocytes in the absence of levamisole in order to produce HMW-CSA resulted in three HMW-CSA moieties after appropriate fractionation (5). After 10 days of drug administration, no increase in peripheral granulocyte was observed; since the drug was poorly tolerated by the patient, levamisole was then discontinued.

Of seven patients with RAEM, six produced one moiety; four of these six have progressed to acute myeloid leukemia. Of 10 patients with preleukemia syndrome (15,17), 7 produced a single moiety, and only one of this group has progressed to a clinical state of acute leukemia. Eight of these 10 patients are still at risk, including the 3 patients producing three moieties of HMW-CSA. For the high-risk group of IASA patients, 12 of 19 patients had only a single HMW-CSA moiety detectable in fractionated leukocyte conditioned medium; 2 of these have developed acute leukemia. Of the 19 IASA patients, 11 have died and 8 remain at risk, including 3 of the 7 patients in which three moieties were detected. For related control groups (no increased risk to develop leukemia) of SSA and HSA, all four patients expressed three HMW-CSA moieties.

The follow-up of these patients now varies from approximately 1 to more than 7 years. No patient in which three moieties of HMW-CSA have been detected after fractionation has as yet developed acute leukemia. Five patients assessed as producing a single moiety of CSA have died without any evidence of acute leukemia at death. In summary, 13 patients assessed as producing a single moiety of HMW-CSA and 7 patients with 3 HMW-CSA moieties remain at risk. The association of HMW-CSA moieties with clinical diagnosis of leukemia or preleukemia syndrome is imperfect, and the *in vivo* relevance is still undetermined. The disease associations and modification by immunostimulants suggest that expression of HMW-CSA moieties will be found to be dependent upon a complex series of cellular interactions in the hemopoietic system (lymphoid and myeloid).

TABLE 7. *Summary of hemopoietic regulatory growth factors in peripheral leukocyte conditioned medium[a]*

Disease status (number of patients)	Modification[b] *(in vitro/in vivo)*	HMW-CSA moieties[c]
Nonleukemia		
(18)[d]	None/none	3
Leukemia		
(18)	None/Cx[c]	1
(2)	PHA[c]/Cx	3
(2)[e]	LMS[c]/Cx	3
(1)[e]	None/LMS	3
Leukemia in remission		
(4)	None/Cx	3
(1)	None/none	1
RAEM[c]		
(1)	None/none	3
(6)	None/none	1
Preleukemia syndrome		
(3)	None/none	3
(7)	None/none	1
Preleukemia syndrome (1 HMW-CSA moiety)		
(3)	LMS/none	3
IASA[c]		
(7)	None/none	3
(12)	None/none	1
SSA[c]		
(3)	None/none	3
HSA[c]		
(1)	None/none	3

[a]Details of preparation and purification of factors in human peripheral leukocyte conditioned medium have been described previously. (14,20,23). The three HMW-CSA are of approximate MWs 93,000, 36,500, and 14,700. With but one exception in the leukemia group, all single species were of approximate molecular weight 36,500.

[b]Modification of conditioned medium production *in vitro* is described elsewhere (14,25).

[c]Abbreviations: HMW-CSA, high molecular weight colony stimulating activity; Cx, chemotherapy; PHA, phytohemagglutinin; LMS, levamisole; RAEM, refractory anemia with excess myeloblasts; IASA, idiopathic acquired sideroblastic anemia; SSA, secondary sideroblastic anemia; HSA, hereditary sideroblastic anemia.

[d]Nonleukemic patients include both normal volunteers and patients with nonmalignant hematological disorders such as hemochromatosis, polycythemia rubra vera, and megaloblastic anemia.

[e]Two of 18 patients with leukemia and one HMW-CSA moiety were used to test *in vitro* modification by LMS of HMW-CSA production. One patient was also given *in vivo* LMS (25).

DISCUSSION

Our previous findings indicated a significant similarity and association of various molecular weight species of macrophage products which stimulate myeloid and lymphoid cell populations (13,18). In the mouse, these macrophage products, at least for the lymphostimulatory function, were demonstrably MHC restricted. The 70 to 90K MW factor restriction was coded for by genes in the K/D ends of the MHC, while the 30 to 45K MW factor restriction was coded for in the IA and/or IB region of the MHC; the 15,000 MW factor was observed to stimulate across histocompatibility barriers.

Affinity chromatography using anti-β_2m removed up to 90% of the activity in macrophage culture supernatants capable of inducing a T lymphocyte cytotoxic response and removed up to 100% of the colony stimulating activity (18). Anti-I antisera used with relevant recombinant strains as a source of responder cells and tested for effects on both 70 to 90K and 30 to 45K stimulatory activities showed inhibition of 30 to 45K activities upon CFU-C, and induction of T lymphocyte cytotoxic responses was not due to cytotoxicity directed against the cells (13). While CFU-C stimulation by these factors was less evidently genetically restricted than the induction of T lymphocyte cytotoxicity or antibody-producing cells (13), the ability to remove colony stimulating activity with an anti-I region antiserum suggests that the same molecules, at least in the 30 to 45K moiety, are responsible for CFU-C colony formation and lymphostimulation. The potential association of components of the mouse MHC with reactive lymphostimulatory molecules has previously been suggested for genetically restricted factors for T helper cell induction (6) and allogeneic effect factor (5), which also reportedly contained β_2-microglobulin determinants (1), and a factor involved in T cell maturation and differentiation *in vitro* (3), which also contained I-region coded determinants in the mouse.

In contrast to these observations of lymphostimulatory and hemopoietic factor association with MHC coded and β_2m-determinants, Fitchen et al. (7) recently reported a lack of cross-reactivity of two anti-β_2m antisera with colony stimulating activity from the conditioned medium of a human T cell line and pregnant mouse uterus extract. They suggested that the difference in reported results could be related to the technical factors of different sources of CSA and anti-β_2m antiserum which were used. In the absence of further information, we would agree that these factors may account for the different observations. We ourselves have observed that L cell colony stimulating activity is unaffected by anti-β_2m. However, as reported in Price et al. (24), Gorczynski and Price (13), and Price and Gorczynski (18), our anti-β_2m antiserum gave no evidence of activity through a direct cytotoxicity upon either CFU-C or effectors of cytotoxic T lymphocytes under the conditions of assay.

The heterogeneity in mouse macrophage populations *in vivo* or produced *in vitro* from progenitors, CFU-C, has been demonstrated using antigen-presentation assays for TNP-coupled carbohydrate antigens (Table 6 and Fig. 1). Although not shown here, a heterogeneity of macrophage ability to release lymphostimulatory products to replace certain macrophage functions can also be observed (10). Further, the appearance of cells able to present immunogenic stimuli to lymphocytes and release lymphostimulatory molecules is not correlated.

Supplemental to previous observations of heterogeneity in molecular weight species of HMW-CSA of human peripheral leukocyte conditioned medium as produced and purified from leukocytes of patients in various disease categories, we report in Table 7 an update and extension of previous results (20,26). Lymphostimulatory reagents, PHA and levamisole (25), have been shown to potentiate the release of granulopoietic colony stimulating activities. We suggest that these observations of disease-associated perturbation and effects of lymphostimulatory mitogens in human cultures may further reflect some common denominator between those cellular interactions and growth factors associated with lymphopoiesis and myelopoiesis. The observations of macrophage heterogeneity and the MHC association of some hemopoietic factors in mouse suggest the need for similar studies of genetic restriction and accessory cell heterogeneity in human hemopoiesis (myelopoiesis and lymphopoiesis).

ACKNOWLEDGMENTS

This research was supported by the Medical Research Council, Grant #MA-6677 (JSS), Grant #MA-5440 (RMG), and the National Cancer Institute of Canada (GBP, RMG).

REFERENCES

1. Amerding, D., Kubo, R. T., Grey, H. M., and Katz, D. H. (1975): Activation of T and B lymphocytes *in vitro*. Presence of β_2-microglobulin determinants on allogeneic effect factor. *Proc. Natl. Acad. Sci. U.S.A.*, 72:4577–4581.
2. Austin, P. E., McCulloch, E. A., and Till, J. E. (1976): Characterization of the factor in L-cell conditioned medium capable of stimulating colony formation by mouse marrow cells in culture. *J. Cell. Physiol.*, 177:121–134.
3. Beller, D. I., Farr, A. G., and Unanue, E. R. (1978): Regulation of lymphocyte proliferation and differentiation by macrophages. *Fed. Proc.*, 37:91–96.
4. Chen, C., and Hirsch, J. G. (1972): The effects of mercaptoethanol and of peritoneal macrophages on the antibody forming capacity of non-adherent spleen cells *in vitro*. *J. Exp. Med.*, 136:604–617.
5. Delovitch, T. L., and McDevitt, H. O. (1977): *In vitro* analysis of allogeneic lymphocyte interaction. I. Characterization and cellular origin of an Ia-positive "helper" factor allogeneic effect factor. *J. Exp. Med.*, 146:1019–1032.
6. Erb, P., and Feldmann, M. (1975): The role of macrophages in the generation of T helper cells. III. Influence of macrophage-derived factors in helper cell function. *Eur. J. Immunol.*, 5:759–766.
7. Fitchen, J. H., Ferrone, S., Lusis, A. J., and Cline, M. J. (1980): Cytotoxicity of anti-β_2-microglobulin xenoantisera to human and murine myeloid progenitor cells and lack of cross-reactivity with colony-stimulating activity. *J. Immunol.*, 124:2906–2908.
8. Gorczynski, R. M. (1976): Control of the immune response. Role of macrophages in regulation of antibody and cell-mediated immune responses. *Scand. J. Immunol.*, 5:1031–1047.
9. Gorczynski, R. M. (1977): Role of macrophage derived factors in generation of cytotoxic antibody responses. *Scand. J. Immunol.*, 6:665–674.
10. Gorczynski, R. M., Benzing, K., MacRae, S., and Price, G. B. (1980): *In vitro* generation from murine bone marrow cells of accessory cells with discrete antigen presentation capacity and ability to release lymphostimulatory molecules. *Immunopharmacology*, 2:327–339.

11. Gorczynski, R. M., MacRae, S., and Jennings, J. J. (1979): A novel role for macrophages: antigen discrimination of distinct carbohydrate bonds. *Cell. Immunol.*, 45:276–294.

12. Gorczynski, R. M., Miller, R. G., and Phillips, R. A. (1973): Reconstitution of T cell depleted spleen cell populations by factors derived from T cells. I. Conditions for the production of active T cell supernatants. *J. Immunol.*, 110:968–983.

13. Gorczynski, R. M., and Price, G. B. (1979): The role of macrophages in stimulation of immune induction and myelopoiesis. II. Analysis of genetic restriction involved in the stimulation of granulocyte colony precursors or mature lymphocytes using factors prepared from different recombinant inbred strains of mice. *Immunopharmacology*, 1:187–201.

14. Lau, L., McCulloch, E. A., Till, J. E., and Price, G. B. (1978): The production of hemopoietic growth factors by PHA-stimulated leukocytes. *Exp. Hematol.*, 6:597–600.

15. Linman, J. W., and Bagby, G. C. (1976): The preleukemic syndrome: clinical and laboratory features, natural course, and management. *Blood Cells*, 2:11–31.

16. Miller, R. G., and Phillips, R. A. (1967): Separation of cells by velocity sedimentation. *J. Cell. Physiol.*, 73:191–202.

17. Pierre, R. V. (1974): Preleukemic states. *Semin. Haematol.*, 11:73–92.

18. Price, G. B., and Gorczynski, R. M. (1979): The role of macrophages in stimulation of immune induction and myelopoiesis. I. Comparison of activity of macrophage-derived factors in granulopoiesis and immunostimulation. *Immunopharmacology*, 1:175–185.

19. Price, G. B., and Krogsrud, R. L. (1978): Use of molecular probes for detection of human hemopoietic progenitors. In: *Differentiation of Normal and Neoplastic Hemopoietic Cells*, edited by B. D. Clarkson, P. A. Marks, and J. E. Till, pp. 371–381. Cold Spring Harbor Laboratory, Cold Spring Harbor, N.Y.

20. Price, G. B., Krogsrud, R. L., Stewart, S., and Senn, J. S. (1978): Heterogeneity and biochemistry of colony stimulating activities. In: *Hemopoietic Cell Differentiation*, edited by D. W. Golde, M. J. Cline, D. Metcalf, and C. F. Fox, pp. 417–431. Academic Press, New York.

21. Price, G. B., and McCulloch, E. A. (1978): Cell surfaces and the regulation of hemopoiesis. In: *Leukemia and Lymphoma*, edited by E. J. Freireich, E. M. Hersh, P. A. Merscher, and E. R. Jaffe, pp. 304–321. Grune & Stratton, New York.

22. Price, G. B., McCulloch, E. A., and Till, J. E. (1975): Cell membranes as sources of granulocyte colony stimulating activities. *Exp. Hematol.*, 3:227–233.

23. Price, G. B., Senn, J. S., McCulloch, E. A., and Till, J. E. (1975): The isolation and properties of granulopoietic colony stimulating activities from human peripheral leukocyte conditioned medium. *Biochem. J.*, 148:209–217.

24. Price, G. B., McCulloch, E. A., and Till, J. E. (1976): Cross reactivity of human β_2-microglobulin with human granulocyte colony-stimulating activity. *J. Immunol.*, 117:416–418.

24a. Rittenberg, M. B., and Pratt, K. L. (1969): Anti-trinitrophenyl (TNP) plaque assay. Primary response of BALB/c mice to soluble and particulate immunogen. *Proc. Soc. Exp. Biol.*, 132:575–581.

25. Senn, J. S., Lai, C. C., and Price, G. B. (1980): Levamisole: evidence for activity on human hemopoietic progenitor cells. *Br. J. Cancer*, 41:40–46.

26. Senn, J. S., Pinkerton, P. H., Price, G. B., Mak, T. W., and McCulloch, E. A. (1976): Human preleukemia cell culture studies in sideroblastic anemia. *Br. J. Cancer*, 33:299–306.

27. Senn, J. S., Price, G. B., Mak, T. W., and McCulloch, E. A. (1976): An approach to human preleukemia using cell culture studies. *Blood Cells*, 2:161–166.

28. Stanley, E. R., and Heard, P. M. (1977): Factors regulating macrophage production and growth. Purification and some properties of the colony stimulating factor from medium conditioned by mouse cells. *J. Biol. Chem.*, 252:4305–4312.

29. Till, J. E., Mak, T. W., Price, G. B., Senn, J. S., and McCulloch, E. A. (1976): Cellular subclasses in human leukemic hemopoiesis. In: *Modern Trends in Human Leukemia II*, edited by R. C. Gallo, K. Mannweiler, and W. C. Moloney, pp. 33–45. J. F. Lehrmans Verlag, Munich.

30. Till, J. E., Price, G. B., Senn, J. S., and McCulloch, E. A. (1977): Cell interactions in the control of hemopoiesis. In: *Growth Kinetics and Biochemical Regulation of Normal and Malignant Cells*, edited by B. Drewinko and R. M. Humphrey, pp. 223–235. Williams & Wilkins, Baltimore.

31. Worton, R. G., McCulloch, E. A., and Till, J. E. (1969): Physical separation of hemopoietic stem cells from cells forming colonies in culture. *J. Cell. Physiol.*, 74:171–182.

Maturation Factors and Cancer,
edited by Malcolm A. S. Moore.
Raven Press, © New York 1982.

Characterization of Hemopoietic Cells Which Bind Radioiodinated Colony Stimulating Factor

Richard K. Shadduck, Abdul Waheed, Giuseppe Pigoli, and Cecilia Caramatti

Department of Medicine, Montefiore Hospital, University of Pittsburgh School of Medicine, Pittsburgh, Pennsylvania 15213

Colony stimulating factor (CSF) is a glycoprotein material or class of materials which induces certain bone marrow progenitor cells to proliferate and differentiate into identifiable hemopoietic cells (5). When added to bone marrow cells immobilized in soft agar gels, CSF leads to the development of large colonies containing 50 to 500 cells of the granulocyte and macrophage series. Based on the high fraction of the responsive cells in DNA synthesis (9), as well as the apparent restriction to two common pathways of differentiation, it is widely believed that CSF acts on stem cells committed to the granulocyte-macrophage pathway.

Although the colony assay for CSF has been well characterized, only limited information is available concerning the interaction of CSF with marrow progenitor cells. This factor is continuously required for both survival of the progenitor cells as well as differentiation into identifiable cells of the granulocytic and macrophage series (3,4,6).

Recently, the purification of several sources of murine CSF has permitted further study of the interaction of these materials with responsive cells in the marrow (1,14,15). Purified murine lung CSF stimulates a marked increase in bone marrow RNA synthesis with apparent action on both immature as well as mature cells of the granulocytic series (2). In addition, purified iodinated CSF from murine fibroblasts (L cells) has been shown to specifically bind to marrow cells (8). In this chapter, we outline an initial characterization of this binding phenomenon with emphasis on the kinetic type of hemopoietic cells involved.

MATERIALS AND METHODS

Bone marrow cells were obtained from the femurs of female CF_1 mice. Each femur was removed by aseptic technique and cleansed; cells were forcibly flushed into 2 ml of McCoy's modified 5A medium using a syringe and 23 gauge needle. Suspensions of dispersed cells were prepared by repeated pipetting. Binding to the bone marrow was compared to that using spleen cells or fetal liver cells. The latter were obtained from 17 to 18 day embryos. The spleen and fetal liver cell suspensions were prepared by finely mincing the tissues with scissors into medium and sequentially passing the resultant cell suspensions through 19 and 21 gauge needles. Fibrous connective tissue and debris were allowed to settle for 5 min prior to the use in binding assays. Cell counts were obtained manually to assure complete dispersion of the cell suspensions. After preliminary studies, 10^7 marrow, spleen, or fetal liver cells were dispensed into 1 ml volumes of McCoy's medium supplemented with additional vitamins, amino acids, 15% fetal calf serum, and DEAE dextran, 75 µg/ml (8).

Binding assays were performed by incubating the cell suspensions for various time intervals in the presence of saturating doses of ^{125}I labeled CSF. Control tubes contained an 80-fold excess of unlabeled CSF as a measure of nonspecific binding. After 3 to 24 hr incubation at 37°C in a 7.5% CO_2 atmosphere, tubes were washed and centrifuged at 1,000g for 7 min. Binding was measured by the degree of cellular radioactivity. Specific binding was calculated by subtraction of the counts obtained in tubes containing excess "cold" CSF. Triplicate tubes were used for each determination.

L-cell CSF was prepared by the growth of murine fibroblasts in serum free medium as previously described (15). After 7 days of incubation, the supernatant conditioned media were harvested and kept at 4°C prior to purification. Working pools of 10 liters of conditioned media were concentrated 250-fold by ultrafiltration using an Amicon ultrafiltration cell and PM-10 membrane. Highly purified CSF was obtained by alcohol precipitation and chromatography on DEAE cellulose and Con-A Sepharose. In the latter step, two-thirds of the CSF was adherent and was subsequently eluted with alpha-methyl glucoside. This material was further fractionated on Sephadex G-150, and the CSF was separated from trace contaminants by sucrose density centrifugation. The final material was increased greater than 1,000-fold in specific activity to approximately 5×10^7 units/mg of protein. This purified CSF appeared homogeneous as judged by its electrophoretic migration in varying concentrations of acrylamide, in SDS-acrylamide, and by reaction with anti-CSF in Ouchterlony gel diffusion (15).

Highly purified CSF was iodinated by a modified chloramine T technique with full retention of biologic activity (12). Iodinated CSF was separated from free iodine using a column of Sephadex G-150. Most of the tracers prepared by this technique contained 3 to 5 moles of ^{125}I per mole of CSF. This variation in iodination as well as differences in the quantity of tracer used in each study contributed to differences in the total cellular radioactivity which was bound by the cells. The iodinated material was used for 2 to 3 weeks, during which time there was only minimal loss of biologic activity.

The time course of CSF binding was examined using both bone marrow and spleen cell cultures incubated for intervals of 3 to 24 hr after preparation. Once it was established that 24 hr represented an optimal time for interaction of CSF with marrow cells, further studies explored the effect of various metabolic inhibitors in the binding reaction. Cultures were incubated in varying concentrations of vincristine (Eli-Lilly Co.) or cytosine arabinoside (ARA-C; The Upjohn Co.) for intervals of 24 hr. Similar studies explored the effect of cobalt irradiation on the marrow and spleen cell suspensions. Cultures were treated with 300 to 1,200 rads immediately after preparation. They were subsequently incubated for 24 hr and cellular uptake of radioactivity was determined.

In several experiments designed to determine whether CSF binds only to colony forming cells, marrow cells were separated by Ficoll-Hypaque density gradient cell centrifugation. A total of 10^8 marrow cells in 5 ml of medium were overlayed onto 25 ml of Ficoll-Hypaque, specific gravity 1.077, and centrifuged at $400g$ for 45 min. Cells from the interface (top layer) and bottom of the gradient were examined morphologically and assessed for CFU-C content and binding capability. CSF and CFU-C assays were performed as previously described (11). In brief, 10^5 marrow cells were incubated in 1 ml of McCoy's agar in the presence of 5% L-cell CSF. Cultures were held for 7 days in a 37°C, 7.5% CO_2 atmosphere prior to counting. Colonies of 50 or more cells were scored using a dissecting microscope. The number of colonies (CFU-C) was used as a measure of granulocyte-macrophage progenitor cell content.

RESULTS

Preliminary studies showed that virtually no binding occurred at early time intervals after incubation of marrow cells with tracer. With prolongation of the incubation time to 24 hr, there was a marked increase in cellular radioactivity. In most studies, 10^7 marrow cells bound 15,000 to 40,000 cpm when incubated with 250,000 to 400,000 cpm of tracer. The binding reaction was inhibited by an 80-fold excess of unlabeled CSF but was not influenced by a variety of unrelated proteins. All subsequent experiments therefore included control tubes with "cold" CSF as a measure of nonspecific binding.

A typical study of the saturability of the binding reaction is shown in Table 1. Cells were exposed to incremental quantities of tracer, and cell-associated radioactivity was determined after 24 hr of incubation. A plateau in binding was observed using 377,271 to 686,947 cpm of tracer. Saturation of the reaction occurred with the 377,271 cpm dose of tracer wherein 9.7% of the radioactivity was bound. This represented the specific binding of 4.6 units or 91 pcg of CSF.

Several additional parameters were explored for their effect on CSF binding. The cellular uptake of radioactivity was measured using cultures incubated in McCoy's medium supplemented with a variety of additives. As shown in Table 2, modest binding was detected using serum free medium. The addition of supplemental vitamins and amino acids increased binding with maximal radioactivity incorporated in those cultures fully supplemented with the addition of fetal calf serum and DEAE dextran. Variation in the pH of the cultures from 7.0 to 8.0 had virtually no effect; using saturating quantities of tracer, radioactivity varied between 25,383 and 29,934 cpm/10^7 cells. The binding reaction was due to incorporation of [125]I

TABLE 1. *Effect of increasing dose of* [125]*I CSF on marrow cell binding*[a]

Dose of tracer	[125]I CSF bound	Nonspecific binding	Specific binding
24,545	5,584 ± 194	546 ± 32	5,038 ± 216
86,793	16,968 ± 775	1,441 ± 34	15,528 ± 754
171,860	27,470 ± 1,112	5,495 ± 9	21,975 ± 1,103
377,271	40,608 ± 1,560	3,903 ± 65	36,704 ± 1,624
509,100	39,649 ± 1,587	6,292 ± 149	33,357 ± 1,735
686,947	43,970 ± 1,957	7,597 ± 254	36,372 ± 1,968

[a]Values represent the cpm of ^{125}I CSF which were added and subsequently bound using 10^7 marrow cells/culture. Nonspecific counts were obtained using cultures with an 80-fold excess of unlabeled CSF. Specific counts were calculated by subtraction of nonspecific binding. Cultures were incubated for 24 hr using triplicate tubes for each point. Values are means ±1 SE.

TABLE 2. *The effect of various media on the binding reaction*[a]

Culture medium	[125]I CSF bound	Nonspecific binding	Specific binding
McCoy's 5A medium	10,057 ± 1,365	1,975 ± 94	8,082 ± 1,460
McCoy's supplemented with vitamins and amino acids.	14,531 ± 1,480	1,740 ± 93	12,791 ± 1,530
McCoy's supplemented plus FCS + DEAE dextran.	17,087 ± 828	2,382 ± 213	14,704 ± 843

[a]Values depict the total nonspecific and specific cpm bound after 24 hr incubation of 10^7 marrow cells in the various media. Cultures were incubated with 370,000 cpm of tracer. Numbers are means ±1 SE from triplicate cultures.

CSF rather than free ^{125}I as it was not inhibited by addition of a marked excess(100 ng) of unlabeled sodium iodide. Moreover, incubation of the radioactive sodium iodide with marrow cells did not lead to a cellular accumulation of radioactivity.

The time course of CSF binding to 10^7 bone marrow or spleen cells is shown in Fig. 1. Virtually no cellular radioactivity could be detected in marrow cultures after 10 min to 3 hr exposure to the tracer. Thereafter, a marked increase in radioactivity was observed between 3 and 15 hr. No further increase in binding was apparent between 15 and 24 hr. In contrast, a gradual increase in spleen cell radioactivity occurred between 1 and 24 hr of incubation. Total cellular uptake was approximately 10% of that in marrow cultures, which is in accord with the lower content of colony forming cells in this organ.

In similar studies, fetal liver cells were compared to bone marrow cells for their uptake of radiolabeled CSF. Cultures were incubated with 275,000 cpm of tracer for 1, 6, and 24 hr. As shown in Fig. 2, there was minimal binding at 1 and 6 hr,

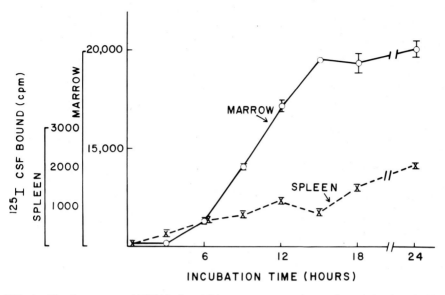

FIG. 1. The time course of CSF binding: 10^7 bone marrow or spleen cells were incubated with 400,000 cpm of tracer for various intervals, and cellular radioactivity was determined. Nonspecific binding seen in cultures with an 80-fold excess of unlabeled CSF was subtracted from total counts to obtain specific binding. Values are means ± SE from triplicate cultures.

with a marked increase at the 24 hr time point. Fetal liver cells showed only one-third the binding capacity of adult marrow cells. Although this may reflect differences in the content of colony forming cells, differential counts indicated marked differences between the two sources of hemopoietic cells. Fetal liver contained 45% normoblasts, 20% lymphocytes, and 13.5% proliferative and 14.5% nonproliferative granulocytes. The marrow suspension had fewer normoblasts (15%), similar numbers of lymphocytes (22%), and less proliferative granulocytes, but it had a substantially greater number of nonproliferative cells of the granulocytic series (53%).

To determine whether CSF binds primarily to proliferative or nonproliferative cells, further marrow cell cultures were established in the presence of vincristine and cytosine arabinoside. As shown in Fig. 3, 0.01 to 1 µg of vincristine had no effect on binding, whereas a 24% decrease was observed in cultures exposed to 10 µg of this metaphase blocking agent. Similar results were obtained in three studies with cytosine arabinoside, wherein there was a 20 to 46% reduction in binding using 10 µg of ARA-C per culture. The inhibition of binding by ARA-C was nearly identical in both the bone marrow and fetal liver (Table 3). This cycle active agent caused a 46% decrease in binding with bone marrow and a 38% reduction with fetal liver.

The effect of irradiation on marrow and spleen cell binding is shown in Table 4. Marrow cultures were unaffected by 300 to 900 rads. There was, however, a

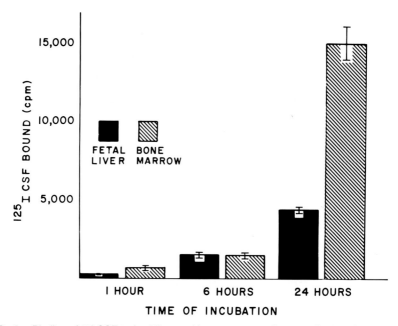

FIG. 2. Binding of ^{125}I CSF to fetal liver and bone marrow cells: 10^7 cells were incubated with 275,000 cpm of tracer for 1, 6, and 24 hr, and specific uptake of radioactivity was determined. Values are means $\pm$ 1 SE from triplicate cultures.

12% reduction in binding at the 1,200 rad dose level ($p < 0.01$). Spleen cell cultures showed a significant reduction in binding at all doses of irradiation which suggests that a higher proportion of CSF responsive cells may have been in an active phase of the cell cycle.

Further characterization of the cell types involved was undertaken using marrow cells separated by Ficoll-Hypaque density gradient centrifugation. Differential counts and colony forming assays are shown in Table 5. Increased numbers of lymphocytes were found in the top layer of the gradient, whereas red cell precursors and mature cells of the granulocytic series were partially concentrated in the bottom layer. A twofold increase in CFU-C was detected in the top layer; however, none were cultured from cells from the bottom of the gradient. CSF binding is depicted in Fig. 4. Despite the concentration of CFU-C in the top layer, a greater degree of binding was apparent in the denser cell population. A repeat study evaluated the effect of ARA-C on the CSF responsive cells in each layer (Fig. 5). A 21% reduction in binding was seen with unseparated cells. Although less total ^{125}I CSF was incorporated into cells from the top layer of the gradient, a much higher percentage (70%) of these cells appeared to be in DNA synthesis as judged by inhibition by ARA-C. Cells from the bottom of the gradient, which did not contain detectable CFU-C, showed a greater degree of cellular binding but only a 19% decrease with ARA-C.

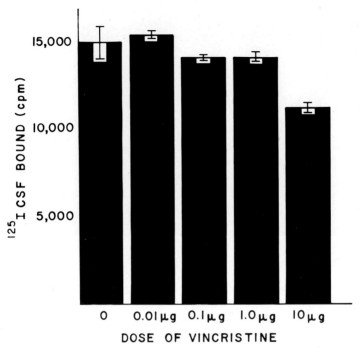

FIG. 3. The effect of vincristine on binding of ^{125}I CSF to bone marrow. Triplicate cultures were incubated with a saturating dose of tracer for 24 hr in the presence of varying doses of vincristine. Values are means ± 1 SE.

TABLE 3. *Effect of cytosine arabinoside on CSF binding[a]*

| Cell source | Specific binding (cpm) | |
	Control	ARA-C
Bone marrow	14,950 ± 909	8,125 ± 440
Fetal liver	2,101 ± 265	1,292 ± 149

[a]Values depict the cpm bound after 24 hr incubation with or without 10 μg/ml of cytosine arabinoside (ARA-C). Numbers are means ±1 SE from triplicate cultures.

DISCUSSION

The studies presented in this chapter show that CSF binds in a specific fashion to certain cells in murine bone marrow, spleen, and fetal liver suspensions. These findings extend our previous observations of marrow cell binding in which the interaction of CSF with marrow cells is both saturable and specific (8). The latter conclusion derives from control studies in which CSF does not bind to lymph node, thymic, hepatic, or renal cells. Moreover, the incorporation of marrow cell radio-

TABLE 4. *The effect of irradiation on marrow and spleen binding of* ^{125}I *CSF[a]*

Dose of irradiation (rads)	Specific binding (cpm)	
	Marrow cells	Spleen cells
0	14,034 ± 98	1,938 ± 113
300	13,970 ± 181	1,432 ± 71[b]
600	12,983 ± 1,302	1,355 ± 18[c]
900	13,703 ± 377	1,139 ± 65[c]
1,200	12,542 ± 190[c]	926 ± 133[c]

[a]Numbers denote the specific cpm bound after 24 hr incubation. All cultures were prepared simultaneously and irradiated prior to incubation. Values are means ±1 SE from triplicate cultures.
[b]$p < 0.05$.
[c]$p < 0.01$.

TABLE 5. *The morphology and colony forming potential of marrow cells separated by Ficoll-Hypaque centrifugation[a]*

Marrow source	Lymphocyte	Normoblast	Blast	Pro	Myelo	Meta	Poly	CFU-C/10^5 cells
Unseparated cells	26.5	30.5	1.5	1.0	7.5	5.5	26.0	151 ± 6
Top layer FH	73.5	3.5	4.0	0	2.5	10.0	5.5	359 ± 8
Bottom layer FH	36.5	30.0	0.5	1.5	5.0	8.0	15.5	0

[a]Counts were determined using 200 cell differentials. Numbers represent the percent of each cell type. CFU-C assays were performed in agar gel using five samples per point. Values are means ±1 SE. Colonies from the top layer of Ficoll-Hypaque (FH) were calculated from assays done using 5×10^4 cells/plate.

activity is blocked by purifed CSF but not by a variety of unrelated proteins. Further control observations have shown no binding of iodinated CSF to human marrow (which is unresponsive to L-cell CSF) and only limited binding to peritoneal exudate macrophages. Further specificity studies are presented herein which indicate that cellular accumulation of radioactivity is not due to ingestion or binding of radio-labeled sodium iodide. In addition, the binding is not blocked by addition of excess cold iodide.

The binding of CSF to bone marrow, spleen, and fetal liver cells differs from the binding of other types of polypeptide hormones to their specific target cells. In the case of insulin and related hormones, cellular binding occurs at 4°C with maximal binding over a 15 min to 1 hr interval (10). In contrast, virtually no CSF binding occurs at reduced temperatures. This time delay does not appear related to "activation" of the tracer, as unbound radiolabeled CSF removed after 24 hr incubation with marrow cells still requires a 24 hr time delay for binding to fresh marrow cells (8). Instead, the delay in binding appears to be a cellular phenomenon. Preincubation of marrow cells for 12 to 15 hr prior to addition of the tracer leads to a rapid binding of CSF at 4°C over a 5 min to 3 hr interval (13). Recent studies suggest that this increase in binding sites may be due to synthesis of receptors as subsequent binding

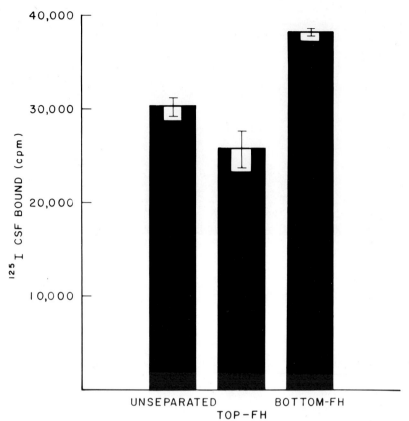

FIG. 4. The binding of ^{125}I CSF to bone marrow cells separated by Ficoll-Hypaque density gradients: 10^7 unseparated cells as well as those from the top and bottom of the gradient were incubated with tracer for 24 hr. Values represent specific binding from triplicate cultures. Numbers are means ± 1 SE.

is blocked if cycloheximide (a potent inhibitor of protein synthesis) is included during the preincubation phase. Thus as described in the present studies, CSF binding appears to require both the synthesis of binding proteins as well as the specific interaction of CSF with certain hemopoietic cells.

Since bone marrow, spleen, and fetal liver cells are known sources of granulocyte-macrophage colony forming cells (CFU-C), it is tempting to speculate that CSF is binding only to these hemopoietic stem cells. The differences in total binding may, in part, be explained by differences in CFU-C in these various tissues. However, as shown in these studies, there are wide differences in differential counts in these tissues. Large numbers of mature granulocytic cells are found in the bone marrow with a relative paucity of these cells in the fetal liver. Since CFU-C are rapidly cycling with approximately 40% of the cells in DNA synthesis over 2 hr (9), drugs which specifically act on proliferative cells would be expected to inhibit binding to the CFU-C if included during the 24 hr period of incubation. As shown in these

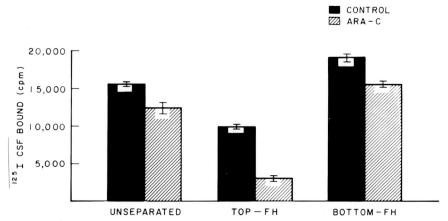

FIG. 5.   The effect of ARA-C on bone marrow cell binding. Unseparated as well as top and bottom layer cells from the Ficoll-Hypaque gradient were incubated with tracer for 24 hr alone or in the presence of 10 μg/ml of ARA-C. Values are means ± 1 SE from triplicate cultures.

studies, vincristine and cytosine arabinoside yielded modest reductions in cellular binding; however, the degree of inhibition was less than would be anticipated if all CFU-C had entered the cell cycle during the 24 hr period of incubation. In addition, irradiation with 900 to 1,200 rads, which is known to kill all CFU-C, did not markedly reduce the cellular uptake of bone marrow radioactivity. The finding of a greater reduction in spleen binding with irradiation as compared to marrow cell binding may be due to a greater ratio of CFU-C to mature cells in this organ as compared to the marrow.

Further characterization of the hemopoietic cells which bind CSF was conducted using bone marrow cells separated by Ficoll-Hypaque density gradient centrifugation. Although all CFU-C were selectively concentrated in the upper portion of the gradient, CSF bound to both the top and bottom layer of cells. Differential counts showed an increase in mature cells of the granulocytic series in the bottom layer, suggesting that these cells are also capable of binding CSF. Incubation of both top and bottom layer cells with cytosine arabinoside confirmed the impression that CSF indeed binds to different classes of cells. The top layer of cells appeared to be a highly proliferative population as judged by a 70% reduction in binding when incubated with ARA-C. In contrast, cells from the bottom layer, which did not contain any detectable CFU-C, had only a slight reduction of binding in the presence of ARA-C.

These findings clearly indicate that CSF binds to both proliferative and nonproliferative cells, but they do not indicate which of the many cells in the marrow, spleen, and fetal liver are involved in the binding reaction. Recent autoradiographic studies done in collaboration with Dr. Lewis Schiffer of Allegheny General Hospital in Pittsburgh help to resolve this question (7). Autoradiographs show that, after 6 hr of incubation, binding to bone marrow and fetal liver cells is confined to large mononuclear cells and proliferative elements of the granulocytic series. With incubation for 24 hr to achieve plateau binding, all blasts and promyelocytes are labeled, with as many as 50% of later cells in the granulocytic series incorporating the label. It is noteworthy that no binding is detected with lymphocytes, erythroblasts, megakaryocytes, or eosinophils.

Although CSF is believed to function primarily as a regulator of granulocyte and macrophage production, there are several observations which suggest that this material may also act on more mature cells of the granulocyte-macrophage series. First, CSF is known to induce RNA synthesis in suspensions of mature neutrophilic granulocytes (2). Secondly, recent studies in our laboratory have shown specific activation of mature macrophages to induce tumoristatic and tumoricidal activity in response to CSF (16). When coupled with the data reported herein, it appears that CSF may act on all levels of maturation in the granulocyte and macrophage series. Using the model systems outlined in this report, further study of receptor binding in normal as well as leukemic populations may help to unravel the many defects which exist in granulocyte maturation.

ACKNOWLEDGMENTS

The authors gratefully appreciate the excellent technical assistance of Mrs. Florence Boegel, Mrs. Donna Hodge, and Mrs. Ellen Turpening. These studies were supported in part by NIH Grant no. RO1CA15237.

REFERENCES

1. Burgess, A. W., Camakaris, J., and Metcalf, D. (1977): Purification and properties of colony-stimulating factor from mouse lung-conditioned medium. *J. Biol. Chem.*, 252:1998–2003.
2. Burgess, A. W., and Metcalf, D. (1977): The effect of colony stimulating factor on the synthesis of ribonucleic acid by mouse bone marrow cells in vitro. *J. Cell. Physiol.*, 90:471–483.
3. Metcalf, D., and Foster, R. (1967): Behavior on transfer of serum stimulated bone marrow colonies. *Proc. Soc. Exp. Biol. Med.*, 75:89–100.
4. Metcalf, D. (1970): Studies on colony formation in vitro by mouse bone marrow cells. II. Action of colony stimulating factor. *J. Cell. Physiol.*, 76:89–100.
5. Metcalf, D. (1973): Regulation of granulocyte and monocyte-macrophage proliferation by colony stimulating factor (CSF): a review. *Exp. Hematol.*, 1:185–201.
6. Paran, M., and Sachs, L. (1968): The continued requirement for inducer for the development of macrophage and granulocyte colonies. *J. Cell. Physiol.*, 72:247–250.
7. Pigoli, G., Shadduck, R. K., and Schiffer, L. M. (1980): Binding of radiolabeled colony stimulating factor to bone marrow and fetal liver cells: autoradiographic studies. *Clin. Res.*, 28:320A.
8. Pigoli, G., Waheed, A., and Shadduck, R. K. (1982): Observations on the binding and interaction of radioiodinated colony stimulating factor with murine bone marrow cells in vitro. *Blood*, 59:408–420.
9. Rickard, K. A., Shadduck, R. K., and Stohlman, F., Jr. (1970): A differential effect of hydroxyurea on hemopoietic stem cell colonies in vitro and in vivo. *Proc. Soc. Exp. Biol. Med.*, 134:152–156.
10. Roth, J. (1973): Peptide hormone binding to receptors: a review of direct studies in vitro. *Metabolism*, 22:1059–1073.
11. Shadduck, R. K., and Nagabhushanam, N. G. (1971): Granulocyte colony stimulating factor. I. Response to acute granulocytopenia. *Blood*, 38:559–568.
12. Shadduck, R. K., Waheed, A., Porcellini, A., Rizzoli, V., and Pigoli, G. (1979): Physiologic distribution of colony stimulating factor in vivo. *Blood*, 54:894–905.
13. Shadduck, R. K., Waheed, A., and Caramatti, C. (1981): The effect of pre-incubation of bone marrow cells on the binding of colony stimulating factor. *Clin. Res.*, 29:522A.

14. Stanley, E. R., and Heard, P. M. (1977): Factors regulating macrophage production and growth. Purification and some properties of the colony stimulating factor from medium conditioned by mouse L-cells. *J. Biol. Chem.*, 252:4305–4312.
15. Waheed, A., and Shadduck, R. K. (1979): Purification and properties of L-cell derived colony stimulating factor. *J. Lab. Clin. Med.*, 94:180–194.
16. Wing, E. J., Waheed, A., Shadduck, R. K., Nagle, L. S., and Stevenson, K. (1928): Effect of colony stimulating factor on murine macrophages: Induction of antitumor activity. *J. Clin. Invest.*, 69:270–276.

Maturation Factors and Cancer,
edited by Malcolm A. S. Moore.
Raven Press, © New York 1982.

Potential Therapeutic Value of Endogenous Stem Cell Proliferation Regulators

B. I. Lord and E. G. Wright

Paterson Laboratories, Christie Hospital and Holt Radium Institute, Manchester M20 9BX, England

It is well recognized that hemopoietic tissue is one of the most sensitive tissues in the body to cytotoxic therapy procedures, particularly when the therapy is administered in a fractionated manner over a period of time. Experimentally, it is known that in mice, hemopoietic stem cells, defined here as spleen colony forming units, CFU-S (23), are normally insensitive to S-phase toxic agents such as hydroxyurea, cytosine arabinoside, or tritiated thymidine, because under normal steady state conditions, the proportion of stem cells in DNA synthesis is < 10% (1). However, due to the concomitant damage to their more rapidly proliferating differentiated progeny, the normally quiescent stem cells enter a proliferation phase and become sensitive to subsequent doses of the cytotoxic agent. For example, four successive doses of hydroxyurea (1 mg/g) given 7 hr apart reduce CFU-S numbers to <10% of normal (10).

Damage to this tissue is therefore a most important consideration when developing therapeutic regimes which are suitable for tackling the various proliferative and neoplastic disorders. This is especially true when chemotherapy is indicated since it is likely that all regions of hemopoiesis will be affected. Thus dosages required for the destruction of a disordered growth are necessarily limited by the damage expected to accrue to hemopoiesis. An understanding of the normal physiological regulatory processes operative in hemopoietic tissue can, therefore, potentially lead to a means of protecting, selectively, the stem cell population during cytotoxic therapy procedures.

In the narrower, though no less important, field of leukemia, understanding of the regulation of hemopoietic stem cell behavior is also of paramount importance both from the theoretical and, potentially, the therapeutic points of view. The studies reviewed below illustrate our current understanding of the regulation of hemopoietic stem cell proliferation and illustrate some possible potential uses in the control and/or normalization of proliferative and neoplastic disorders.

LOCAL CONTROL OF STEM CELL PROLIFERATION

Several publications have demonstrated that the control of stem cell proliferation is essentially a local phenomenon. In 1970, Croizat et al. (3), shielding one limb of a mouse while irradiating the rest of the animal, found complementary changes in the number and kinetics of the CFU-S in the shielded and nonshielded bone marrow. This work was extended and confirmed by Gidali and Lajtha (7), who gave 600 rads X-rays to a similarly shielded mouse. They observed an early reduction in CFU-S numbers in the shielded leg accompanied by a rise in the proliferation rate of those remaining. This loss of CFU-S was almost certainly due to migration for reestablishing hemopoiesis in the heavily irradiated marrow spaces. The interesting feature of this experiment, however, was that within 5 days, the CFU-S number and proliferation in the shielded limb had returned to normal, while in the irradiated regions, regeneration was far from complete: what CFU-S were present were few in number and proliferating rapidly. Thus local control of CFU-S proliferation had determined, in the shielded limb, that the marrow population was now normal with no further need for proliferation despite the overall excess demands of the animal.

At about the same time, Rencricca et al. (22), and later Wright and Lord (26), showed that in an acute phenylhydrazine induced hemolytic anemia, CFU-S migrated to the spleen from the marrow. This led to a rapidly proliferating though diminished marrow CFU-S population concomitant with an enlarged, quiescent splenic CFU-S population. Here again, therefore, the direct regulation of CFU-S proliferation is clearly governed by the local rather than by circulating systemic factors. The nature of these local conditions, the cellular environment, etc., thus became the subject of investigation into the regulation of hemopoietic stem cell proliferation.

MANIPULATION OF CFU-S PROLIFERATION BY ENDOGENOUS FACTORS IN HEMOPOIETIC TISSUE

Two basic approaches were made in this study. In the first phase, simple saline washings of hemopoietic cell suspensions were partially purified by passing through Amicon Diaflo ultrafiltration membranes to give a series of fractions with nominal molecular weight cutoff values of 10,000, 30,000, 50,000, and 100,000 daltons. Two particular fractions, the 30,000 to 50,000 daltons (fraction III) and the 50,000 to 100,000 (fraction IV) daltons, proved interesting, and for the purposes of this chapter, results on other fractions will be omitted.

The fractions were assayed for their effect on CFU-S proliferation by the tritiated thymidine (^{3}HTdR) suicide technique (1,15). Full details of the experimental procedures have been published previously (19). In essence, the assessment of inhibition was made by reduction in ^{3}HTdR kill of rapidly proliferating regenerating bone marrow CFU-S following a period of 4½ hr of incubation with the test extract.

The second approach utilized the different rates of CFU-S proliferation in phenylhydrazine (PHZ) treated mice described above. Again, the details of the experimental methods have been published previously (26). In brief, either proliferating PHZ-treated bone marrow CFU-S were incubated with a suspension of irradiated

PHZ-treated spleen cells or nonproliferating PHZ-treated spleen CFU-S were incubated with PHZ-treated bone marrow cells. These mixtures were assayed, respectively, for proliferation, inhibition, and stimulation as above.

The results of these assays are summarized in Table 1. Normal bone marrow extract fraction-IV (NBME-IV) and spleen cells from PHZ-treated mice both protect rapidly proliferating CFU-S from the lethal effect of a large dose (200 μCi/ml) of ^{3}HTdR. The equivalent fraction from regenerating bone marrow containing rapidly proliferating CFU-S does not inhibit. Conversely, regenerating bone marrow extract fraction III (RBME-III) and bone marrow from PHZ-treated mice both stimulate slowly proliferating CFU-S, leaving them sensitive to the incorporation of ^{3}HTdR. Fraction III from normal bone marrow does not similarly stimulate.

Dose response studies showed that 20 to 40 μg of dried NBME-IV and 10 μg of dried RBME-III per ml of incubation mixture containing 5×10^6 regenerating or normal bone marrow cells, respectively, were found to be the minimum effective doses. In neither case is there any effect on the number of CFU-S in the target population, so the extracts can be considered noncytotoxic. All other fractions affected neither CFU-S number nor ^{3}HTdR kill.

NBME-IV was further found to be specific for CFU-S. A similar ^{3}HTdR suicide assay carried out on the more rapidly proliferating direct progeny of CFU-S, the GM-CFC (the granulocyte/macrophage committed colony-forming cell), assayed by culture in agar (2,21), was unaffected by treatment with the inhibitor (19). A direct specificity assay for the stimulator is more difficult to carry out, but it has proved negative as a colony stimulating activity in the GM-CFC assay and negative also as a lymphocyte mitogen (14).

TABLE 1. *Stimulation and inhibition of CFU-S by hemopoietic tissue extracts[a]*

Target CFU-S	Treatment	CFU-S/10^6 cells	Percent CFU-S in DNA synthesis
Regenerating bone marrow	—	206 ± 17	31.3 ± 1.0
	RBME-IV	201 ± 15	29.2 ± 0.6
	NBME-IV	187 ± 14	4.5 ± 1.0
PHZ treated bone marrow	—	123 ± 15	41.8 ± 8.0
	PHZ treated spleen cells[b]	117 ± 10	9.2 ± 5.3
Normal bone marrow	—	250 ± 16	8.8 ± 5.3
	NBME-III	246 ± 24	4.4 ± 13.2
	RBME-III	249 ± 17	36.5 ± 6.9
PHZ treated spleen	—	22 ± 2	6.4 ± 5.1
	PHZ treated bone marrow cells[b]	24 ± 2	38.8 ± 6.1

[a]NBME, normal bone marrow extract; RBME, regenerating bone marrow extract; III, 30,000–50,000 daltons fraction; IV, 50,000–100,000 daltons fraction; PHZ, phenylhydrazine.
[b]Cells irradiated with 900 rads; ^{137}Cs-γ rays.

A similarly active inhibitor and stimulator of CFU-S proliferation has been reported by Frindel and her colleagues. Apart from its ability to trigger CFU-S into the ^{3}HTdR sensitive phase, no details are available for their stimulator, which was described simply as a diffusible factor present in cytotoxically damaged bone marrow (5). More information is available for their inhibitor, which was obtained as the dialysable product of a frozen fetal bone marrow extract (6). Thus it appears to be a considerably smaller molecule than that reported above. Nevertheless, it has been reported to be noncytotoxic and specifically inhibitory to CFU-S. The differences are not yet understood, but it seems probable that they may lie in the methods of preparation and handling.

To date, extracts from a number of different sites of hemopoietic tissue have been tested (27), and as shown in the generalized Table 2, when the source is one containing rapidly proliferating CFU-S, then stimulator is present. In reverse, when the source contains slowly proliferating CFU-S, then inhibitor is present.

It appears, therefore, that these endogenously derived factors are capable of switching CFU-S proliferation on and off more or less at will. A study designed to investigate this possibility was, therefore, carried out using NBME-IV and RBME-III in competition experiments (18). The results summarized in Table 3 show that the excess inhibitor prevents the stimulation of resting CFU-S when applied at the same time as stimulator or abrogates the stimulation when applied 1 hr later. Similarly, excess stimulator will either prevent inhibition of rapidly proliferating CFU-S or restimulate them, depending on the times of application. The successful application of these experiments depended on the careful selection of dosages, and the appropriate dose response studies have, of course, been carried out (17,27).

Based on these results, it is tempting to speculate that NBME-IV and RBME-III represent physiological factors and that the level of stem cell proliferation is regulated by the balance of inhibitor and stimulator present. More complete studies of extracts from fractionated hemopoietic cell populations show, in fact, irrespective of the proliferative status of the CFU-S, that all hemopoietic tissue contains both

TABLE 2. *Effect of interaction between various grades of hemopoietic tissue on CFU-S proliferation*

Target CFU-S	Source of factor	Effect on CFU-S
Normal bone marrow	Regenerating bone marrow	Stimulation
	Regenerating spleen	
PHA treated spleen	PHZ treated bone marrow	
	Fetal liver	
(Low CFU-S proliferation)	(High CFU-S proliferation)	
Regenerating bone marrow		Inhibition
Regenerating spleen	Normal bone marrow	
PHZ treated bone marrow	PHZ treated spleen	
Fetal liver		
(High CFU-S proliferation)	(Low CFU-S proliferation)	

TABLE 3. *Interaction of CFU-S proliferation stimulator and inhibitor*

Target CFU-S	Treatment	% CFU-S in DNA synthesis
Normal bone marrow	—	8.0 ± 4.5
	RBME-III + NBME-IV (applied together)	2.5 ± 4.5
	RBME-III	39.1 ± 6.1
	RBME-III + NBME-IV (applied 1 hr separated)	1.3 ± 2.2
Regenerating bone marrow	—	26.4 ± 7.2
	NBME-IV + RBME-III (applied together)	44.6 ± 5.1
	NBME-IV	5.8 ± 5.6
	NBME-IV + RBME-III (applied 1 hr separated)	28.6 ± 11.0

inhibitor and stimulator producing cells (27) in quantities approximately related to the level of CFU-S proliferation (27). Furthermore, recent studies with an inhibitor of protein synthesis (cycloheximide) have shown that the inhibitor, at least, is actively and continuously produced in the cells (25).

SPECIES SPECIFICITY

Originally, the inhibitor was made from mouse bone marrow and, of course, assayed against mouse CFU-S. However, in the search for a more abundant supply of material, extracts have been made also from rat, rabbit, and pig marrow. The French group used fetal calf marrow. All yield active inhibitory material, and our standard source is now pig marrow. (One set of pig ribs yields as much inhibitor as about 400 mice, and much extra material can also be obtained from other parts of the skeleton.) Since all these extracts must necessarily be assayed against mouse CFU-S, inhibitor is clearly not species-specific. In addition, human marrow, fresh or grown in long term culture (20) for 2 and 6 weeks, also produces the inhibitor in equivalent proportions to the other sources (16,29). It should be noted that the human extract, like the others, is specific for the stem cells. It is, of course, not practicable to assay it against human stem cells, but it is active against mouse CFU-S while not affecting either murine or human GM-CFC (16,29).

Sources of actively proliferating hemopoietic stem cells are less common, with the result that studies of species specificity for the stimulator have so far been minimal. However, it has recently been shown that human fetal liver is a very rich source of stimulator (A. Riches, personal communication). It seems probable, therefore, that the stimulator is equally not species-specific.

EFFECTS IN LONG TERM MARROW CULTURES

Having established the efficiency of the factors in modifying the proportion of CFU-S in DNA synthesis as a result of a short exposure to the extracts, the next step was to investigate their role in the long term culture of hemopoietic cells as developed by Dexter et al. (4). It had already been established (5,28) over a period of two feeding cycles for the culture (14 days) that within 1 day of feeding, CFU-S were cycling rapidly, 40 to 50% being killed by ^{3}HTdR. This high level of proliferation was maintained to day 4 postfeeding, after which it fell to nonsignificant levels by day 5 and remained at this low quiescent level until the culture was refed on day 7. This pattern was clearly repeated for each subsequent feeding cycle (5,29).

Assay of the spent medium from day 7 cultures, when CFU-S cycling was low, readily showed the presence of inhibitor, which could be extracted, fractionated, and used as for normal marrow extracts (24). This was also true for the human marrow cultures as mentioned above (16,29). Medium from cultures fed 1 day previously, on the other hand, contained stimulator, which also could be harvested and used in the same way as RBME-III (24). Thus CFU-S proliferation in the culture appears to be regulated in the same way as in freshly obtained marrow preparations.

Over the longer term, application of the extracts directly to the cultures modified the patterns of CFU-S proliferation very markedly. Table 4 shows the effect of treating cultures, 1 day after feeding with NBME-IV. While the untreated cultures behave as described above, giving a wave of CFU-S cycling from day 1 to 4, the treated cultures rapidly slow down and become fully quiescent within 1 day (24). Similarly, CFU-S in quiescent cultures treated, without feeding at 7 days, on day 8 are rapidly triggered into DNA synthesis, and the high rate of cycling is maintained for at least the next 5 days (24) (Table 5). The control cultures remain quiescent.

These changes in proliferation characteristics have not yet been fully related to changes in cell number, but it should be remembered that the cultures pass through

TABLE 4. *Proportion of CFU-S killed by*
^{3} HTdR in long term marrow cultures treated with NBME-IV[a]

Time postfeeding[b] (days)	% CFU-S in DNA synthesis	
	Control	NBME-IV treated[c]
0	7 ± 6	7 ± 6
1	40 ± 7	40 ± 7
1.25		27 ± 4
1.5		17 ± 6
1.75		5 ± 8
2		5 ± 2
3	37 ± 2	7 ± 5
4	29 ± 8	12 ± 6
5	4 ± 9	
7	10 ± 4	
8	4 ± 5	

[a]Combined data for adherent and nonadherent culture cells. Adapted from Toksöz et al. (24).
[b]Culture fed at 7 days after the previous feeding.
[c]Cultures treated with NBME-IV at 1 day postfeeding.

TABLE 5. *Proportion of CFU-S killed by [3]HTdR in long term marrow cultures treated with RBME-III[a]*

Time postfeeding[b] (days)	% CFU-S in DNA synthesis	
	Control	RBME-III treated[c]
7	2 ± 11	2 ± 11
8	4 ± 3	4 ± 3
8.3		36 ± 10
9		38 ± 8
9.3		41 ± 9
10	8 ± 5	40 ± 9
11		46 ± 9
12	4 ± 4	40 ± 8
13	8 ± 5	47 ± 9

[a]Combined data for adherent and nonadherent culture cells. Adapted from Toksöz et al. (25).
[b]Cultures were left unfed at the normal 7 day interval.
[c]Cultures treated with RBME-IV at 8 days postfeeding.

this active growth phase in each feeding cycle for many weeks with differentiation from the stem cell taking place continuously. An increased CFU-S proliferation rate does not, therefore, necessarily mean an increase in CFU-S number. Nevertheless, the changes in proliferation rates observed do indicate the possibility of externally controlling proliferation over extended periods of time.

ACTIVITY OF NBME-IV *IN VIVO*

While NBME-IV and RBME-III may well contain physiological regulators of hemopoietic stem cell proliferation as illustrated by the above *in vitro* experiments, they can have no practical value unless they are equally effective *in vivo*. In fact, there is no *a priori* reason to believe that they can be made to work *in vivo*. Bearing in mind the initial premise for the investigation of bone marrow extracts, i.e., the highly localized nature of stem cell proliferation control, it might be expected that following administration, their activity would be destroyed or removed before reaching any appropriate sites of hemopoietic tissue. Nevertheless, the inhibitory extract NBME-IV has been tested *in vivo*. Initially, it was tested for a direct effect on CFU-S proliferation. Phenylhydrazine treated mice, in which the bone marrow CFU-S were proliferating rapidly (i.e., 7 days post-PHZ treatment; ref. 26), were injected intravenously with 1 mg of NBME-IV. Four hours later, an *in vivo* suicide measurement was made. The results (Table 6) show a reduction in the proportion of cells in DNA synthesis, clearly indicating that in spite of the local control phenomenon, NBME-IV can be effective *in vivo*. The dose used was large by comparison with that used in the *in vitro* experiments, and the explanation for its effectiveness may lie simply in that excess, a sufficiently large pool proving enough for an adequate dose to reach the marrow.

Also shown in Table 6 are the original results of Frindel and Guigon (6). These were for mice irradiated with 150 rads, 22 hr before injecting two doses of their

TABLE 6. *In vitro effects of bone marrow extracts on the proportion of CFU-S in DNA synthesis*

	CFU-S per femur	% CFU-S in DNA synthesis
PHZ control mice	2,999 ± 385	24 ± 4
PHZ mice treated with NBME-IV	2,876 ± 185	3 ± 7
Irradiated control mice[a]	34 ± 5[b]	44 ± 5
Irradiated mice treated with bone marrow extract	38 ± 6[b]	3 ± 12

[a]Data from Frindel and Guigon (6).
[b]CFU-S per 10^6 cells injected.

TABLE 7. *Effect of NBME-IV on the recovery of the CFU-S population in vivo following cytotoxic S-phase treatment with hydroxyurea (HU)*

Time (hrs)		Inoculation		
0		HU	HU	HU
3			NBME-IV[a]	NBME-IV[b]
6				NBME-IV
7		HU	HU	HU
CFU-S/femur	~4,000	630 ± 20	1,100 ± 40	1,360 ± 60

[a]1 mg/mouse.
[b]0.5 mg/mouse.

extracts, and they indicate a reduction in kill from 44 to 3%. Again, it may well have been the very large dose (a total of 4 mg protein) which permitted the extract to be effective. In neither case was there any sign of CFU-S toxicity from the extracts, CFU-S per femur and per 10^6 cells injected remaining unaffected.

The *in vivo* observations were then extended, utilizing the results obtained by Hodgson and Blackett (10,11). They showed that while a single injection of hydroxyurea (HU) at 900 mg/kg killed very few CFU-S, the subsequent HU block of entry into DNA synthesis (which lasts for about 4 hr at this dose) caused a partial synchronization of the population. A second dose of HU at 7 hr thus killed a large proportion of CFU-S. NBME-IV was, therefore, injected during the HU induced blockage in an attempt to extend it beyond the period of the second HU injection. Assay of the CFU-S population was delayed 2 days after the HU injection so that rather than measure any direct protection against the second HU kill, one could measure the potential recovery effected by the use of NBME-IV. Table 7 shows the results. Two doses of HU resulted in 630 CFU-S/femur 2 hr later. A single dose of NBME-IV at 3 hr resulted in 1,100 CFU-S per femur, while giving the NBME-IV as two half doses at 3 and 6 hr improved the yield further to 1,360 per femur. Thus NBME-IV injected before CFU-S are released from the HU block significantly delays further their release, so that fewer CFU-S are killed by the second dose and a better recovery is effected. In these experiments, the efficiency of the protection afforded by NBME-IV was not good. Fractionating the dose improved the efficiency, and no doubt the time-dose relationships can be refined to give more complete protection.

Guigon and Frindel (9) have also shown that their bone marrow extract, injected into mice together with cytosine arabinoside, ARA-C, prevented the production of a stimulating factor assayed *in vitro*. More recently, they have also presented preliminary results which indicate that the bone marrow extract increases CFU-S survival after ARA-C treatment (8). Thus it seems probable that an endogenously derived hemopoietic stem cell proliferation could be used to manipulate the level of CFU-S cycling.

POTENTIAL THERAPEUTIC USE

The above experiments will of course be instantly recognizable as a simple chemotherapeutic regime and thus indicate the most obvious potential use. Protection of the hemopoietic stem cell could allow intensification of protracted treatment schedules which may normally be severely limited by excessive damage to hemopoiesis. In order to develop this aspect of its use, detailed *in vivo* experiments exploring the hemopoietic stem cell responses to NBME-IV *in vivo* are essential.

At the same time, it should be recognized, as Dr. Mertelsman suggested (elsewhere in this volume), that cell kill is not necessarily the sole factor of interest. It is, in fact, often not recognized that the simple assumption that to cure cancer it is necessary to destroy all cancer cells is not tenable. As pointed out by Lajtha and Oliver (13), in a population of tumors, each containing 10^n cells, one would have to kill 10^{n+1} cells to obtain a 90% cure rate. Unfortunately, there is not enough sensitivity difference between normal and cancer cells to allow any drug or radiation dose to permit anything like this degree of tumor cell kill to be tolerated by the normal tissues. The fact that cures are obtained at all suggests that many other factors are involved. The growth of a tumor depends on the balance between proliferation, differentiation, and cell death. One can only assume that the various sophisticated treatments may not only kill and sterilize tumor cells but may in a variety of ways alter the balance so that the net rate of growth of the tumor is decreased. In some cases, differentiation and death may outrun proliferation, and the tumor then declines. This change in balance can be effected by increasing the differentiation (or death) rate, as several groups have tried to exploit (this volume), or by decreasing the proliferation rate. The question is: Do the tumor cells respond at all to the normal proliferation regulators? There are in fact several chapters in this volume showing that tumor cell lines still carry many of the characteristics of the normal cell. It would not be surprising, therefore, if the tumor cells carry some vestige of their normal control, and a neoplastic growth should perhaps not be considered so much as *completely uncontrolled* but rather *incompletely controlled*. An example of this might be the abnormal Philadelphia clone of chronic granulocytic leukemia, which apparently exhibits a lowered sensitivity to the normal inhibitory control processes. Its growth is less restricted, and as a result it eventually becomes the dominant clone (12).

It is conceivable in cases like this that the inhibitory factors could be effective in slowing down the proliferation rate of the abnormal clone to the extent that the tumor growth rate will become negative. In this sense, it will be necessary to study, in detail, the relative responsiveness of normal and abnormal cell types to the normal physiological regulators specific for that cell type.

ACKNOWLEDGMENTS

We would like to thank Mrs. Lorna Woolford for excellent technical assistance. Mrs. A. P. Sheridan maintained the human bone marrow cultures. The work was supported by grants from the Cancer Research Campaign and the Medical Research Council.

REFERENCES

1. Becker, A. J., McCulloch, E. A., Siminovitch, L., and Till, J. E. (1965): The effect of differing demands for blood cell production on DNA synthesis by haemopoietic colony forming cells of mice. *Blood*, 26:296–308.
2. Bradley, T. R., and Metcalf, D. (1966): The growth of mouse bone marrow cells *in vitro*. *Aust. J. Exp. Biol. Med. Sci.*, 44:287–300.
3. Croizat, H., Frindel, E., and Tubiana, M. (1970): Proliferative activity of the stem cells in the bone marrow of mice after single and multiple irradiations (total or partial body exposure). *Int. J. Radiat. Biol.*, 18:347–358.
4. Dexter, T. M., Allen, T. D., and Lajtha, L. G. (1977): Conditions controlling the proliferation of haemopoietic stem cells. *J. Cell. Physiol.*, 91:335–344.
5. Frindel, E., Croizat, H., and Vassort, F. (1976): Stimulating factors liberated by treated bone marrow: in vitro effect on CFU kinetics. *Exp. Hematol.*, 4:56–61.
6. Frindel, E., and Guigon, M. (1977): Inhibition of CFU entry into cycle by a bone marrow extract. *Exp. Hematol.*, 5:74–76.
7. Gidali, J., and Lajtha, L. G. (1972): Regulation of haemopoietic stem cell turnover in partially irradiated mice. *Cell. Tissue Kinet.*, 5:147–157.
8. Guigon, M., Enouf, J., and Frindel, E. (1980): Inhibition of bone marrow cell proliferation. X[th] meeting, Eur. Study Group for Cell Proliferation. Knokke, Belgium. Abstr. No. 36. *Cell Tissue Kinet.*, 13:201.
9. Guigon, M., and Frindel, E. (1978): Inhibition of CFU-S entry into cell cycle after irradiation and drug treatment. *Biomedicine*, 29:176–180.
10. Hodgson, G. S., and Blackett, N. M. (1977): *In vivo* synchronisation of haemopoietic stem cells with hydroxyurea. *Exp. Hematol.*, 5:423–426.
11. Hodgson, G. S., Bradley, T. R., Martin, R. F., Sumner, M., and Fry, P. (1975): Recovery of proliferating haemopoietic progenitor cells after killing by hydroxyurea. *Cell Tissue Kinet.*, 8:51–60.
12. Lajtha, L. G., Lord, B. I., Mori, K. J., and Wright, E. G. (1977): Growth regulations in normal and leukaemic haemopoietic stem cells. *Leukaemia Res.*, 1:153–156.
13. Lajtha, L. G., and Oliver, R. (1961): Some radiobiological considerations in radiotherapy. *Br. J. Radiol.*, 34:252–257.
14. Lord, B. I. (1979): Proliferation regulators in haemopoiesis. In: *Clinics in Haematology: Cellular Dynamics of Haemopoiesis*, edited by L. G. Lajtha, pp. 435–451. W. B. Saunders, London.
15. Lord, B. I., Lajtha, L. G., and Gidali, J. (1974): Measurement of the kinetic status of bone marrow precursor cells: three cautionary tales. *Cell Tissue Kinet.*, 7:507–515.
16. Lord, B. I., and Wright, E. G. (1980): Sources of haemopoietic stem cell proliferation stimulators and inhibitors. *Blood Cells*, 6:581–593.
17. Lord, B. I., Wright, E. G., and Lajtha, L. G. (1979): Actions of the haemopoietic stem cell proliferation inhibitor. *Biochem. Pharmacol.*, 28:1843–1848.
18. Lord, B. I., Mori, K. J., and Wright, E. G. (1977): A stimulator of stem cell proliferation in regenerating bone marrow. *Biomed. Exp.*, 27:223–226.

19. Lord, B. I., Mori, K. J., Wright, E. G., and Lajtha, L. G. (1976): An inhibitor of stem cell proliferation in normal bone marrow. *Br. J. Haematol.*, 34:441–445.
20. Moore, M. A. S., and Sheridan, A. P. (1979): Pluripotential stem cell replication in continuous human, prosimian and murine bone marrow culture. *Blood Cells*, 5:297–311.
21. Pluznik, D. H., and Sachs, L. (1965): The cloning of normal 'mast' cells in tissue culture. *J. Cell. Comp. Physiol.*, 66:319–324.
22. Rencricca, N. J., Rizzoli, V., Howard, D., Duffy, P., and Stohlman, F., Jr. (1970): Stem cell migration and proliferation during severe anaemia. *Blood*, 36:764–771.
23. Till, J. E., and McCulloch, E. A. (1961): A direct measurement of the radiation sensitivity of normal mouse bone marrow cells. *Radiat. Res.*, 14:213–222.
24. Toksöz, D., Dexter, T. M., Lord, B. I., Wright, E. G., and Lajtha, L. G. (1980): The regulation of haemopoiesis in long term bone marrow cultures II. Stimulation and inhibition of stem cell proliferation. *Blood*, 55:931–936.
25. Wright, E. G., Garland, J. M., and Lord, B. I. (1980): Specific inhibition of haemopoietic stem cell proliferation:characteristics of the inhibitor producing cells. *Leuk. Res.*, 4:537–545.
26. Wright, E. G., and Lord, B. I. (1977): Regulation of CFU-S proliferation by locally produced endogenous factors. *Biomed. Exp.*, 27:215–218.
27. Wright, E. G., and Lord, B. I. (1979): Production of stem cell proliferation regulators by fractionated haemopoietic cell suspensions. *Leuk. Res.*, 3:15–22.
28. Wright, E. G., Lord, B. I., Dexter, T. M., and Lajtha, L. G. (1979): Mechanisms of haemopoietic stem cell proliferation control. *Blood Cells*, 5:247–258.
29. Wright, E. G., Sheridan, P., and Moore, M. A. S. (1980): An inhibitor of murine stem cell proliferation produced by normal human bone marrow. *Leukaemic Res.*, 4:309–319.

Maturation Factors and Cancer,
edited by Malcolm A. S. Moore.
Raven Press, © New York 1982.

Cell Contact Modulation by Adherent Cells of Granulopoietic Proliferation and Differentiation

Gary Spitzer, Dharmvir S. Verma, and Miloslav Beran

The University of Texas System Cancer Center, M.D. Anderson Hospital and Tumor Institute, Houston, Texas 77030

Numerous experiments (1) report on the essential role of soluble factors called colony stimulating activity (CSA) for the *in vitro* growth of human or murine granulopoietic colonies (CFU-C). However, the *in vivo* experiments of Queensberry and co-workers (2,3) question the relevance of CSA for the granulopoietic response to repeated endotoxin injections and the granulopoietic growth observed in *in vivo* diffusion chambers. Moreover, the long term growth of murine bone marrow in tissue culture flasks does not appear to require CSA for maintenance of granulopoiesis (4,5).

We, therefore, initiated studies *in vitro* to determine whether marrow cell contact with adherent cells realized a different result from that mediated by factors released by adherent cells *in vitro*. We examined the survival of human normal CFU-C and leukemic CFU-C after short term exposure to adherent cell monolayers derived from human peripheral blood mononuclear cells. Murine CFU-C survival was also tested after short term exposure to adherent cell layers derived from thioglycollate mobilized peritoneal adherent cells.

MATERIAL AND METHODS

Collection and Storage of Human Marrow and Blood

Marrow from patients with acute myeloid leukemia and with greater than 90% myeloblasts was collected by aspiration from previously untreated patients and frozen as previously described (6). To examine normal granulocyte-macrophage colonies (GM-CFC) or eosinophilic colonies (E-CFC), approximately 5 cc of marrow was collected into preservative free heparin from patients with lung cancer who had had no prior chemotherapy or any marrow involvement. Approximately 100 to 200 cc blood from normal volunteers was collected into syringes which had been previously rinsed with preservative free heparin.

Collection of Murine Marrow and Peritoneal Cells

BDF_1 mice, 8 to 10 weeks old, were used for all experiments. Donor mice were sacrificed by cervical dislocation, and both femora were dissected free. The distal femur tip was cut with scissors, 2 ml of Hanks' balanced salt solution (HBSS) was forcefully injected through the needle into the proximal end of the femur, and the expelled marrow was collected and passed through a stainless steel filter. To obtain peritoneal cells, these same age mice were injected intraperitoneally with 2 to 3 ml aged 3% thioglycollate media (Difco, Detroit, Mich.). Four days after injection, cells were harvested into 5 ml of Hanks' balanced salt solution with heparin.

Preparation of Peripheral Blood or Peritoneal Adherent Cell Monolayers

To deplete blood of neutrophils and erythrocytes, human blood was subjected to density centrifugation over Ficoll-isopaque (7). Adherent cell monolayers were then prepared from either washed interface cells or from freshly harvested murine peritoneal cells by incubating 2×10^6 cells/ml, 2 ml total volume, in α-MEM with 15% FCS in Corning #25000 (35 mm) petri dishes for 3 hr. Nonadherent cells were removed by aspirating the media and rinsing the dish two times with phosphate buffered saline (PBS) solution. The number of adherent cells in each dish was calculated by counting the total number of cells recovered, counting the number of cells in $\frac{1}{40}$ of the surface area using an inverted microscope; the count was also confirmed by lysing parallel plates with acetic acid and counting residual nuclei in a coulter counter.

Coincubation Experiments

Nonadherent leukemic cells were prepared by thawing, diluting, washing, and then centrifugation over Ficoll-isopaque to remove nonviable cells. Leukemic cells, now 100% viable as assessed by trypan blue, were then incubated for 3 hr in plastic petri dishes. At the end of this time, nonadherent leukemic cells were removed by several washes with alpha modification of minimal essential media (α-MEM) and pooled. Human bone marrow was first subject to density centrifugation over Ficoll isopaque as described above, and then nonadherent cells were prepared from these interface cells. Marrow nonadherent cells from whole murine bone marrow were similarly prepared.

The first type of coincubation experiment involved preparing various cell fractions (from normal peripheral blood mononuclear cells) and incubating them in 1 ml of α-MEM with 15% FCS containing 5×10^5 target cells (leukemic bone marrow or normal light density bone marrow). Adherent cells were prepared by removing adherent cells from plastic surfaces with a PBS-EDTA-lidocaine solution, and T cell depleted suspensions were prepared by removing E rosette positive cells from mononuclear cell preparations with neuraminidase treated erythrocytes (8).

Immediately upon preparing the cell mixture, half the culture (0.5 ml, 2.5×10^5 target cells) was centrifuged to remove the media. The cells were resuspended in a 5 ml volume of α-MEM with 15% FCS and 0.3% agar and plated on three or four dishes with a final target cell concentration of 0.5×10^5 per dish. The remaining 0.5 ml of the cell mixture was incubated for 4 hr at 37°C in a conical tissue culture tube and then cultured as described above. In these experiments, the number of effector cells was varied to create ratios of mononuclear cells to target cells from 0:1 to 10:1. This kind of coincubation experiment was not complicated by growth from normal mononuclear cells on the seventh day of culture. Clusters from mononuclear cells alone did not occur in numbers greater than 2 per 5×10^5 cells, the maximum number of normal cells present in agar culture in these experiments. Growth of peripheral blood clusters and colonies usually occurs during the second week of culture (9).

In the second experimental protocol for coincubation experiments (Fig. 1), nonadherent leukemic cells or nonadherent normal marrow cells were added in varying numbers to petri dishes with and without normal peripheral blood adherent cells. Nonadherent murine marrow was added at differing cell numbers to petri dishes with and without adherent peritoneal cells. In order to determine the number of nonadherent target cells to be added, the number of adherent cells had to be first calculated. Cells were then added to achieve ratios of 0.5:1, 2:1, and 5:1 adherent normal cells to nonadherent target cells. Cells were then allowed to coincubate for usually 4 hr. Nonadherent cells were then extracted by first removing the supernatant

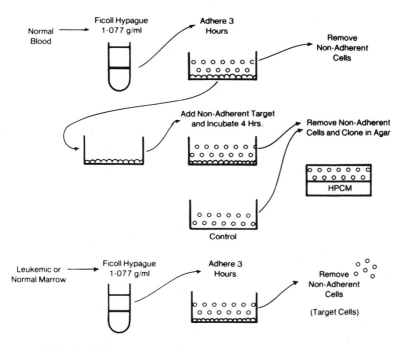

FIG. 1. Coincubation experiments: experimental protocol number 2.

and washing once with α-MEM. The cells were then centrifuged and resuspended to a suitable working volume in single strength media. Cell recoveries at the end of the 4 hr incubation were equivalent to the number of nonadherent cells originally added, suggesting that cells were not lost by adherence and that adherent cells did not lose their adherence during the period of coincubation. Target cells were also 100% viable as assessed by trypan blue and contained 2% or less latex positive cells.

Nonadherent target cells from identical experiments were pooled and cultured at 0.5×10^5 cells/ml in 0.3% agar α-MEM as previously described (10). Human placental conditioned media (HPCM) was used as a source of colony stimulating activity (CSA) for human growth and fibroblast conditioned media (FCM) for murine growth. All cultures were plated in triplicate and leukemic cluster growth (aggregates of 3–39 cells) or normal human or murine GM-CFC (aggregates of 40 cells or greater) were counted after 5 or 8 days of incubation. To exclude any entrapment of leukemic cluster growing cells or GM-CFC in the monolayers, the following controls were performed. The monolayers were overlaid with 0.3% agar α-MEM and HPCM or FCM. No leukemic clusters or GM-CFC could be detected. To eliminate the possibility that prostaglandin E secretion prevented the appearance of leukemic clusters, monolayers were also overlaid with 10^{-6} M indomethacin or monolayer cells were removed with a PBS-EDTA-lidocaine solution and cultured in agar with HPCM at low cell numbers. Again, no leukemic clusters or GM-CFC could be detected.

RESULTS

We initially investigated the possibility that normal peripheral blood contained cells capable of inhibiting leukemic cluster growth by nonspecific mechanisms. The cell populations used were light density (Ficoll-Hypaque < 1.077 g/ml), unfractionated, T cell depleted, adherent cell depleted, and adherent normal mononuclear peripheral blood cells. These were either immediately cocultured with 0.5×10^5 human leukemic cells or, prior to agar culture, preincubated for 4 hr in α-MEM with 15% FCS (experimental protocol 1). Table 1 shows an experiment representative of the effects of normal peripheral mononuclear cells on the growth of leukemic clusters in immediate agar culture. The inhibition of leukemic growth was usually noted with the addition of high numbers of unfractionated mononuclear cells (10:1) and was exaggerated by the removal of T cells or the addition of adherent cells.

Table 2 shows two experiments in which the various mononuclear fractions from normal peripheral blood were preincubated at various normal to leukemic cell ratios for 4 hr in liquid culture prior to agar culture, a procedure that significantly lessened the ratio of normal to leukemic cells required to produce significant inhibition of leukemic growth. In both these coincubation experiments, marked inhibition of leukemic cluster growth was produced by whole mononuclear cells (< 50% inhibition) at mononuclear cell to leukemic cell ratios of 0.5:1. Experiment 2 in Table 2 is the same normal cell-leukemic cell mixture as in Table 1 but with a liquid

TABLE 1. *Effect of coculturing human peripheral blood mononuclear cells with human leukemic cells without coincubation on human leukemic cluster growth[a]*

Ratio normal/leukemic	Cell fractions added from normal mononuclear cells			
	Whole mononuclear	T cell depleted	Adherent cell depleted	Adherent cells
Control	25.3 ± (1.8)[b]	25.3 ± (1.8)	25.3 ± (1.8)	25.3 ± (1.8)
0.2:1	19 ± 4.4	21.6 ± 4	26.6 ± 1.8	32 ± 0
0.5:1	24.6 ± 3.3	19.3 ± 2[c]	32.6 ± 2.4	32.6 ± 2.8
1:1	25.6 ± 4.3	13.3 ± 1.3[d]	27.3 ± 3.2	13.0 ± 2.2[d]
2:1	24.3 ± 2.6	13.0 ± 0.6[e]	30.6 ± 0.7	
10:1	11.6 ± 1.5[d]		25 ± 5.9	

[a]Varying numbers of human peripheral blood mononuclear cells or fractions derived therefrom were cocultured in agar culture with 0.5 × 10[5] leukemic cells. All cultures were cultured in triplicate. Control is 0.5 × 10[5] leukemic cells alone.
[b]Mean ± SEM.
[c]$p < 0.05$.
[d]$p < 0.005$.
[e]$p < 0.001$.

preincubation. If one compares these two sets of data, it is obvious that the inhibition of leukemic cluster growth by populations of whole mononuclear cells and those depleted in T and adherent cells is more marked when preceded by a liquid preincubation. Only in a high cell dose is any inhibition with an adherent cell depleted population obtained.

To assess the specificity of this inhibition, identical experiments were performed to examine the effect of mononuclear cells on normal allogeneic bone marrow growth. Table 3 gives two examples of the results obtained when various mononuclear fractions are cocultured immediately with normal bone marrow. In experiment 2, some inhibition of normal bone marrow growth was produced at ratios of 10:1 (mononuclear cells to normal cells) from both whole mononuclear cell and T cell depleted mononuclear cells suspensions. This inhibition was not produced by mixtures of adherent cells and normal bone marrow at ratios of 2:1, and there was no differential effect on clusters, as colony-to-cluster ratios remained constant at all experimental points. Mononuclear cell fractions were cocultured with normal marrow in liquid prior to agar culture, and some moderate inhibition of colony growth was detected in one of the experiments at a ratio of 1:1 (mononuclear cells to bone marrow) (Table 4). This inhibition was not as marked as that observed on leukemic growth, it occurred at a higher ratio of mononuclear cells to normal cells, and at no experimental points was the ratio of colonies to clusters changed.

The finding that greater inhibition of leukemic growth occurred with liquid preincubation led to further experiments. In the previous coculture experiments, inhibition of leukemic growth could have been due to mechanisms such as direct cell-to-cell contact during the liquid preincubation period and further inhibition by factors released from mononuclear cells during the period of agar culture. To test the

TABLE 2. The effect of four hour preincubation of normal donor peripheral blood mononuclear cells with leukemic cells on leukemic cluster growth[a]

Experiment no.	Ratio normal/leukemic	Cell fractions added from normal mononuclear cells			
		Whole mononuclear	T cell depleted	Adherent cell depleted	Adherent cells
1	0:1	500 ± 55.7[b]	500 ± 55.7	500 ± 55.7	500 ± 55.7
	0.2:1	200 ± 5.7[c]		406.6 ± 6.7	
	0.5:1	53.5 ± 12[d]	181.6 ± 6.7[d]	318 ± 25.9[e]	
	1:1	20.3 ± 0.33[d]	0	360 ± 11.5[e]	
	2:1			201.6 ± 14.8[c]	
2	0:1	23.3 ± 1.3	23.3 ± 1.3	23.3 ± 1.3	23.3 ± 1.3
	0.2:1	16.6 ± 1.3[e]	16.6 ± 1.3[e]	23.3 ± 1.3	16 ± 1[e]
	0.5:1	9.7 ± 1.4[c]	11 ± 3[e]	31.6 ± 3.3	12.6 ± 1.7[c]
	1:1	8.3 ± 1.3[c]	6.3 ± 2.3[f]	23.5 ± 3.3	8 ± 0.6[d]
	2:1	5.0 ± 0.6[d]	4 ± 1.5[c]	24.6 ± 6	
	10:1	4.7 ± 0.3[d]		8.7 ± 1.8[c]	

[a]Varying numbers of mononuclear cells or cell fractions derived from peripheral blood of normal volunteers were incubated with 5 × 10⁵ Ficoll-isopaque concentrated leukemic cells for 4 hr in α-media and 15% FCS. At the end of this incubation period, 0.1 ml cell volumes of resuspended cultures were plated per dish in agar culture. This would give a constant number of 0.5 × 10⁵ leukemic cells in all culture plates. All experimental points were cultured in triplicate. Control is leukemic cells alone.
[b]Mean ± SEM.
[c]p < 0.005.
[d]p < 0.001.
[e]p < 0.05.
[f]p < 0.01.

TABLE 3. *The effect of coculturing human peripheral blood mononuclear cells with normal human marrow cells without preincubation on normal colony growth[a]*

Experiment no.	Ratio blood/marrow	Cell fractions added from normal mononuclear cells				
		Whole mononuclear	T cell depleted	T cell concentrated	Adherent cell depleted	Adherent cells
1	0:1	4 ± 1[b]	4 ± 1	4 ± 1	4 ± 1	4 ± 1
	0.2:1	4 ± 0.8	5.3 ± 0.7	4.3 ± 1	4.3 ± 0.9	3.7 ± 0.3
	0.5:1	4 ± 1.1	4.3 ± 0.9		2.7 ± 0.9	4 ± 0.6
	1:1	4.3 ± 0.6	4 ± 1.5	6 ± 0.6	5.7 ± 0.9	3.3 ± 0.7
	2:1	5 ± 1	3.7 ± 0.3	5.3 ± 0.3	4.3 ± 0.3	5 ± 1
2	0:1	40.6 ± 2.3	40.6 ± 2.3	40.6 ± 2.3	40.6 ± 2.3	40.6 ± 2.3
	0.2:1	50.3 ± 4.3	42 ± 0.6	47.6 ± 0.9	48 ± 1.0	51.6 ± 1.2
	0.5:1	40.3 ± 3.2		48.3 ± 4.3	48.6 ± 1.2	47.3 ± 1.7
	1:1	37 ± 2.1	46 ± 2.9		48.3 ± 5.7	35 ± 4.6
	2:1	38 ± 1.0	34 ± 3.6	42.6 ± 0.3	47.6 ± 4.3	40.6 ± 1.0
	10:1	31 ± 3.0[c]	18.6 ± 2.3[d]	39.6 ± 1.9	44.3 ± 4.5	

[a]Varying numbers of human peripheral blood mononuclear cells or fractions derived therefrom were cocultured in agar culture with 0.5×10^5 light density normal bone marrow cells (<1.078 g/ml). All cultures were in triplicate. Control is normal bone marrow cells alone.
[b]Mean ± SEM.
[c]$p < 0.05$.
[d]$p < 0.001$.

TABLE 4. The effect of four hour preincubation of normal donor peripheral blood mononuclear cells with normal marrow cells on normal colony growth[a]

Experiment no.	Ratio blood/marrow	Cell fractions added from normal mononuclear cells				
		Whole mononuclear	T cell depleted	T cell concentrated	Adherent cell depleted	Adherent cells
1	0:1	5 ± 0.6[b]	5 ± 0.6	5 ± 0.6	5 ± 0.6	5 ± 0.6
	0.2:1	8 ± 1.5	5.7 ± 0.6	8 ± 1.7	4.7 ± 0.8	6 ± 0.4
	0.5:1	4.3 ± 1.4	6 ± 0.6		4 ± 1	5 ± 1
	1:1	5.3 ± 0.7	5.7 ± 1.4	7.7 ± 0.7	3 ± 0.9	6 ± 1.5
	2:1	4.6 ± 1.4	3.7 ± 0.3	6.3 ± 0.7	3 ± 0[e]	6.5 ± 0.4
2	0:1	50 ± 2.6	50 ± 2.6	50 ± 2.6	50 ± 2.6	50 ± 2.6
	0.2:1	54.3 ± 4.2	51 ± 4.4	49 ± 1	51.6 ± 2.6	47 ± 6.0
	0.5:1	46.3 ± 2.9	48 ± 4	48 ± 2.4	47.3 ± 2.4	45.6 ± 3.2
	1:1	39 ± 1.5[c]	31.3 ± 1.9[e]		40.3 ± 1.5[f]	40.3 ± 2.0[f]
	2:1	45.6 ± 0.3	29.3 ± 3.8[c]	42 ± 1.3	41.6 ± 2.4[f]	
	10:1	17.6 ± 0.3[d]	30 ± 0[d]	47.3 ± 3.2	28 ± 3.2[e]	

[a]Varying numbers of mononuclear cells or cell fractions derived from the peripheral blood of normal volunteers were incubated with 5×10^5 Ficoll-isopaque normal bone marrow cells for 4 hr in α-medium and 15% fetal calf serum. At the end of this incubation period, 0.1 ml cell volumes of resuspended cultures were plated per dish in agar culture. This would give a constant number of 0.5×10^5 normal marrow cells in all culture plates. All experimental points were cultured in triplicate. Control is normal bone marrow cells alone.
[b]Mean ± SEM
[c]$p < 0.01$.
[d]$p < 0.001$.
[e]$p < 0.005$.
[f]$p < 0.05$.

involvement of adherent cells in the preincubation phase, adherent cell monolayers from normal peripheral blood were prepared as described above under Material and Methods and incubated with nonadherent leukemic target cells at ratios of adherent cells to leukemic cells of 2:1 and 5:1. After varying periods of incubation, nonadherent cells, which were probably only leukemic (see Material and Methods) were cultured at 0.5×10^5 cells in agar culture with HPCM either with or without adherent cell underlayers. The purpose of this design was to avoid the transfer of normal adherent cells to the solid phase and to allow dissection of the contribution of leukemic growth inhibition mediated by cell-to-cell contact and that mediated by inhibitory factors during the agar phase of culture. When 0.8 to 1×10^6 normal adherent cells (a number not used in the solid phase in the previous coculture experiments) are added to agar culture, inhibition of approximately 60% of leukemic growth occurred (Table 5). However, when leukemic cells were preincubated for 4 hr or overnight with normal adherent cell monolayers and cultured in agar with only HPCM, an 80 to 90% inhibition of leukemic growth occurred (Table 5). This inhibition increased only slightly with the addition of adherent cells in the solid phase, suggesting that most of the inhibition observed in these experiments is mediated by cell-to-cell contact.

A total of 10 normal donors have been used to examine the effect of the adherent cells on this one frozen leukemic sample. When leukemic cells were incubated with adherent cells from 9 of these donors at varying ratios of adherent to leukemic

TABLE 5. *Effect of incubation of nonadherent leukemic cells with normal peripheral blood adherent cells on leukemic cluster formation[a]*

| Ratio normal/leukemic | After preincubation nonadherent cells cultured in agar | | | |
| | With HPCM + | | Without HPCM + | |
	0	Adherent cells from normal blood	0	Adherent cells from normal blood
0:1[b]	1,275	455	0	385
2:1[b]	180	110	0	115
5:1[b]	70	85	0	55
0:1[c]	915	565	0	260
2:1[c]	275	225	0	140
5:1[c]	130	140	0	60

[a]Monolayers containing approximately 1×10^6 cells per 35 mm³ tissue culture petri dish were prepared from human peripheral blood. Nonadherent leukemic cells were incubated in control tissue culture petri dishes or in petri dishes with adherent cells to give final ratios of adherent cells to leukemic cells of 2:1 and 5:1. After 4 or 15 hr incubation, nonadherent leukemic cells were removed and cultured at 0.5×10^5 cells in agar over either human placental conditioned media (HPCM), 1×10^6 adherent mononuclear cells from normal blood, none of these, or combinations of these. Cultures were scored for clusters after 7 days of culture.
[b]Four hr coincubation.
[c]Fifteen hr coincubation.

TABLE 6. *Human peripheral blood adherent cell enhancement of leukemic cluster growth through factors[a]*

Experiment	+HPCM	−HPCM	HPCM + adherent cells	HPCM + adherent cells + 10^{-6} M indomethacin	adherent cells	Adherent cells + 10^{-6} M indomethacin
A	280 ± 30	0	1,100 ± 25	1,255 ± 40	310 ± 23	240 ± 44
B	163 ± 12	0	1,573 ± 55	1,533 ± 60	1,450 ± 39	
C_1	433 ± 21	0	536 ± 29		220 ± 40	
C_2	433 ± 21	0	550 ± 39			

[a]To exclude the possibility of a macrophage soluble factor as the cause of the reduced cluster growth, adherent cells at the same numbers as those used for the coincubation experiments were overlaid with 0.5% agar and α-MEM with or without HPCM or indomethacin, 10^{-6} M. Nonadherent leukemic cells (0.5×10^5 cells) were then cultured in a 0.3% agar α-MEM upper layer, and cultures were scored for leukemic clusters at day 8. Experiments A to C_1 involved adherent cells which had not been previously coincubated with leukemic cells. Experiment C_2 involved using adherent cells from the same donor as in experiment C_1, but which had been used for the leukemic coincubation experiment. Results are means ± SEM. HPCM = human placental conditioned media.

cells, suppression of cluster growth was marked (up to 96%), occurring at low adherent cell to leukemic cell ratios (0.5:1), and this suppression of growth was greater with higher numbers of adherent cells. Only one donor did not show leukemic cell cluster suppression. Because no cluster growing cells were isolated from the adherent monolayers (see Material and Methods), it is unlikely that the mechanism of inhibition of cluster growth is secondary to the entrapment of viable cluster forming cells by the adherent cell layer. To exclude the possibility that this inhibition of leukemic growth was unique to the target cell used, adherent cells from one donor were tested against two different leukemic targets and both were inhibited. With further experiments using three different fresh leukemic cell suspensions, it was shown that inhibition of cluster growth is not unique to frozen cells.

The short period of incubation needed to produce this effect probably indicated a direct cell-to-cell contact mechanism rather than a rapid production of a possible growth inhibitory soluble factor. To partly exclude a soluble factor mechanism, the adherent cell monolayers from three of the donors were overlaid with 0.5% agar α-MEM with and without HPCM or indomethacin at 10^{-6} M. In one experiment, adherent cells that had been previously exposed for 4 hr to leukemic cells were also used. Adherent cells tested in this fashion and at these numbers were frequently more stimulatory to leukemic growth than that achieved with HPCM alone (Table 6). It must be remembered that these underlayers contained a lesser number of adherent cells (range $2-4 \times 10^5$) than those represented in Table 1 (1×10^6). Indomethacin, an inhibitor of prostaglandin synthesis, had no further enhancing effect on leukemic growth. Media was also harvested after coincubation. Fresh nonadherent marrow cells were cultured with this media or media harvested from control cultures for periods of 4 to 15 hr. No difference in survival of leukemic clusters was detected between cultures growing in media from coincubated cultures or that from control cultures.

TABLE 7. *Human peripheral blood adherent cell inhibition of GM-CFC[a]*

Experiment	Ratio mΘ/nonadherent marrow cells	Colonies coincubation	Colonies control	Percent inhibition
Autologous				
1. (a)	0.5:1	13 ± 1[a]	31 ± 3	58
(b)	2:1	7 ± 1	32 ± 2	78
Allogeneic				
2. (a)	0.5:1	25 ± 1	23 ± 1	−9
(b)	2:1	8 ± 1	26 ± 4	69

[a]Mean ± SEM. Experiment 1: Donor (A) adherent cells coincubated with donor (A) nonadherent marrow cells (autologous mix). Experiment 2: Donor (A) adherent cells coincubated with donor (B) nonadherent marrow cells (allogeneic mix). All suppressions are significant $p < 0.05$ (two-sided Student *t*-test). MΘ = monocyte.

TABLE 8. *Effect of peripheral blood adherent cells after coincubation with nonadherent marrow on GM-CFC growth when separated by an agar layer[a]*

Source of adherent cells[b]	Colonies in cultures with adherent cells	Colonies in cultures without adherent cells
1 (a)	33 ± 1	31 ± 3
1 (b)	39 ± 3	32 ± 2

[a]Nonadherent bone marrow cells from control cultures in experiments depicted in Table 7 were cultured in agar with HPCM ± adherent underlayers derived from monolayers after coincubation with nonadherent marrow from the same source. The purpose of this experiment was to determine if interaction between adherent cells and marrow induced the adherent cells to release a suppressive factor for CFU-C growth.
[b]See Table 7.

Since the total coincubation period was only 4 hr and after this resumption of growth did not appear, a mechanism other than cytostasis appeared likely. The cloning efficiency of leukemic cells in these systems ranges from 0.2 to 10%, but in these particular experiments, it was 0.3 to 4%. If the adherent cell effect on leukemic cells is only directed at this subpopulation, that is, clonogenic, then such an effect may not be detected in a cytotoxicity assay such as chromium release. We therefore compared chromium release to inhibition of cluster growth. In two experiments, the percent inhibition of cluster growth was 89 and 42%, respectively, at ratios of adherent cells to leukemic cells of 0.5:1, but the chromium release was insignificant. It appears, therefore, that inhibition of cluster growth is a much more sensitive indicator of modulations on leukemic growth than chromium release. This suggests that the adherent cell effect may be directed at only a subpopulation (clonogenic) or leukemic cells or that considerable growth inhibition can occur without early membrane damage and chromium release.

To further examine whether human peripheral blood adherent cells specifically modified leukemic clonogenic cells, we tested their effect on normal human marrow GM-CFC cloning efficiency. Table 7 shows an experiment using adherent cells from the one donor and coincubating these cells with nonadherent bone marrow cells from that of the same person (autologous mix) and a second experiment with an unrelated donor (allogeneic mix). As can be seen, suppression of GM-CFC did occur and, if anything, was more marked with the autologous combination. Like the leukemic data, these adherent cells were stimulatory to GM-CFC growth when used as underlayers and separated from the nonadherent marrow target by an agar underlayer (Table 8).

From cumulative data of experiments using normal marrow with adherent cells usually prepared from unrelated donors, the following conclusions can be made. GM-CFC suppression has occurred in most experiments (approximately 80–90%).

TABLE 9. *Peritoneal macrophage inhibition of GM-CFC[a]*

Ratio MΘ/nonadherent marrow cells	Colonies coincubation	Colonies control	Percent inhibition
0.5:1	130 ± 10[b]	122 ± 2	
2:1	72 ± 7	111 ± 7	35
5:1	74 ± 3	110 ± 3	35

[a]Inhibition was significant at $p < 0.01$ (two-sided Student t-test). MΘ = monocyte.
[b]Mean ± SEM.

However, at higher marrow numbers (lower adherent cells to marrow ratios) some stimulation occurred in some experiments. Morphological analysis has revealed that only granulocytic colonies are suppressed and not eosinophilic colonies. Moreover, adherent cells prepared from human bone marrow do not suppress but instead stimulate GM-CFC growth. This indicates the specificity of the source of adherent cells and argues against technical artifacts. These data certainly suggest that adherent cells suppress both normal and leukemic GM-CFC. The comparable sensitivity of these clonogenic cells to this mechanism of suppression still needs to be determined.

To examine the species specificity of this phenomenon, thioglycollate mobilized peritoneal cells were used as adherent monolayers. Syngeneic nonadherent marrow cells were used as targets. Table 9 shows one such experiment. GM-CFC inhibition occurred at ratios of 2:1. Mixing experiments were performed to eliminate the possibility that this suppression of GM-CFC was secondary to the induction of suppressor cells within the nonadherent marrow target after its exposure to adherent monolayers. Nonadherent marrow cells after coincubation were mixed with equal numbers of nonadherent marrow cells which had not been previously coincubated on adherent peritoneal cells. CM-CFC incidence was compared with that expected from the summation of the colony counts of these specimens plated separately. Mixtures of coincubated and fresh marrow did not significantly suppress over that expected. This would suggest that the mechanism of GM-CFC suppression is due to direct cell contact modulation of GM-CFC growth rather than the rapid induction of suppressor cells, causing a factor mediated GM-CFC suppression.

DISCUSSION

This study represents the first demonstration of human or murine adherent cell contact inhibition of hematopoietic progenitor cells. This may represent a mechanism similar to monocytic or macrophage cytotoxicity or cytostasis of tumor cell lines. Studies are in progress to determine if these two phenomena parallel each other.

These studies demonstrated that despite inhibition by cell contact, stimulation could still be effected by probable factors secreted by the same cells. Because of the preliminary nature of these experiments, we as yet do not know all the differences in the behavior of adherent cell populations derived from marrow, blood, perito-neum, spleen, etc., on cell contact with GM-CFC. Similarly, data is lacking as to whether adherent cell contact is inhibitory to other progenitor cell populations or even true stem cell populations.

Eosinophilic-CFC are the predominant circulating-CFC in human peripheral blood (9). The inhibition of granulocytic but not eosinophilic colonies by peripheral blood adherent cells suggests that these findings may have *in vivo* relevance. In marrow, GM-CFC are the predominant colony type detected, and adherent cells from this source were not inhibitory of GM-CFC survival, further suggesting that the ex-perimental protocol reported may be useful in examining the microenvironment of different tissues.

It has been postulated that different differentiation tendencies in different organs, such as myelopoiesis in marrow, erythropoiesis in spleen, and lymphopoiesis within lymph nodes, are determined by a different microenvironment (11–15). This in-ductive microenvironment is thought to be related to different fibroblastic popu-lations (16,17). It is conceivable, however, that different directions of differentiation could be due to negative or positive controls exerted by adherent cell populations within different organs. This adherent cell population is highly likely to be pre-dominately monocytic or macrophage. These cells are well known to interact by cell-to-cell contact mechanisms with lymphocytes and as a consequence finally regulate lymphopoiesis. (18). Alternatively, the *in vivo* significance of any of these phenomena may be simply one mechanism to limit hematopoiesis to the marrow where it may be finally regulated. At the same time, soluble factors from these same cells may enhance hematopoiesis, a long range regulatory mechanism. This would allow tissue invasion by microorganisms to be recognized and be translated into increased marrow hematopoiesis.

The variable inhibition of human marrow GM-CFC by peripheral blood adherent cells could be related to HLA or Ia compatible or incompatible requirements. Alternatively, a necessity for a certain stage of monocytic activation or maturity which may vary between donors may explain the varying results. Nevertheless, the inhibition of leukemic GM-CFC is not specific. The possible greater sensitivity of leukemic GM-CFC to this process may be secondary to an extreme sensitivity of clonogenic cells at this stage of differentiation. These leukemic clonogenic cells may have a surface structure differentiation antigen making them peculiarly sus-ceptible to growth modulation by adherent cell contact.

In conclusion, we believe that cell contact modulation of hematopoietic growth and differentiation is a previously unexplored area of intense importance. Experi-mental protocols such as described in this chapter may be used to study the normal microenvironmental control of different progenitor cell populations. Numerous ex-periments are proposed to examine (a) the role of subsets of lymphocytes on this cell contact regulation and (b) the effect of various immunoadjuvants and other pharmacological reagents. Also, such an experimental protocol may be useful for delineating hostile marrow microenvironments which may occur in potential transplant recepients and in pathological conditions such as aplastic anemia, congenital neutropenia, and leukemia.

ACKNOWLEDGMENTS

This paper was supported in part by grants CA-11520 and CA-14528, from the National Institutes of Health, Bethesda, Maryland. Gary Spitzer is the recipient of a scholarship from the Leukemia Society of America, Inc.

REFERENCES

1. Metcalf, D. (1977): Haemopoietic colonies, in vitro cloning of normal and leukemic cells. *Recent Results Cancer Res.*, 61:37.
2. Queensberry, P., Halperin, J., Ryan, M., and Stohlman, F., Jr. (1975): Tolerance to the granulocyte releasing and colony-stimulating factor elevating effects of endotoxin. *Blood*, 45:789–800.
3. Sullivan, R., Zuckerman, K. S., and Queensberry, P. (1980): The role of colony stimulating activity in modulating murine diffusion chamber granulopoiesis. *Br. J. Haematol.*, 44:365–374.
4. Dexter, T. M., and Shadduck, R. K. (1980): The regulation of haemopoiesis in long-term culture: 1. Role of L-cell CSF. *J. Cell. Physiol.*, 102:279–286.
5. Williams, N., and Burgess, A. W. (1980): The effect of mouse lung granulocyte-macrophage colony-stimulating factor and other colony-stimulating activities on the proliferation and differentiation of murine bone marrow cells in long-term culture. *J. Cell. Physiol.*, 102:287–295.
6. Dicke, K. A., and Schaefer, U. M. (1979): Preparation of hematopoietic stem cells in primates. In: *Cryopreservation of Normal and Neoplastic Cells*, edited by R. Weiner, R. Oldham, and L. Schwartzenberg, p. 81. INSERM Symposium, Paris.
7. Boyum, A. (1968): Separation of leukocytes from blood and bone marrow. *Scand. J. Clin. Lab. Invest.*, 21(Suppl. 97):77.
8. Weiner, M. S., Bianco, C., and Nussenzwerg, J. (1973): Enhanced binding of neuraminidase sheep erythrocytes to human T lymphocytes. *Blood*, 42:939–946.
9. Verma, D. S., Spitzer, G., Zander, A. R., Fisher, R., McCredie, K. B., and Dicke, K. A. (1980): The myeloid progenitor cell: a parallel study of subpopulations in human marrow and peripheral blood. *Exp. Hematol.*, 8:32–43.
10. Spitzer, G., Verma, D. S., Dicke, K. A., Smith, T., and McCredie, K. B. (1979): Subgroups of oligoleukemia as identified by in vitro agar culture. *Leuk. Res.*, 3:29–39.
11. Curry, J. L., and Trentin, J. J. (1967): Hemopoietic spleen colony studies: growth and differentiation. *Dev. Biol.*, 15:395–413.
12. Wolf, N. S., and Trentin, J. J. (1968): Effect of hemopoietic organ stroma in differentiation of pluripotent stem cells. *J. Exp. Med.*, 127:205–214.
13. Trentin, J. J. (1970): Influence of hematopoietic organ stroma (hematopoietic inductive microenvironments) in stem cell differentiation. In: *Regulation of Hematopoiesis*, edited by A. S. Gordon, pp. 161–186. Appelton-Century-Crofts, New York.
14. Tavassoli, M. (1975): Studies on hemopoietic microenvironments. *Exp. Hematol.*, 3:213–226.
15. Boggs, D. R. (1980): The hematopoietic microenvironment. *New Engl. J. Med.*, 302:1359–1360.
16. Friedenstein, A. T., Chailakhyan, R. K., Latsinik, N. V., Panasyuk, A. F., and Keilliss-Berek, I. V. (1974): Stromal cells responsible for transferring the microenvironment of the hemopoietic tissue: cloning in vitro and retransplantation in vivo. *Transplantation*, 17:331–340.
17. Friedenstein, A. J., Gorskaja, U. F., and Kulagina, N. N. (1976): Fibroblast precursors in normal and irradiated mouse hematopoietic organs. *Exp. Hematol.*, 4:267–274.
18. Rosenthal, A. S., Thomas-Black, J., Ellner, J. J., Greineder, D. K., and Lipsky, P. E. (1976): Macrophage function in antigen recognition by T lymphocytes. In: *Immunobiology of the Macrophages*, edited by D. S. Nelson, pp. 131–160. Academic Press, New York.

Maturation Factors and Cancer,
edited by Malcolm A. S. Moore.
Raven Press, © New York 1982.

Myelopoietic Maturation and Human Leukocyte Interferon

D. S. Verma, G. Spitzer, and M. Beran

Department of Developmental Therapeutics, The University of Texas System Cancer Center, M.D. Anderson Hospital and Tumor Institute, Houston, Texas 77030

Since its discovery as an antiviral agent (11), interferon has been demonstrated to be involved in various vital cellular interactions that regulate immune responses (7,12,13,23,26,29,30). It has also been documented to affect macrophage functions, natural killer cell activity, and the expression of membrane surface antigens of various cells (5,25,32,39). These findings tend to suggest that interferon may primarily be a humoral mediator of various intercellular messages that are essential for an appropriate homeostasis of various tissues.

Recently, methods have been developed to produce human leukocyte interferon (HLIF) in larger quantities (3). This has made it possible to use HLIF for the therapeutic trials in the treatment of some viral infections and neoplastic conditions (8,17,18,19). These trials have almost invariably been associated with granulocytopenia. This finding and the fact that variable quantities of interferon are elaborated in response to almost any antigenic stimulus (10) prompted us to examine the role of HLIF in granulopoietic regulation. The present chapter describes some of the findings of our *in vitro* experiments that suggest an inhibitory role for HLIF in the granulopoietic maturation.

MATERIALS AND METHODS

Collection of Light-Density Human Marrow Cells

Bone marrow specimens obtained from normal human volunteers were collected in polystyrene centrifuge tubes (Corning Glass Works, Corning, N.Y.) containing a solution of preservative-free heparin (1,000 units/ml; Gibco Laboratories, Grand Island, N.Y. in phosphate-buffered saline (PBS). To obtain light-density marrow cells, the specimen was centrifuged over a column of Ficoll-Hypaque solution (density 1.077 g/ml) at 200g for 35 min. The interface cells were aspirated with a Pasteur pipette and washed twice with PBS and once again with single strength α-MEM (alpha modification of minimum essential medium) plus 15% fetal calf serum (FCS). Subsequently, the cells were resuspended in α-MEM plus 15% FCS at an approximate concentration of 1 to 1.5 $\times$ 10^6 cells/ml. These cells were then used as target cells for granulocyte-macrophage progenitor cell (GM-CFC) assay.

Granulocyte-Macrophage Progenitor Cell Assay in Semisolid Agar

One ml underlayers of a mixture of 0.5% bactoagar (Difco Laboratories, Detroit, Mich.) and α-MEM plus 15% FCS were prepared in 35-mm plastic petri dishes (Corning Glass Works, Corning, N.Y.) and allowed to dry. To stimulate GM-CFC proliferation and differentiation, HPCM was incorporated in the underlayers at an optimum concentration of 20% (v/v). Subsequently, these underlayers were overlaid with a 1-ml mixture of 0.3% bactoagar, α-MEM, and 15% FCS containing 1 or 2 $\times$ 10^5 human marrow target cells. These cultures were then incubated at 37°C in a fully humidified atmosphere of 5% CO_2 in air. After 8 days of incubation, the dishes were scored under an Olympus dissecting microscope ($\times 25$ magnification) for the number of colonies (aggregates of $\geqslant 40$ cells) and clusters (3 to 39 cells) per dish. The final results were noted as the mean from triplicate dishes $\pm$ one standard deviation.

Morphological Examination of Cell Aggregates

Individual colonies or clusters were picked up with a Unopette pipette (Becton Dickinson Co., Rutherford, N.J.) and placed on egg albumin-smeared microscopic slides that were etched in small squares by a diamond pencil (one cell aggregate per square) as described by Verma et al. (36). After they were dried, the slides were stained with Luxol Fast Blue MBS (Hartman-Leddon Co., Philadelphia, Pa.) for 2 hr, then rinsed in distilled water for 2 hr more and counterstained with Harris's hematoxylin for 2 min. The percentage differential counts were calculated from the cumulative data on differentials of 50 clusters from each pertinent observation.

Use of HLIF

The preparation of HLIF was obtained from Dr. K. Cantell (Finnish Red Cross, Kivihaantie, Helsinki). It was provided in 0.5 ml vials containing a total of 3 $\times$ 10^6 international reference units (IRU) of interferon and 4 mg of protein with no preservative chemicals. For use, a whole vial was thawed and stored at 4°C as a stock solution in α-MEM at a concentration of 10^5 IRU per ml for up to 2 weeks.

RESULTS

Effects of HLIF on GM-CFC Growth *In Vitro*

The various concentrations of HLIF were incorporated in the upper layers of the agar culture dishes, and the target marrow cells were stimulated by HPCM present in the underlayers. Table 1 presents the numbers of colonies and clusters noted in the presence of 0, 10, 100, 1,000, and 10,000 IRU/ml. A progressive decrease in the size of cell aggregates was noted with increasing concentrations of HLIF in the

TABLE 1. *Effect of human leukocyte interferon on colony and cluster formation when incorporated in agar overlayers with HPCM[a]*

Experiment	Cell aggregates scored	Plating efficiency without interferon (control)	Number of colonies and clusters as percent of control at various concentration of interferon per dish (IRU/ml)			
			10	100	1,000	10,000
1	Colonies[b]	171.3 ± 3.5	24.7	9.5	0.6	0.0
	Clusters[c]	370.0 ± 10.0	124.3	138.0	138.7	155.4
	Total	541.3	93.0	97.0	95.0	106.0
2	Colonies	124.3 ± 5.1	16.6	1.8	0.0	0.0
	Clusters	326.7 ± 15.0	135.7	135.0	122.0	119.4
	Total	451.0	103.0	98.0	88.7	86.5
3	Colonies	35.0 ± 4.6	14.2	2.8	0.0	0.0
	Clusters	68.0 ± 6.5	139.7	147.0	152.5	147.0
	Total	103.0	97.0	98.0	100.0	97.0
4	Colonies	26.7 ± 4.0	87.2	93.6	36.3	37.4
	Clusters	253.0 ± 5.8	102.0	104.0	110.7	109.4
	Total	279.7	101.3	103.0	107.0	102.5

[a]Number of light density (<1.077 g/ml) cells plated per dish was 2×10^5 for the first two experiments and 10^5 for the last two. The colony and cluster incidences are means ± SD from triplicate culture dishes.
[b]Aggregates of ≥ 40 cells.
[c]Aggregates of 3–39 cells.
From Verma et al. (*Blood*, 54:1423–1427, 1979, with permission).

culture dishes, leading to a decline in the colony incidence and corresponding increase in the cluster incidence. This resulted in nearly a constant plating efficiency, regardless of the HLIF concentrations used. The HLIF effect, though variable on different marrow target cells, remained consistent. This variability could be due to a variable sensitivity of marrow cells from different donors to HLIF.

Morphology of the Clusters

Since the HLIF preparations used in these experiments did not stimulate any colony or cluster formation in the absence of HPCM, the increase in clusters noted with increasing HLIF concentrations suggested either an inhibition of proliferation at a latter stage of the granulopoietic maturational process or a prolongation of the generation time of each successive mitosis. When the cultures were incubated for 4 more days, no significant difference in colony or cluster numbers was noted. This suggested that either prolonged generation time was not the cause of our observations or, if it was, the prolongation was of a rather significant degree or was increasing progressively with each successive mitosis. To explore these points further, we examined the clusters morphologically. Table 2 presents the differential counts of clusters from one of these experiments. It is clear from these data that increasing HLIF concentrations induced a progressive differentiation block.

Using liquid suspension cultures, we have similarly demonstrated that HLIF causes differentiation block and leads to an accumulation of granulopoietic pre-

TABLE 2. *Effect of human leukocyte interferon on cell composition of aggregates grown in agar culture*

Interferon concentration (IRU/ml)	Differential count of cells contained in clusters (%) [a]						
	Myeloblasts	Promyelocytes	Myelocytes	Metamyelocytes	Bands	Polymorphs
0	0.0	0.0	5.7	22.8	23.0	48.5
10	3.0	10.0	27.0	27.2	22.4	10.4
100	9.6	19.2	27.0	27.8	10.6	4.8
1,000	6.0	12.7	37.0	30.0	9.2	4.1
10,000	8.4	16.2	40.8	28.0	6.6	0.0

[a]Average percentage from 50 clusters examined for morphologic type. Morphologic examination of the colonies from dishes with and without interferon revealed normally differentiating cells.

From Verma et al. (*Blood,* 54:1423–1427, 1979, with permission).

cursors (38). We have also documented a dose-related competition between HPCM, a source of CSF and HLIF. Further, it has been found that HLIF induces the release of cycloxygenase pathway product that inhibits the GM-CFC proliferation (unpublished data). The studies investigating the effect of various other types of interferons, i.e., human fibroblast interferon (HFIF) and immune interferon (IF II), have revealed that while IF II is as active as HLIF in blocking the granulopoietic maturational process, the HFIF is much less active (unpublished data).

DISCUSSION

The first study relating inhibition of GM-CFC by interferon was reported by McNeill and Killen (16). This study demonstrated that a decrease in the colony-stimulating activity (CSA) in the serum of mice immediately following an intra-peritoneal injection of Poly(I)-Poly(C) was associated with the presence of a factor inhibitory of GM-CFC. Later, McNeill and Fleming (14) also demonstrated that, based on the molecular size and the sensitivity to heat, pH, and trypsin, the CSA inhibitory activity thus produced was possibly due to interferon. Using an *in vitro* agar culture system, Fleming et al. (6) confirmed that mouse interferon inhibited GM-CFC proliferation. Based on the presence of "abnormal multinucleated cells" in these experiments, they suggested that interferon might be involved in normal granulocytic differentiation (6). However, no evidence or details of such a regulatory role of interferon in granulopoiesis were presented. More recently, McNeill and Fleming (15) have emphasized that caution should be exercised in interpreting these data, as occasionally, megakaryocytes microscopically resembling those unusual cells previously found in their experiments can also grow in agar cultures simultaneously with granulocytic colonies (22).

The maturation arrest of granulopoiesis observed in our experiments could be due either to (a) HLIF-induced prolongation of intermitotic period, an action of interferon previously documented using various cell lines and/or to (b) progressively increasing HLIF sensitivity of the granulocyte precursors as they mature down the hierarchy of granulopoiesis from GM-CFC to segmented neutrophils. Using micro-cinematographic analysis of dividing mouse mammary tumor cells, d'Hoogue et al. (4) have shown that interferon treatment induces a progressive prolongation in the intermitotic time as a cell undergoes sequential mitoses, resulting in the final arrest of a significant number of cells by the fourth generation. It is possible that the interferon-treated GM-CFC also behave in a similar manner, resulting in maturation arrest.

The second possibility, a progressively increasing HLIF sensitivity of the granulocyte precursors, may also apply. When the effect of double-stranded RNA (dsRNA) on protein synthesis is examined in cell-free systems, it is found that reticulocyte lysates are as sensitive to the action of dsRNA as normal interferon-primed cells and much more sensitive than normal noninterferon primed cells (24). Considering the fact that priming of normal cells with interferon makes them more sensitive to the action of viral or nonviral (dsRNA) interferon inducers (31,36), this suggests that the erythroid differentiation process may involve the exposure to interferon at some stage of maturation. Also, Rossi et al. (27,28) have demonstrated that interferon can block dimethylsulfoxide-(DMSO)-induced differentiation of Friend virus-induced murine erythroleukemia cells. In the light of these data, there exists a possibility that interferon may be functioning as a regulator of normal erythropoietic differentiation through progressively increasing sensitivity of the cells as they mature from progenitor cells to reticulocytes. The experiments described in this chapter demonstrate that HLIF at the concentrations used does allow GM-CFC proliferation, but only up to a certain stage of the maturation process. This results in formation of cluster-size cell aggregates, consisting predominantly of granulocytic precursors. Similar to the interferon effect on erythropoiesis, we postulate that as GM-CFC proliferate and differentiate, their successive generations become progressively more sensitive to the HLIF effect. Whether this is achieved by "interferon-priming" of successive generations of cells or by genetic predetermination remains an open question. Such a mechanism would allow the differentiation of early granulopoietic precursors to continue at a relatively slower rate; they would not accumulate in large numbers. This, however, would result in a gradually increasing accumulation of successively more differentiated progeny, constituting the late mitotic pool of the myelopoietic hierarchy. This would ultimately result in the formation of small aggregates of cells belonging to the late mitotic pool rather than large aggregates consisting of early granulopoietic precursors. At higher concentrations of HLIF, this effect would manifest itself at even earlier stages of the maturation process.

We have recently reported the involvement of putative helper and suppressor T lymphocytes in CSA elaboration (33–35,37). This makes our finding that IF II, a product of suppressor T lymphocytes, is as potent as HLIF in blocking the granulopoietic maturation process, and HFIF much less so, very intriguing. It is possible that HLIF and IF II do not influence granulopoiesis directly but through an intermediary differentiation-blocking factor released under their influence by some cells contaminating the marrow. These cells could not be monocyte-macrophages, since removal of these cells does not abrogate the HLIF or IF II effect on granulopoiesis. In the light of the data reporting the presence of enhanced suppressor T lymphocyte activity in certain neutropenic disorders that are associated with myeloid maturational arrest in the bone marrow (1,2), it is likely that the cells mediating the maturation-blocking effect of HLIF or IF II are a subpopulation of T lymphocytes. Studies are under way in our laboratory to investigate these questions.

The data on erythropoiesis show that cells forming multiple (burst) erythroid colonies (BFU-E) require much higher erythropoietin concentration than their immediate progeny, the CFU-E, which give rise to small single colonies (9). Analogous to erythropoiesis, the cells giving rise to multiple granulocytic colonies have been found to require a much higher concentration of CSF for their growth than the cells forming single granulomonocytic colonies (21). In turn, the GM-CFC also require higher CSF concentrations than their immediate progeny, the macrophage progenitor cells (M-CFC) (20). Therefore, as depicted in Fig. 1, a model of myelopoiesis could be envisaged with a positive control by CSF and a negative control by interferon; both working competitively at each stage of proliferation and differentiation, with progressively increasing responsiveness of the successive progeny to

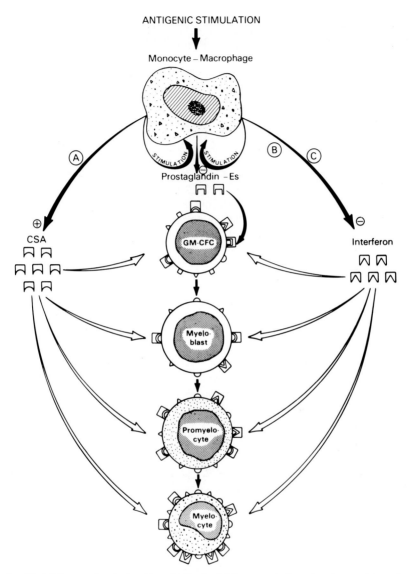

FIG. 1. Model for myelopoiesis. Almost all microbial agents induce interferon elaboration, although to a variable extent. Recently, CSA and interferon have both been shown to stimulate PGE release from MΘ. We propose that the respective quantities of CSA, PGEs, and interferon elaborated could depend upon the degree of stimulus by a microbial agent and/or its immuno-chemical character, thus aligning the myelopoietic "assembly line" according to the needs.

these control mechanisms as they proceed down the hierarchal system of maturation. Such a regulatory process would provide the myelopoietic system with a great flexibility of control in terms of clonal expansion. It is of interest that all the micro-organisms phagocytosed primarily by macrophages induce interferon elaboration

(10). It is possible, therefore, that the dose and/or immunochemical properties of a microorganism may decide the differential elaboration of CSF and interferon to different extents, respectively, and thus align the leukopoietic response according to the needs.

ACKNOWLEDGMENTS

The authors express their gratitude for the gift of human leukocyte interferon preparations by Dr. J. U. Gutterman. They also thank Ms. Sherrie Smith for technical assistance and Ms. Kathi Orsak for her secretarial assistance. This study was supported in parts by Grants CA-14528 and CA-11520 from The National Institutes of Health, Bethesda, Maryland. G. Spitzer is the recipient of a Scholar of the Leukemia Society of America, Inc., Award. D.S. Verma is a recipient of a Special Fellow of the Leukemia Society of America, Inc., Award.

REFERENCES

1. Abdou, N. I., NaPombejara, C., Balentine, L., and Abdou, N. L. (1978): Suppressor cell-mediated neutropenia in Felty's syndrome. *J. Clin. Invest.*, 61:738–743.
2. Bagby, G. C., and Gabourel, J. D. (1979): Neutropenia in three patients with rheumatic disorders. *J. Clin. Invest.*, 64:72–82.
3. Billiau, A., Ioniau, M., and de Sower, P. (1973): Mass production of human interferon in diploid cells by Poly I-C. *J. Gen. Virol.*, 19:1–8.
4. d'Hooghe, M. D., Brount-Boye, D., Malise, E. P., and Gresser, I. (1977): Interferon and cell division. XII. Prolongation by interferon of intermitotic time of mouse mammary tumor cells *in vitro*. Microcinematographic analysis. *Exp. Cell Res.*, 105:73–77.
5. Fellous, M., Kamoun, M., Gresser, I., and Bono, R. (1979): Enhanced expression of HLA antigens and β_2-microglobulin on interferon-treated human lymphoid cells. *Eur. J. Immunol.*, 9:446–449.
6. Fleming, W. A., McNeill, T. A., and Killen, M. (1972): The effects of an inhibiting factor (interferon) on the *in vitro* growth of granulocyte-macrophage colonies. *Immunology*, 23:429–437.
7. Gisler, R. H., Lindahl, P., and Gresser, I. (1974): Effect of interferon on antibody synthesis *in vitro* . *J. Immunol.*, 113:438–444.
8. Greenberg, H. B., Pollard, R. B., Lutwick, L. I., Gregory, P. B., Robinson, W. S., and Merigan, T. C. (1976): Effect of human leukocyte interferon on hepatitis B virus infection in patients with chronic active hepatitis. *N. Engl. J. Med.*, 295:517–522.
9. Gregory, C. J. (1976): Erythropoietin sensitivity as a differentiation marker in the hemopoietic system: studies of three erythropoietic colony responses in culture. *J. Cell. Physiol.*, 89:289–301.
10. Ho, M., and Armstrong, J. A. (1975): Interferon. *Annu. Rev. Microbiol.*, 29:131–161.
11. Isaacs, A., and Lindenmann, J. (1957): Virus interference: 1. The interferon. *Proc. Roy. Soc. Lond. (Biol.)*, 147:258–267.
12. Johnson, H. M., Smith, B. G., and Baron, S. (1975): Inhibition of the primary *in vitro* antibody response by interferon preparations. *J. Immunol.*, 114:403–409.
13. Lindahl-Magnusson, P., Leary, P., and Gresser, I. (1972): Interferon inhibits DNA synthesis induced in mouse lymphocyte suspensions by phytohaemagglutinin or by allogeneic cells. *Nature (New Biol.)*, 237:120–121.
14. McNeill, T. A., and Fleming, W. A. (1971): The relationship between serum interferon and an inhibitor of mouse haemopoietic colonies *in vitro*. *Immunology*, 21:761–766.
15. McNeill, T. A., and Fleming, W. A. (1977): Effect on interferon on hemopoietic colony forming cells. *Interferon Systems*. *Tex. Rep. Bio. Med.*, 35:343–349.
16. McNeill, T. A., and Killen, M. (1971): The effect of synthetic double-stranded polyribonucleotides on haemopoietic colony forming cells *in vivo*. *Immunology*, 21:751–759.
17. Mellstedt, H., Bjorkholm, M., Johansson, B., Ahre, A., Holm, G., and Strander, H. (1979): Interferon therapy in myelomatosis. *Lancet*, 1:245–247.

18. Merigan, T. C., Rand, K. H., Pollard, R. B., Abdallah, P. S., Jordan, G. W., and Fried, R. P. (1978): Human leukocyte interferon for the treatment of herpes zoster in patients with cancer. *N. Engl. J. Med.*, 298:981–987.

19. Merigan, T. C., Sikora, K., Breeden, J. H., Levy, R., and Rosenberg, S. A. (1978): Preliminary observations on the effect of human leukocyte interferon in non-Hodgkin's lymphoma. *N. Engl. J. Med.*, 299:1449–1453.

20. Metcalf, D. (1978): The control of neutrophil and macrophage production at the progenitor cell level. In: *Experimental Hematology Today*, edited by S. J. Baum and G. D. Ledney, pp. 35–46. Springer-Verlag, New York.

21. Metcalf, D., and MacDonald, H. R. (1975): Heterogeneity of *in vitro* colony- and cluster-forming cells in the mouse marrow. Segregation by velocity sedimentation. *J. Cell. Physiol.*, 85:643–653.

22. Metcalf, D., MacDonald, H. R., Odartchenko, N., and Sordat, B. (1975): Growth of mouse megakaryocyte colonies *in vitro*. *Proc. Natl. Acad. Sci., U.S.A.*, 72:1744–1748.

23. Miorsser, H., Landstrom, L. E., Larner, E., Larsson, I., Lundgven, E., and Strannegard, O. (1978): Regulation of mitogen-induced lymphocyte DNA synthesis by human interferon of different origins. *Cell. Immunol.*, 35:15–24.

24. Morser, J., and Burke, D. (1979): Interferon and double-stranded RNA. *Nature*, 277:435.

25. Rabinovitch, M., and Manejias, R. E. (1978): Anti-interferon globulin inhibits macrophage phagocytic enhancement *in vivo* by Tilorone or Newcastle disease virus. *Cell. Immunol.*, 39:402–406.

26. Rasmussen, L., and Merigan, T. C. (1978): Role of T lymphocytes in cellular immune responses during herpes simplex virus infection in humans. *Proc. Natl. Acad. Sci., U.S.A.*, 75:3957–3961.

27. Rossi, G. B., Dolei, A., Cico, L., Benedetto, A., Matarese, G. P., Belardelli, F., and Rita, G. (1977): Interferon and Friend leukemia cells in culture. *Interferon Systems, Tex. Rep. Biol. Med.*, 35:420–428.

28. Rossi, G. B., Matarese, G. P., Grappelli, C., and Belardelli, F. (1977): Interferon inhibits dimethylsulphoxide-induced erythroid differentiation of Friend leukemia cells. *Nature*, 267:50–52.

29. Sonnenfeld, G., Mandel, A. D., and Merigan, T. C. (1977): The immunosuppressive effect of Type II mouse interferon preparations on antibody production. *Cell. Immunol.*, 34:193–206.

30. Sonnenfeld, G., Mandel, A. D., Merigan, T. C. (1978): Time and dosage dependence of immunoenhancement by murine Type II interferon preparations. *Cell. Immunol.*, 285–293.

31. Stewart, W. E., II, Gosser, L. B., and Lockart, R. Z., Jr. (1971): Priming: a nonantiviral function of interferon. *J. Virol.*, 7:792–801.

32. Trinchieri, G., and Santoli, D. (1978): Antiviral activity induced by culturing lymphocytes with tumor-derived or virus-transformed cells. Enhancement of human natural killer cell activity by interferon and antagonistic inhibition of susceptibility of target cell to lysis. *J. Exp. Med.*, 147:1314–1333.

33. Verma, D. S., Spitzer, G., Beran, M., Zander, A. R., Smith, S., McCrady, A., McCredie, K. B., and Dicke, K. A. (1979): The T-lymphocyte-mediated augmentation and suppression of colony-stimulating activity elaboration and abrogation of the suppression by lithium in man (abstract). *Blood*, 54(1):163a.

34. Verma, D. S., Spitzer, G., Zander, A. R., Fisher, R., McCredie, K. B., and Dicke, K. A. (1979): T-lymphocyte and monocyte-macrophage interaction in colony-stimulating activity elaboration in man. *Blood*, 54:1376–1383.

35. Verma, D. S., Spitzer, G., Zander, A. R., Beran, M., Smith, S., McCrady, A., Dicke, K. A., and McCredie, K. B. (1980): The human monocyte-macrophage and helper and suppressor T-lymphocyte interaction in colony-stimulating activity elaboration. *Exp. Hematol.*, 8(9):9 (abstract # 14).

36. Verma, D. S., Spitzer, G., Zander, A. R., McCredie, K. B., and Dicke, K. A. (1980): The myeloid progenitor cell: a parallel study of subpopulations in human marrow and peripheral blood. *Exp. Hematol.*, 8:32–43.

37. Verma, D. S., Spitzer, G., Zander, A. R., Beran, M., Dicke, K. A., and McCredie, K. B. (1981): Monocyte-macrophage interaction with putative helper and suppressor T lymphocytes in colony-stimulating activity elaboration. In: *Experimental Hematology Today*, edited by S. J. Baum G. D. Ledney and A. Khan, pp. 139–150, Springer-Verlag, New York.

38. Verma, D. S., Spitzer, G., Zander, A. R., Gutterman, J. U., McCredie, K. B., Dicke, K. A., and Johnston, D. A. (1981): Human leukocyte interferon preparation-mediated block of granulopoietic differentiation *in vitro*. *Exp. Hematol.*, 9:63–76.

39. Vignaux, F., and Gresser, I. (1977): Differential effect of interferon on the expression of H-2K, H-2D, and Ia antigens on mouse lymphocytes. *J. Immunol.*, 118:721–723.

Maturation Factors and Cancer,
edited by Malcolm A. S. Moore.
Raven Press, © New York 1982.

The Role of Proliferation and Maturation Factors in Myeloid Leukemia

Malcolm A. S. Moore and Alice P. Sheridan

*Department of Developmental Hematopoiesis, Memorial Sloan-Kettering Cancer Center,
New York, New York 10021*

Hematopoietic regulation from the earliest multipotential stem cell through to the mature end cell involves progressive loss of self-renewal, in most but not all cell lineages, with sequential restriction of differentiation potential. Earlier dogma of a programmed transit to post-mitotic differentiated end cells is clearly no longer tenable, as greatly extended proliferative potential is now evident in highly differentiated cell populations such as T cells (1), B cells (2), macrophages (3), mast cells (4), and neutrophil granulocyte precursors (5). Thus, the ability to use extended proliferative capacity as a marker for neoplastic transformation is clearly not valid. The concept of dedifferentiation associated with hematopoietic malignancy also lacks experimental support as evidence points to the bi- or multipotent stem cells as preferential targets for leukemic transformation. Morphological approaches to analysis of the pathophysiology of leukemia have led to the erroneous concept that malignant transformation involves an irreversible block in the maturation process, and has favored the view that leukemia involves "escape" from normal growth control. Although it is true that many leukemic cell lines have been adapted to culture and in the process have lost responsiveness to exogenous regulators, extensive *in vitro* studies involving primary culture of human myeloid leukemic cells emphasize a remarkable homogeneity with respect to retention of a requirement for growth stimulating factors (6) with varying degrees of impairment in responsiveness to normal growth inhibitory factors (7). Unlike many other growth-factor dependent systems, the various hemopoietic regulators are not simply inducers of differentiation but, rather are required continuously for both proliferation and differentiation. Indeed there are examples of the same regulatory factor acting on an early hemopoietic stem cell population and on mature post-mitotic end cells (8). To place the current state of knowledge of the action of growth control and maturation factors in myeloid leukemia in perspective, a brief summary of normal myelopoietic regulation is necessary.

REGULATION OF NORMAL MYELOPOIESIS

The development of an agar culture technique that supported the clonal proliferation and differentiation of bone marrow progenitors of the granulocyte-macrophage (GM) lineage (9,10) provided evidence for a compartment of lineage committed cells intermediate between pluripotent stem cells and morphologically identifiable myeloid cells, and provided evidence of humoral regulators of granulopoiesis and monocyte-macrophage proliferation. Two types of heterogeneity can be defined within the myelopoietic system, a) a heterogeneity in the capacity of marrow progenitors to respond to specific stimulators and generate specific progeny, and b) GM-colony-stimulating factor (CSF) molecules exist that have preferential or restricted capacity to stimulate subsets of GM-precursor cells. In the former case, it has proved possible to identify pluripotent progenitors giving rise to colonies of granulocytes and macrophages admixed with erythroid and megakaryocytic cells (CFU-GEMM), neutrophil and macrophage progenitors (CFU-GM), and progenitors restricted to neutrophil (CFU-G), eosinophil (CFU-Eo), basophil-mast cell (CFU-Bas) and monocyte-macrophage (CFU-M) differentiation (11). In the case of regulatory factors, the commonly used nomenclature recognizes various factors with lineage restriction as defined by the types of mature cells found in bone marrow colonies stimulated to grow by CSF-containing preparations (e.g., GM-CSF, G-CSF, M-CSF, Eo-CSF). This approach is somewhat subjective owing to variations imposed by culture conditions and by the fact that many CSF preparations contain more than one CSF subspecies. Colony-stimulating factor subclass specific assays now exist for some species of CSF and utilize sterospecific recognition by specific antibody or specific receptor (12).

GM-CSF

Sources of GM-CSF in man and mouse are varied, but macrophages, mitogen-stimulated lymphocytes, endothelial cells, and certain fibroblast populations are particulary active sources (8,12). It is possible that all tissues contain and synthesize GM-CSF, since production of detectable activity occurs at a basal rate in many adult and fetal tissues. Table 1 summarizes the current status of the biochemical and functional status of GM-CSF. As can be seen, GM-CSF has both a proliferation-inducing activity and a differentiation-inducing action which extends to an ability

TABLE 1. *Properties of GM-CSF[a]*

1. Activates noncycling GM-CFC into cycle.
2. Shortens doubling time of GM cells.
3. High concentrations favor granulocyte differentiation and low concentrations macrophage ("differentiation downgrading").
4. Colony size increases with CSF concentration
5. Increases RNA and protein synthesis in polymorphs.
6. Induces increased macrophage phagocytosis, cytolysis, protease, and prostaglandin synthesis.
7. Stimulates initial proliferation of multipotential cells and early erythroid progenitors.
8. Induces differentiation in myeloid leukemic cells.

[a]Mouse: 23,000 MW; human: 40,000–50,000 MW.
Refs. 8, 11, and 13.

to influence RNA and protein synthesis in mature post-mitotic neutrophil granulocytes (8).

Macrophage CSF (M-CSF, CSF-1)

This species of CSF was the first to be completely purified from a human (urine)
or murine (L-cell) source and is characterized by its selective ability to induce the
formation of colonies composed exclusively or predominantly of monocytes and
macrophages (12,14). The properties of M-CSF are shown in Table 2. Although
both mouse and human purified M-CSF are active on mouse bone marrow CFU-
M and on subpopulations of phagocytic mononuclear cells, species restriction exists
since murine CSF is inactive on human cells and colonies of macrophages of human
origin stimulated by human M-CSF are much smaller than their murine counterparts
(12). The M-CSF is capable of acting as a macrophage growth factor as well as
inducing a variety of macrophage secretory products and in this respect is similar
to GM-CSF; however, although nearly 100% of macrophages have receptors for
M-CSF, there is no competition between GM-CSF and M-CSF for binding to
macrophages, implying the existence of different receptors (8,12).

Neutrophil CSF (G-CSF) and Eosinophil CSF (Eo-CSF)

These activities have not been purified to homogeneity but have been sufficiently
characterized to distinguish them from the preceding CSF species, and each other.
An activity separable from Eo-CSF and from GM- and M-CSF was reported in
conditioned media obtained from the WEHI-3 myelomonocytic cell line (15). This
factor was characterized by a low affinity for DEAE Sephadex and capacity to
stimulate increasing proportions of pure neutrophil colonies as the activity was
serially diluted (15). Subsequently, G-CSF was identified in mouse postendotoxin
serum (8,16) and could be distinguished from conventional species of CSF by its
lack of neutralization by anti-L cell CSF antiserum and its apparent molecular weight
(16). Granulocyte-CSF can be distinguished from other CSF species by the selective
unresponsiveness of its target CFU-G to inhibition by prostaglandins of the E series
(PGE). Prostaglandins of the E series inhibit monocyte-macrophage colony for-

TABLE 2. *Macrophage-CSF (CSF-1, M-CSF)*

1. Acidic, sialic acid-containing glycoproteins of 45,000-86,000 MW.
2. 28,000 MW polypeptide of two identical subunits with approx 50% glycosylation.
3. Source: Heterogeneous but purified from human urine and mouse L-cell CM.
4. Action:
   Stimulates marrow CFU-M to generate 10^9 macrophages.
   Stimulates approx 20% of phagocytic mononuclear cells to proliferate.
   Induces macrophage plasminogen activator and prostaglandin synthesis.
5. All macrophages have CSF-1 receptors (70,000 per peritoneal macrophage).
6. GM-CSF does not compete with CSF-1 for binding to macrophages.
7. Active *in vitro* at 25 pM and inactivated by receptor-mediated endocytosis.

Refs. 12 and 14.

mation by human and murine CFU-M, at concentrations as low as 10^{-8} to 10^{-9} M (17). The PGE is significantly less inhibitory to CFU-GM, and neutrophil or eosinophil colonies stimulated by G-CSF or Eo-CSF, respectively, are not inhibited even by pharmacological, rather than physiological, concentrations of PGE (17). Since the biosynthesis of PGE by normal and neoplastic macrophages is intrinsically linked to their synthesis of and/or their exposure to myeloid CSF (18), we further investigated the selective capacity of different species of CSF to induce macrophage PGE production. Purified M-CSF and GM-CSF both induced a striking increase in macrophage PGE biosynthesis within 24 hr, whereas semipurified G-CSF did not (18).

Evidence exists for genetic restriction in responsiveness to G-CSF which is not seen when other species of CSF are studied (19). A particular abnormality was evident in NZB marrow cultures when conditioned media from WEHI-3 leukemic cells were used as CSF sources. This involved a greatly reduced incidence of colonies relative to the incidence in other strains (Table 3). When a semipurified G-CSF preparation was used, colony formation by NZB marrow was even further reduced. Indeed the residual colony formation observed was not of granulocytic type and could be eliminated by addition of PGE to the cultures. The incidence of colony formation seen with F_1 hybrid bone marrow was intermediate between the normal responder parent and the NZB (19). Certain other strains in addition to NZB showed defective G-CSF response, these include the closely related NZC, the C58 which shares with NZB a high incidence of spontaneous leukemia and lymphoma and produces high levels of endogenous xenotropic virus (20), and the RF strain with a high incidence of spontaneous granulocytic leukemia (21). The inability of CFU-G from certain mouse strains to respond to G-CSF derived from a leukemic cell line may involve a defect in the CSF molecule itself or an underlying abnormality in the hematopoietic progenitor population of mouse strains exhibiting autoimmunity, aberrant regulation of endogenous virus production, and high leukemia incidence.

Mast Cell Growth Factor (MCGF)

Long-term *in vitro* culture of murine mast cells from bone marrow or spleen has proved possible using conditioned media from lectin-stimulated spleen cell cultures or WEHI-3 leukemic cells as sources of growth factor (4,22). Proliferating populations of mast cells exhibited the characteristic ultrastructure and histochemistry of tissue mast cells, possessed receptors for IgG and IgE, and were positive for histamine, serotonin, L-DOPA, 5-hydroxytryptophan, and sulfated products. Established mast cell lines have been developed from various tissues devoid of mature mast cells, indicating that the conditioned media (CM) contain an activity capable of inducing mast-cell differentiation from a precursor as well as a mast cell mitogenic factor (4). Purification studies suggest that the mast cell differentiation and proliferation activities reside in the same molecule (22). Established mast-cell lines have been maintained in exponential growth for many months by passage in WEHI-3

TABLE 3. *Influence of conditioned media from WEHI-3 leukemic cells on colony formation by Balb/c and NZB marrow cells*

Concentration of CM[a]	Colonies per 5 × 10⁴ Balb/c marrow				Colonies per 5 × 10⁴ NZB marrow			
	W3B-D⁻CM	W3B-D⁺CM	W3B-D⁻CM + PGE[b]	W3B-D⁺CM + PGE	W3B-D⁻CM	W3B-D⁺CM	W3B-D⁻CM + PGE	W3B-D⁺CM + PGE
1:1	76 ± 11	49 ± 5	46 ± 8	17 ± 7	9 ± 2	16 ± 2	2 ± 1	0
1:2	74 ± 12	29 ± 3	44 ± 6	5 ± 2	5 ± 2	18 ± 8	5 ± 2	0
1:4	57 ± 6	20 ± 4	36 ± 2	2 ± 0	5 ± 1	10 ± 3	0	0
1:8	54 ± 3	13 ± 2	38 ± 14	1 ± 1	6 ± 1	7 ± 6	0	0
1:16	43 ± 2	9 ± 5	19 ± 2	0	6 ± 2	9 ± 3	0	0
1:32	20 ± 1	5 ± 3	11 ± 2	0	2 ± 1	0	0	0

[a]W3B-D⁻CM is a ×10 concentrate of serum-free CM from the nondifferentiating cell line. W3B-D⁺CM is unconcentrated CM from the differentiating line.

[b]PGE: Cultures were exposed to 10^{-6} M PGE_2 or 10^{-7} M PGE_1.

CM every 3 to 7 days. Cultured mast cells are absolutely dependent on the conditioned medium for viability as well as growth, and cell death ensues within 24 hrs in the absence of the factor. In some respects, MCGF resembles T-cell growth factor (IL-2) in being induced by mitogen activation of lymphocytes and by its capacity to promote continuous proliferation of a highly specialized, differentiated cell population. The MCGF can be dissociated from IL-2 after the first stage of purification on a DEAE-cellulose column. The MCGF elutes in the breakthrough fraction, whereas IL-2 binds avidly to DEAE (22). The MCGF also differs from IL-2 with respect to molecular weight (as estimated by Sephadex G-150 chromatography) and sensitivity to trypsin.

The close relationship of mast cells and basophils to the neutrophil series, together with the observation that sources of MCGF are generally potent sources of G-CSF, raises the possibility that the two factors are identical. The G-CSF and MCGF copurify from WEHI-3 CM or concanavalin A (Con A) spleen CM, sharing a low affinity for DEAE and similar molecular weight on Sephadex G-150 (23). Another property shared by MCGF and G-CSF is a genetically determined impairment in responsiveness of NZB bone marrow target cells. Attempts to establish mast cell lines from NZB bone marrow have been unsuccessful using semipurified MCGF from Con A spleen CM or WEHI-3 CM. A common defect in mast cell production and neutrophil granulopoiesis is also seen in long-term bone marrow cultures established using the technique of Dexter (24). As shown in Table 4, long-term marrow cultures of NZB failed to generate any mast cells over a 14-week period of observation and neutrophils disappeared within 2 weeks. In contrast, neutrophil granulopoiesis persisted for 10 weeks, and extensive mast cell production was initiated at 5 to 6 weeks in CBA and (CBA×NZB)F₁ marrow cultures. In the marrow cultures established under the conditions first described by Dexter (24), no exogenous sources of hematopoietic growth factors are provided other than the horse serum component of the culture medium, but the close interactions between

TABLE 4. *Comparison of mast cell and neutrophil production in long-term cultures of NZB, CBA, and (CBA × NZB) F₁ marrow*

Culture	CBA		NZB		(CBA × NZB) F₁	
	Mast[a] × 10⁴	PMN[a] × 10⁴	Mast × 10⁴	PMN × 10⁴	Mast × 10⁴	PMN × 10⁴
1–2	0	14.4	0	105.3	0	85.5
3–4	0	122.3	0	0	0	209.0
5–6	39.2	353.4	0	0	24.0	631.5
7–8	4.9	21.3	0	0	4.3	89.9
9–10	5.3	1.1	0	0	4.1	0.5
11–12	4.9	0	0	0	4.2	0
13–14	1.4	0	0	0	19.0	0

[a]Total mast cells and mature neutrophils per culture × 10⁴.
Cultures were established by inoculation of the contents of a single femur into culture flasks containing 10 ml of Fischer's medium plus 20% horse serum. At weekly intervals the cultures were subjected to demidepopulation and suspension cells were typed for morphology. Neutrophil production assessed by total number of mature PMN per culture.

adherent marrow cells (including macrophages) and hematopoietic progenitor cells may provide the necessary local production of hemopoietic regulators. In this context, preliminary studies have shown that the *in vitro* defect in NZB bone marrow cultures can be overcome by provision of adherent bone marrow cells of WW^v mice, which, although having normal hemopoietic environmental function, are defective in stem cells (23). Although MCGF and G-CSF have many similarities, there are some distinguishing properties including significant quantitative differences in the level of each activity elaborated by spleen cells, peritoneal macrophages, or cell lines. Moreover, lactoferrin, which suppresses G-CSF production by WEHI-3 cells (25), has little effect on production of MCGF.

Lactoferrin—A Negative Feedback Regulator of Myelopoiesis

Lactoferrin is a well-purified and biochemically characterized metal-binding glycoprotein (26), produced in immature granulocytes and stored in secondary granules of mature neutrophilic leucocytes (27). In its fully iron-saturated form, it will bind to specific receptors on monocytes and macrophages (28) and suppress the production and/or release of GM-CSF, G-CSF, and M-CSF from these cells (29,30). Receptor-positive macrophages comprise the Ia antigen-positive subpopulation (31). Although T-lymphocytes are not necessary for the action of lactoferrin, evidence has been presented to suggest that T-lymphocytes may play a role in lactoferrin-monocyte interactions (32). We have suggested that lactoferrin may be a physiological regulator of myelopoiesis (29,30). This is based on its specificity of origin within the neutrophil granulocytes of the hematopoietic system, its specificity of action on target cells possessing receptors for it, the extremely low concentrations (10^{-15} M) needed for activity *in vitro*, and its action *in vivo* in normal mice and mice undergoing rebound myelopoiesis.

Lactoferrin is quantitatively deficient in neutrophils from patients with leukemia, and, even when detected, it is in a relatively inactive form (33). Moreover, monocytes and macrophages from patients with leukemia are relatively insensitive to feedback inhibition by an active preparation of lactoferrin (33). This suggests a double defect in certain forms of leukemia, most notably chronic myeloid leukemia associated with myeloid hyperplasia.

REGULATORY DERANGEMENTS IN MYELOID LEUKEMIA — WEHI-3 AS A LEUKEMIC MODEL

An increased understanding of the pathophysiology of leukemia in man and other species has come from *in vitro* culture studies of leukemic bone marrow and leukemic cell lines. In normal myelopoiesis, CSF is required at each step in the proliferation and differentiation sequence from CFU-GM to mature neutrophil and macrophage; thus it is not possible to distinguish between a proliferation-inducing action versus a differentiation-promoting action. However, in the majority of acute myeloid leukemias, CSF promotes proliferation but not differentiation (6,7). This observation does not necessarily imply that the maturation block in leukemia is irreversible, and much attention has been paid to various myeloid leukemic cell line models that indeed can be induced to terminal differentiation. The most extensively studied has been the mouse myeloid leukemic cell line M-1 (34), which can be induced to granulocyte and/or macrophage differentiation by compounds as diverse as dimethylsulfoxide (DMSO), actinomycin D, endotoxin, phorbol esters, dexamethasone, and various protein inducers (35–38). The human promyelocytic cell line HL-60 (39) can likewise be induced to terminal differentiation to granulocytes following exposure to polar compounds (40,41) or retinoids (42,43), and to macrophages following treatment with phorbol esters (44,45).

The capacity of leukemic cells to produce hematopoietic growth-regulating factors, either constitutively or following appropriate induction is well documented. In this context, cell lines developed from the murine WEHI-3 myelomonocytic leukemia have proved of value in analysis of growth regulator production by neoplastic hematopoietic cells as well as in determining the degree of retention of regulator response of leukemic cells. The myelomonocytic leukemia WEHI-3 originated in a Balb/c mouse. The tumor was composed of a mixed population of monocytic and granulocytic cells which, on transplantation, evolved into four different sublines, two of which retained the original chloroma features but were distinguishable by karyotype (one hypodiploid and one tetraploid) (46,47). Two *in vitro* cell lines have been developed, one by Ralph et al. (48) from the 125th passage of the WEHI-3 subline B (the hypodiploid line); and one, independently developed from the WEHI-3B at an early stage of *in vivo* passages, which, in contrast to the preceding line, retains its hypodiploid karyotype and can be induced to terminal granulocytic and macrophage differentiation (49). The line of Ralph et al. (48) is not inducible to differentiation, although it retains such myelomonocytic features as phagocytosis, Fc and C' receptor positivity and lysozyme production. Although incapable of extensive differentiation, the most significant feature of the cell line (termed WEHI-3B-D$^-$ because of its impaired differentiation capacity) is its capacity to produce a wide spectrum of biologically relevant molecules that influence hemopoiesis and immune responses. The cell line produces GM-CSF (50), macrophage and neutrophil (G) CSF (51), eosinophil CSF (52), megakaryocyte CSF (53), erythroid burst-prompting activity (54), erythropoietin (55), MCGF (22), interleukin I (56), endogenous pyrogen (57), a factor supporting long-term proliferation of early neutrophil granulocyte precursors (5), PGE (58), lysozyme, and plasminogen activator (48). Although it may be argued that production of these various regulatory macromolecules reflects oncogenic transformation, it should be noted that all the features of the cell line are features displayed by subpopulations of macrophages under appropriate conditions. The most abnormal feature of the cell lines is that most of the factors are produced at high levels continuously and constitutively rather than as a result of lymphokine or adjuvant induction.

Retention of Regulatory Responsiveness of WEHI-3 Leukemic Cell Lines to Lactoferrin and PGE

With adaptation to culture, the WEHI-3 leukemic cell line appeared to lose responsiveness to CSF, which in the original studies of the early passages of the tumor greatly increased *in vitro* cloning efficiency and individual colony size (46,47,58). This "autonomy" correlated with increased constitutive production of various CSF species, and thus provides an "autocrine" model of neoplastic progression whereby the leukemic cells acquire the capacity to produce their own growth factor(s). In earlier studies, Broxmeyer and Ralph (25) demonstrated that the *in vitro* cloning of WEHI-3B D$^-$ cells was suppressed by an activity in mature neutrophil granulocytes, and this activity also inhibited CSF production by WEHI-3 leukemic cells and by normal monocytes and macrophages. Subsequent studies identified the inhibitory activity as lactoferrin (29,30), and, as can be seen in Table 5, purified preparations of lactoferrin suppressed colony formation by both differentiating D$^+$ and nondifferentiating D$^-$ variants of WEHI-3. Addition of increasing concentrations of WEHI-3B D$^-$ CM to lactoferrin-depressed WEHI-3B D$^-$ agar cultures resulted in a graded increase in cloning efficiency reaching that of untreated cultures (Table 5). Retention of ability to respond to exogenous lactoferrin is a significant feature of these myeloid leukemic cell lines since it allows the "autocrine" mechanism of self-stimulation of leukemic cell proliferation to be blocked indirectly by inhibition of leukemic cell production of certain CSF species. It should be noted that lactoferrin did not induce differentiation of WEHI-3B D$^+$ leukemic cells.

Retention of responsiveness of myeloid leukemic cells to the antiproliferative action of PGEs has proved variable in studies with human myeloid leukemic bone marrow but in general granulocyte-macrophage colony formation by bone marrow from patients with chronic myeloid leukemia (CML) is virtually insensitive to inhibition by PGE at all stages of the disease and in spite of the presence of substantial numbers of proliferating monocytic clones which are particularly susceptible to PGE inhibition in normal marrow (59,60). Although the demonstration that abnormal regulation contributes to an understanding of the pathophysiology of leukemia it leaves unanswered the mechanism involved in the acquisition of pleiotropic defects in responsiveness to regulators. One mechanism that we have proposed

TABLE 5. *Lactoferrin and PGE inhibition of WEHI-3B leukemic cloning* in vitro

Additives	Colonies per 300 cells			
	W3B-D$^-$	% Δ	W3B-D$^+$	% Δ
Control medium	118 ± 3	—	85 ± 10	—
W3B-D$^-$CM	117 ± 2	−1	—	—
10^{-7}M lactoferrin	57 ± 2	−52	66 ± 5	−22
10^{-7}M lactoferrin + W-3 CM	117 ± 2	0	—	—
PGE 10^{-6}M	26 ± 5	−78	96 ± 6	+13
PGE 10^{-7}M	34 ± 3	−71	89 ± 10	+ 5
PGE 10^{-8}M	56 ± 3	−53	90 ± 6	+ 6
PGE 10^{-9}M	87 ± 6	−26	91 ± 5	+ 7

The differentiating (D$^+$) and nondifferentiating (D$^-$) lines of WEHI-3B myelomonocytic leukemic cells were cloned in semisolid agar for 7 days in the presence or absence of varying concentrations of PGE, a semipurified source of human lactoferrin and/or a source of autologous CSF provided by WEHI-3 conditioned medium. It should be noted that none of the additives induce a significant degree of differentiation of the D$^+$ leukemic cells.

is a linkage between the expression of HLA-DR (Ia-like antigen) on hemopoietic progenitor cells (61) or on hemopoietic regulatory cells such as macrophages (31) and response to regulators. In patients with CML, an absent or decreased expression of Ia antigen on CFU-GM can be demonstrated, and correlates with hyporesponsiveness to PGE-mediated inhibition (62), as well as to impaired responsiveness to other negative feedback mechanisms (63). In Table 5, it can be seen that the clonogenic capacity of the D^+ and D^- variants of WEHI-3 myelomonocytic leukemia differed markedly in response to PGE with significant inhibition seen with as little as 10^{-9} M PGE in cultures of D^- cells, whereas no inhibition was seen at any concentration in the case of D^+ cells. This striking difference may reflect differential expression of Ia antigen, either in terms of an absolute ability to display Ia, or differential modulation of antigen expression. In this context, Pelus (65) has reported that CFU-GM lost Ia antigen by shedding and/or metabolism following *in vitro* culture for 6 hr at 37°C and constitutive expression of Ia is not observed throughout 24 hr of suspension culture. However, incubation of bone marrow cells in suspension with 10^{-6} M PGE for 24 hr resulted in an absolute increase in proliferating CFU-GM expressing Ia antigen and subsequently displaying a sensitivity to PGE-mediated colony inhibition. This suggests that PGE in a limited exposure protocol can modulate CFU-GM Ia antigen expression and subsequent regulator responsiveness, either by a direct action on preexisting CFU-GM or by inducing recruitment of these progenitors from an earlier stem cell compartment. It will be of interest to determine whether PGE-insensitive myeloid leukemic CFU-GM can be induced to express Ia and respond to negative control following such brief exposure to PGE. It is possible that such a reexpression of a normal response to regulator control could explain the differential sensitivity of the D^- and D^+ clones of WEHI-3 to PGE growth inhibition, since the former cell line is a constitutive producer of PGE which may result in retention of Ia antigen expression and thus sensitivity to the antiproliferative effects of PGE.

Induction of Differentiation of WEHI-3 Leukemic Cells

The existence of physiological inducers of myeloid leukemic cell differentiation has been documented in various systems with the most consistent being the observation that serum collected 1.5 to 6 hr following endotoxin treatment of mice could induce terminal granulocyte and macrophage differentiation of the myeloid leukemic cell line M1 and WEHI-3B D^+ (8,16,65–67). Table 6 shows that sera collected 3 hr post-injection of endotoxin into normal $B6D2F_1$ mice neither augmented nor inhibited the cloning of WEHI-3B D^+ cells in agar culture but at higher concentrations converted leukemic colonies from compact undifferentiated to a diffuse type associated with differentiation to segmented neutrophils, macrophages or a mixture of both cell types. This leukemic differentiation is associated with loss of leukemic recloning capacity *in vitro* (8,16,67) and reduced leukemogenicity *in vivo* (67). Since endotoxin also induces a dramatic increase in serum CSF levels with kinetics comparable to those of serum GM-differentiating factor (GM-DF) (Table

TABLE 6. *CSF and differentiation-inducing activity in mouse post-endotoxin sera*

Serum titration[a]	W3B-D⁺CM colonies/ 300 cells	W3B-D⁺CM colonies diffuse %	W3B-D⁺CM colonies differentiated[b]	CFU-C per 5×10^4 BM[c]
1 : 2	108 ± 12	100	87	74 ± 6
1 : 4	113 ± 9	84	44	57 ± 4
1 : 8	113 ± 11	54	25	54 ± 8
1 : 16	105 ± 5	24	26	43 ± 5
1 : 32	113 ± 11	21	9	18 ± 3
1 : 64	105 ± 17	13	3	6 ± 2
0	107 ± 10	1	0	0

[a]Serum collected 3 hr post i.v. injection 5 μg endotoxin. Serum added at 5% vol/vol and at various dilutions.

[b]Percentage of colonies undergoing differentiation to neutrophils and/or macrophages based on morphological analysis of 50 individually isolated colonies.

[c]Colonies per 5×10^4 normal Balb/c marrow cells.

6), and high concentrations of pure murine GM-CSF have been shown to induce leukemic cell differentiation (13), it had been assumed that leukemia differentiation inducing protein was indeed CSF. More recent biochemical characterization of post-endotoxin serum has shown that the differentiation factor could be separated from the bulk of serum GM-CSF (66,68), but may co-purify with a minor species of CSF which stimulates only normal neutrophil-granulocyte colony formation (G-CSF) (16). The cellular origin of endotoxin-induced differentiation protein is unclear, but macrophages are likely candidates; furthermore, certain leukemic cell lines may be capable of generating their own differentiation inducing protein in response to agents such as endotoxin, phorbol esters, and glucocorticoids, which induce leukemic cell differentiation indirectly (67).

To test the possibility that leukemic cells could produce their own differentiation inducing activity, conditioned medium from mass cultures of WEHI-3B D⁺ or D⁻ cells was harvested, concentrated tenfold, and added to agar cultures of WEHI-3B D⁺ cells. As can be seen in Table 7, concentrated W-3 CM was slightly inhibitory to the cloning of WEHI-3B D⁺ cells and only a small degree of colony differentiation was induced. The inability of WEHI-3 CM to induce leukemic cell differentiation was not correlated with low levels of CSF since this latter activity was comparable to the levels in mouse post-endotoxin serum (Tables 3 and 6), which was a potent source of GM-DF. Although it is possible that the appropriate species of CSF was lacking in W-3 CM, it would not be due to a lack of G-CSF considering that this leukemic CM was first identified as a major source of this CSF subspecies (51). A number of possibilities must be considered if the different observations are to be reconciled. The first would recognize that there are two structurally and functionally distinct species of G-CSF, one, the predominant species in W-3 CM causing proliferation and differentiation of normal CFU-G and lacking differentiation inducing ability for leukemic cells and the other, present in post-endotoxin serum retaining the capacity to induce differentiation of both normal and leukemic CFU-G. This

TABLE 7. *The influence of conditioned medium from WEHI-3B-D⁻ leukemic cells on cloning and differentiation of WEHI-B-D⁺*

Concentration of W3B-D⁻CM	Colonies per 300 W3B-D⁺ cells	
	Total	Total diffuse
1 : 1	61 ± 4	10 ± 4
1 : 2	95 ± 2	9 ± 4
1 : 4	115 ± 4	7 ± 3
1 : 8	111 ± 13	7 ± 4
1 : 16	118 ± 20	1 ± 2
1 : 32	134 ± 9	4 ± 1
0	121 ± 11	4 ± 4

W3B-D⁻CM is a ×10 concentrate of serum-free CM from the nondifferentiating line. Colonies were scored at day 7 and typed as compact undifferentiated morphology or diffuse differentiated.

possibility would be particularly attractive if it could be shown that the G-CSF produced by leukemic cell lines was a defective molecule produced as a consequence of leukemic transformation. Although there is no evidence for this in hematopoietic transformation systems, precedents exist in sarcoma transformation systems. A second possibility is that extensive homology exists among various hematopoietic regulatory macromolecules and that some normal regulators may have a limited capacity to induce leukemic cell maturation, and more leukemia-specific molecules may in turn induce maturation of subpopulations of normal hematopoietic cells. A more mundane possibility is that current protein purification and immunological methods have not yet been sufficiently refined to separate functionally distinct but structurally similar polypeptides with biological activity at 10^{-11} M.

CONCLUSIONS

The apparent maturation block associated with neoplastic transformation in a variety of cell systems can be a reversible phenomenon. Terminal (post-mitotic) differentiation can be induced by a variety of factors, both physiological and pharmacological. Where investigated, the proliferation and/or differentiation of renewing cell populations is shown to be controlled by specific growth regulatory factors, generally of a glycoprotein or polypeptide nature. Contrary to earlier beliefs, most transformed cells retain some dependence on growth regulatory factors of exogenous or endogenous origin and thus manipulation of production or action of growth and maturation factors has a role to play in cancer therapy.

In some cell systems, growth factors induce proliferation of target cells without inducing further differentiation. Epidermal-, fibroblast-, and platelet-derived growth factors are well-characterized molecules which can be categorized as mitogenic proteins for their respective target tissues. Inappropriate production of such factors by transformed cells or the production of functionally similar molecules following viral transformation (e.g., sarcoma growth factor) confers a proliferative advantage on the transformed cell. In these instances, therapeutic strategy should be based on blocking the synthesis and/or release of the growth factor on which tumor proliferation depends, or modulating or blocking receptors for growth factors possibly using synthetic peptide antagonists or utilizing monoclonal antibodies against the growth factor or its receptor. An alternative therapeutic strategy for growth factor-dependent tumors could be the use of exogenous growth factors to induce cell cycle synchronization of tumor cells in conjunction with cycle specific chemotherapeutic agents. The recognition of the heterogeneity and species specificity of CSF together with the "dependent" nature of human myeloid leukemia indicates a priority for improved purification and production of large quantities of these factors. A number of human cell lines have been identified as constitutive producers of CSFs and would provide a suitable source for large-scale production. The CSFs may be utilized to cycle-activate G_o leukemic stem cells in conjunction with S-phase-specific chemotherapy. The factors may also be of value in augmenting myelopoiesis in patients receiving intensive chemotherapy and/or radiotherapy for nonhematopoietic malignancy and both GM and M-CSFs may prove to be valuable in activating macrophages and enhancing their capacity to mediate nonspecific tumor-cell killing.

Evidence for the inducibility of terminal maturation of malignant cells is based on extensive use of a relatively small number of tumor cell lines selected for a capacity to differentiate. The generality of this phenomenon requires further investigation in primary tumor culture systems. There is, however, good evidence to suggest that even if terminal differentiation of malignant cells is not obtained, differentiation inducing agents such as retinoids and GM-DF may block self-renewal of malignant clones (68).

Synergism between biological response modifiers has been demonstrated, and, in the context of tumor-cell differentiation, retinoids plus PGE or GM-DF plus low concentrations of actinomycin D are significantly more effective than each agent individually in promoting terminal leukemic-cell differentiation (67). Indeed, leukemic cell lines selected for their inability to differentiate (D⁻ clones) can be induced to differentiate and lose *in vivo* malignancy only when exposed to a combination of actinomycin D as a sensitizer and a differentiation inducer such as GM-DF or retinoic acid (67).

Phase I and II clinical trials of differentiation inducing agents should be considered in patients with malignancies where *in vitro* evidence suggest the possibility of differentiation. Trials with combinations including conventional chemotherapeutic agents are also warranted since the efficacy of certain chemotherapeutic agents may reside not so much in their ability to selectively kill malignant cells but rather in their capacity to induce production of endogenous differentiation factors and/or to sensitize tumor cells to such endogenous influences.

ACKNOWLEDGMENTS

This work was supported in part by grants CA-08748, CA-20194, and CA-17353 awarded by the National Cancer Institute, and by the Gar Reichman Foundation.

REFERENCES

1. Morgan, D. A., Ruscetti, F. W., and Gallo, R. C. (1976): Growth of thymus-derived lymphocytes from normal human bone marrow. *Science*, 193:1007–1010.
2. Sredni, B., Sieckmann, D. G., Kumagai, S., House, S., Green, I., and Paul, W. E. (1981): Long term culture and cloning of non-transformed human B lymphocytes. *J. Exp. Med.*, 154:1500–1516.
3. Moore, M. A. S., Kurland, J., and Broxmeyer, H. (1978): Regulatory interactions in normal and leukemic myelopoiesis. In: *Differentiation of Normal and Neoplastic Hematopoietic Cells*, edited by B. Clarkson, J. Till, and P. Marks, pp. 393–404. Cold Spring Harbor Symposium, Cold Spring Harbor, New York.
4. Tertian, G., Yung, Y-P, Guy-Grand, D., and Moore, M. A. S. (1981): Long-term in vitro culture of murine mast cells. I. Description of a growth factor-dependent culture technique. *J. Immunol.*, 127:788–794.
5. Dexter, T. M., Garland, J., Scott, D., Scolnick, E., and Metcalf, D. (1980): Growth of factor-dependent hemopoietic precursor cell lines. *J. Exp. Med.*, 152:1036–1047.
6. Moore, M. A. S., Spitzer, G., Williams, N., Metcalf, D., and Buckley, J. (1974): Agar culture studies in 127 cases of untreated acute leukemia: The prognostic value of reclassification of leukemia according to in vitro growth characteristics. *Blood*, 44:1–12.
7. Moore, M. A. S. (1979): Humoral regulation of granulopoiesis. *Clin. Haematol.* 8:287–309.
8. Burgess, A. W., and Metcalf, D. (1980): Review: The nature and action of granulocyte-macrophage colony stimulating factors. *Blood*, 56:947–958.
9. Bradley, T. R., and Metcalf, D. (1966): The growth of mouse bone marrow cells in vitro. *Aust. J. Exp. Med. Sci.*, 44:287–300.
10. Pluznik, D. H., and Sachs, L. (1965): The cloning of normal mast cells in tissue culture. *J. Cell. Physiol.*, 66:315–324.
11. Metcalf, D. (1977): Hemopoietic colonies. In vitro cloning of normal and leukemic cells. Springer Verlag, Berlin.
12. Stanley, E. R. (1981): Colony stimulating factors. In: *The Lymphokines: Biochemistry and Biological Activity*, edited by J. W. Hadden and W. E. Stewart, pp. 101–132. Humana Press, New Jersey.
13. Metcalf, D. (1979): Clonal analysis of the action of GM-CSF on the proliferation and differentiation of myelomonocytic leukemic cells. *Int. J. Cancer*, 24:616–623.
14. Guilbert, L. J., and Stanley, E. R. (1980): Specific interaction of murine colony stimulating factor with mononuclear phagocytic cells. *J. Cell Biol.*, 85:153.
15. Williams, N., Jackson, H., Ralph, P., and Nakoinz, I. (1981): Cell interactions influencing murine marrow megakaryopoiesis: Nature of the potentiating cell in bone marrow. *Blood*, 57:157–163.
16. Burgess, A. W., and Metcalf, D. (1980): Characterization of a serum factor stimulating the differentiation of myelomonocytic leukemic cells. *Int. J. Cancer*, 26:647–654.
17. Pelus, L. M., Broxmeyer, H. E., Kurland, J. I., and Moore, M. A. S. (1979): Regulation of macrophage and granulocyte proliferation: Specificities of prostaglandin E and lactoferrin. *J. Exp. Med.*, 150:277–292.
18. Kurland, J. I., Pelus, L. M., Ralph, P., Bockman, R. S., and Moore, M. A. S. (1979): Induction of prostaglandin E synthesis in normal and neoplastic macrophages: Role for colony-stimulating factor(s) distinct from effects on myeloid progenitor cell proliferation. *Proc. Natl. Acad. Sci. USA*, 76:2326–2330.
19. Kincade, P. W., Lee, G., Fernandes, G., Moore, M. A. S., Williams, N., and Good, R. A. (1979): Abnormalities in clonable B lymphocytes and myeloid progenitors in autoimmune NZB mice. *Proc. Natl. Cancer. Inst.*, 76:3464–3468.
20. Moore, M. A. S. (1981): Genetic and oncogenic influences on myelopoiesis. *Hematology and Blood Transfusion*, 26:237–242.
21. Horland, A. A., McMarrow, L., and Wolman, S. R. (1980): Growth of granulopoietic bone marrow cells of RF mice. *Exp. Hematol.*, 8:1024–1030.
22. Yung, Y-P., Eger, R., Tertian, G., and Moore, M. A. S. (1981): Long term in vitro culture of murine mast cells: Purification of a mast cell growth factor and its dissociation from TCGF. *J. Immunol.*, 127:794–799.
23. Moore, M. A. S. (1982): G-CSF: Its relationship to leukemia differentiation-inducing activity and other hematopoietic regulators. *J. Cell. Physiol. (in press)*.

24. Dexter, T. M., Scott, D., and Teich, N. M. (1977): Infection of bone marrow cells in vitro with FLV: Effects on stem cell proliferation, differentiation and leukemogenic capacity. *Cell*, 12:355.

25. Broxmeyer, H. E., and Ralph, P. (1977): Regulation of a mouse myelomonocytic leukemia cell line in culture. *Cancer Res.*, 37:3578–3584.

26. Aisen, P., and Listowski, I. (1980): Iron transport and storage proteins. *Am. Rev. Biochem.*, 49:357–362.

27. Baggiolini, M., De Duve, C., Masson, P. L., and Heremans, J. F. (1970): Association of lactoferrin with specific granules in rabbit heterophil leukocytes. *J. Exp. Med.*, 131:559–568.

28. Van Snick, J. L., and Masson, P. L. (1976): The binding of human lactoferrin to mouse peritoneal cells. *J. Exp. Med.*, 144:1568–1576.

29. Broxmeyer, H. E., Smithyman, A., Eger, R. R., Meyers, P. A., and De Sousa, M. (1978): Identification of lactoferrin as the granulocyte-derived inhibitor of colony stimulating activity (CSA)-production. *J. Exp. Med.*, 148:1052–1067.

30. Broxmeyer, H. E., De Sousa, M., Smithyman, A., Ralph, P., Hamilton, J., Kurland, J. I., and Bognacki, J. (1980): Specificity and modulation of the action of lactoferrin, a negative feedback regulator of myelopoiesis. *Blood*, 55:324–333.

31. Broxmeyer, H. E. (1979): Lactoferrin acts on Ia-like antigen positive subpopulations of human monocytes to inhibit production of colony stimulatory activity in vitro. *J. Clin. Invest.*, 64:1717–1720.

32. Bagby, G. C., Rigas, V. D., Bennett, R. M., Vandenbark, A. S., and Garewal, H. S. (1981): Interaction of lactoferrin, monocytes, and T-lymphocyte subsets in the regulation of steady state granulopoiesis in vitro. *Clin. Invest.*, 68:56–61.

33. Broxmeyer, H. E., Mendelson, N., and Moore, M. A. S. (1977): Abnormal granulocyte feedback regulation of colony forming and colony stimulating activity-producing cells from patients with chronic myelogenous leukemia. *Leukemia Res.*, 1:3–12.

34. Ichikawa, Y. (1969): Differentiation of a cell line of myeloid leukemia. *J. Cell. Physiol.*, 74:223–224.

35. Sachs, L. (1978): Control of normal cell differentiation and the phenotypic reversion of malignancy in myeloid leukemia. *Nature*, 274:535–539.

36. Weiss, B., and Sachs, L. (1978): Indirect induction of differentiation in myeloid leukemic cells by lipid A. *Proc. Natl. Acad. Sci. USA*, 75:1374–1378.

37. Honma, Y., Kasukabe, T., Okabe, J., and Hozumi, M. (1977): Glucocorticoid-induced differentiation of cultured mouse myeloid leukemia cells. *Gan.* 68:241–246.

38. Honma, Y., Kasukabe, T., and Hozumi, M. (1978): Relationship between leukemogenicity and in vivo inducibility of normal differentiation in mouse myeloid leukemia cells. *J. Natl. Cancer Inst.*, 61:837–841.

39. Collins, S. J., Gallow, R. C., and Gallagher, R. E. (1977): Continuous growth and differentiation of human myeloid leukemic cells in suspension culture. *Nature*, 270:347–349.

40. Collins, S. J., Ruscetti, F. W., Gallagher, R. E., and Gallo, R. C. (1979): Normal functional characteristics of cultured human promyelocytic leukemia cells (HL-60) after induction of differentiation by dimethylsulfoxide. *J. Exp. Med.*, 149:969–974.

41. Fontana, J. A., Wright, D. G., Shiffman, E., Corcoran, B. A., and Deisseroth, A. B. (1980): Development of chemotactic responsiveness in myeloid precursor cells: Studies with a human leukemia cell line. *Proc. Natl. Acad. Sci. USA*, 77:3664–3668.

42. Breitman, T., Selanick, S., and Collins, S. (1980): Induction of differentiation of the human promyelocytic leukemia cell line (HL-60) by retinoic acid. *Proc. Natl. Acad. Sci. USA*, 77:2936–2940.

43. Honma, Y., Takenage, K., Kasukabe, T., and Hozumi, M. (1980): Induction of differentiation of cultured human promyelocytic leukemia cells by retinoids. *Biochem. Biophys. Res. Commun.*, 95:507–512.

44. Rovera, G., O'Brien, T. G., and Diamond, L. (1979): Induction of differentiation in human promyelocytic leukemia cells by tumor promotors. *Science*, 204:868–870.

45. Territo, M. C., and Koeffler, H. P. (1981): Induction by phorbol esters of macrophage differentiation in human leukaemia cell lines does not require cell division. *Br. J. Haematol.*, 47:479–483.

46. Warner, N., Moore, M. A. S., and Metcalf, D. (1969): A transplantable myelomonocytic leukemia in Balb/c mice: Cytology, karyotype and muramidase content. *J. Natl. Cancer Inst.*, 43:963–968.

47. Metcalf, D., Moore, M. A. S., and Warner, N. (1969): Colony formation in vitro by myelomonocytic leukemic cells. *J. Natl. Cancer Inst.*, 43:983–1001.

48. Ralph, P., Moore, M. A. S., and Nilsson, K. (1976): Lysozyme synthesis by established human and murine histiocytic lymphoma cell lines. *J. Exp. Med.*, 143:1528–1533.
49. Metcalf, D. (1980): Clonal extinction of myelomonocytic leukemic cells by serum from mice injected with endotoxin. *Int. J. Cancer*, 25:225–233.
50. Ralph, P., Broxmeyer, H. E., Moore, M. A. S., and Nakoinz, I. (1978): Induction of myeloid colony-stimulating activity in murine monocyte tumor cell lines by macrophage activators and in a T-cell line by concanavalin A. *Cancer Res.*, 38:1414–1419.
51. Williams, N., Eger, R. R., Moore, M. A. S., and Mendelsohn, N. (1978): Differentiation of mouse bone marrow precursor cells into neutrophil granulocytes by an activity separated from WEHI-3 conditioned medium. *Differentiation*, 11:59–63.
52. Metcalf, D., Parker, J., Chester, H. M., and Kincade, P. W. (1974): Formation of eosinophilic-like granulocytic colonies by mouse bone marrow cells in vitro. *J. Cell. Physiol.*, 84:275–289.
53. Williams, N., Jackson, H. M., Eger, R. R., and Long, M. W. (1982): The different roles of factors in murine megakaryocyte colony formation. In: *Megakaryocytes In Vitro*, edited by R. Levine, N. Williams, and B. Evatt. Elsevier New York, *(in press)*.
54. Axelrod, A., Burgess, A., Iscove, N., and Wagemaker, G. (1981): Culture of hematopoietic cells: Workshop report. In: *Progress in Clinical and Biological Research, Vol. 66B, Control of Cellular Division and Development*, edited by D. Cunningham, E. Goldwasser, J. Watson, and F. C. Fox, pp. 421–425. Liss, New York.
55. Kubanek, B., Heit, W., and Rich, I. N. (1981): Continuous erythropoietin production by macrophages. *Exp. Hematol.*, 9 (Suppl. 9):59 (Abs.).
56. Lachman, L. B., Hocker, M. P., Blyden, G. T., and Handschumacher, T. (1977): Preparation of lymphocyte-activating factor from continuous murine macrophage cell lines. *Cell. Immunol.*, 34:416–419.
57. Bodel, P. (1978): Spontaneous pyrogen production by mouse histiocytic and myelomonocytic tumor cell lines in vitro. *J. Exp. Med.*, 147:1503–1516.
58. Kurland, J., and Moore, M. A. S. (1977): Modulation of hemopoiesis by prostaglandins. *Exp. Hematol.*, 5:357–373.
59. Pelus, L. M., and Moore, M. A. S. (1982): Regulation of monocyte-macrophage differentiation by colony stimulating factor and prostaglandin E. In: *Immunopharmacology and Immune Regulation*, edited by D. R. Webb and J. S. Goodwin. Marcel Dekker, New York *(in press)*.
60. Pelus, L. M., Broxmeyer, H. E., Clarkson, B. D., and Moore, M. A. S. (1980): Abnormal responsiveness of granulocyte-macrophage committed colony-forming cells from patients with chronic myeloid leukemia to inhibition by prostaglandin E. *Cancer Res.*, 40:2512–2515.
61. Moore, M. A. S., Broxmeyer, H. E., Sheridan, A., Meyers, P., Jacobsen, N., and Winchester, R. (1980): Continuous human bone marrow culture: Ia antigen characterization of probable human pluripotential stem cells. *Blood*, 55:682–690.
62. Pelus, L. M., Saletan, S., Silver, R., and Moore, M. A. S. (1982): Expression of Ia-antigen on normal and chronic myeloid leukemic human granulocyte-macrophage colony forming cells (CFU-GM) is associated with the regulation of cell proliferation by prostaglandin E. *Blood (in press)*.
63. Broxmeyer, H. E., Gentile, P., Bognaki, J., and Ralph, P. (1982): A role for lactoferrin, transferrin, acidic isoferritins and Ia-like antigen positive target cells in the regulation of myelopoiesis during health and leukemia: Potential possibilities for new treatment modalities using normally occurring molecules. *Blood Cells (in press)*.
64. Pelus, L. M. (1982): A direct association between CFU-GM expression of HLA-DR antigen and control of granulocyte and macrophage production. A new role for prostaglandin E in the maintenance of granulocyte-macrophage progenitor cell response in vitro. *(to be published)*.
65. Lotem, J., Lipton, J. H., and Sachs, L. (1980): Separation of different molecular forms of macrophage and granulocyte-inducing proteins for normal and leukemic myeloid cells. *Int. J. Cancer*, 25:763–771.
66. Falk, A., and Sachs, L. (1980): Clonal regulation of the induction of macrophage and granulocyte-inducing proteins for normal and leukemic myeloid cells. *Int. J. Cancer*, 26:595–601.
67. Hozumi, M. (1982): A new approach to chemotherapy of myeloid leukemia: Control of leukemogenicity of myeloid leukemia cells by inducers of normal differentiation. In: *Cancer Biology Reviews, Vol. 3*, edited by J. J. Marchalonis, M. G. Hanna, and I. J. Fiedler. Marcel Dekker, New York *(in press)*.
68. Moore, M. A. S., Mertelsmann, R., and Pelus, L. (1981): Phenotypic evaluation of chronic myeloid leukemia. *Blood Cells*, 7:217–136.

Subject Index

A431 cells, growth factors, 119–126
A673 cells
  immunosuppression, 207–210
  transforming growth factors, 119–126
A2058 cells, growth factors, 119–126
ABE-8 B-cell line, 225,232
Acetylcholine, neuron plasticity, 36
Acid phosphatase
  HL60 cells, TPA, 276–280
  T lymphocytes, 160–162
Actinomycin D
  HL60 cells, differentiation, 261,267
  leukemic cell differentiation, 373
  T lymphomas, factor production,
    245–246,252
  transforming factor block, 126
Acute lymphoblastic leukemia
  plating efficiency, 296
  T-cell growth factor, 153–164,187–201
  TPA treatment, 282–283
Acute myeloid leukemia
  blast progenitors, therapy, 293–297
  colony stimulating activity, 265
  retinoic acid therapy, 261
  TPA, 282–283
Acute nonlymphocytic leukemia, TCGF,
    187–201
Acute promyelocytic leukemia
  retinoic acid therapy, 261
  TPA, 282–284
Adenosine deaminase, treatment, 109–110
Adherent cells, granulopoietic
  modulation, 335–349
Adrenergic neuron plasticity, 36
Adriamycin
  HL60 cells, terminal differentiation,
    267
  and plating efficiency, AML, 296–297
Agar growth assay, 121–124
m-AMSA and plating efficiency, AML,
    296–297
Anchorage-dependent cells, proliferation,
    73–101
Anemia, hemopoietic growth factors,
    306–309
Anergic cancer, thymosins, 145
Anti-Ia treatment, B cells, 219–220

Anti-IgG antisera, B cells, 219–220
Anti-Thy 1 treatment, B cells, 219–220
Antibody production
  suppression by IL-1 and TCGF,
    217–220
  thymosins, 135–140
Anticancer drugs
  and polar solvents, 107–109
  therapy issues, 331–332
Antigens; *see also specific antigens*
  B-cell maturation, 213–215
  macrophages, 303–304
  and polar solvent treatment, 112
  and T-cells, growth factor, 159,161
  tumor cell differentiation, 223–240
Arabinosylcytosine, terminal
  differentiation, 267
ARA-C, *see* Cytosine arabinoside
ASL-1 cells, interleukin-2 activity, 174
Ataxia-telangiectasia, thymosin therapy,
    142
Athymic mice, IL-1 and TRF, B cells,
    218–221
Autocrine model
  neoplasms, 369
Autoimmune approach, 1–6
Autoimmune disorders, thymosin
  therapy, 141–143
Autostimulation, cells
  interleukin-2 production, 180–181
  and T-cell growth factor, 200
  transforming growth factors, 126
8-Azaadenosine treatment, polar
  solvents, 110
8-Azaguanine treatment, polar solvents,
    110

B cell tumors, differentiation stages, 224
B lymphocytes
  differentiation, factors, 213–221
    red blood cell model, 217
  Ig secretion induction, 246–247
B phenotype, leukemia, T-cell growth
  factor, 201
B9.8.1 antibodies, 279–280
B13.4.1 antibodies, 279–280
B10 macrophage factors, 302

377